POWER AND CHARITY
A Chinese Merchant Elite
in Colonial Hong Kong

Echoes: Classics of
Hong Kong Culture and History

Series General Editor: Robert Nield

The life of Hong Kong and its region has been explored in a vast number of books. They include ground-breaking scholarly studies of great standing, and literary works that shed light on people, places and events. Many of these books unfortunately are no longer available to the general reader.

The aim of the Echoes series is once more to make available the best of those books that would otherwise be lost. The series will embrace not only history, but also memoirs, fiction, politics, natural history and other subjects. The focal point will be Hong Kong, but the series will extend to places connected with the city or sharing some of its experiences. In this way we hope to bring a growing number of classic publications to a new and wider readership.

———————————————————

Other titles in the Echoes series:

Thistle and Bamboo: The Life and Times of Sir James Stewart Lockhart
Shiona Airlie

A Biographical Sketch-book of Early Hong Kong
G. B. Endacott

Chinese Christians: Elites, Middlemen and the Church in Hong Kong
Carl T. Smith

Edge of Empires: Chinese Elites and British Colonials in Hong Kong
John M. Carroll

Anglo-China: Chinese People and British Rule in Hong Kong, 1841–1880
Christopher Munn

City of Broken Promises
Austin Coates

Macao and the British, 1637–1842: Prelude to Hong Kong
Austin Coates

A Macao Narrative
Austin Coates

The Road
Austin Coates

The Taking of Hong Kong: Charles and Clara Elliot in China Waters
Susanna Hoe and Derek Roebuck

POWER AND CHARITY
A Chinese Merchant Elite
in Colonial Hong Kong

ELIZABETH SINN

HKU
PRESS
香港大學出版社

Hong Kong University Press
The University of Hong Kong
Pokfulam Road
Hong Kong
https://hkupress.hku.hk

© 2003 Hong Kong University Press

ISBN 978-962-209-669-1 (*Paperback*)

First published in 1989 by Oxford University Press under the title
Power and Charity: The Early History of the Tung Wah Hospital, Hong Kong

British Library Cataloguing-in-Publication Data
A catalogue record for this book is available from the British Library.

10 9 8 7 6 5 4 3

Printed and bound by J&S Printing Co., Ltd. in Hong Kong, China

To the Memory of My Parents

Contents

Plates

Preface to the Paperback Edition

THE re-issue of a book provides a welcome opportunity for the author to re-engage readers in the discussions that she has left off when the book first went to print. When *Power and Charity* appeared in 1989, it was very well received.[1] It broke new ground in a number of ways. Unlike most of the earlier histories of Hong Kong which had primarily focused on governors and the colonial administration, or those that only treated Hong Kong as an issue in Anglo-Chinese diplomacy, the book examines in depth the nature of Hong Kong society by scrutinizing the history of a local institution, the Tung Wah Hospital, and illustrating the Hospital's historical significance on several levels. Far from being merely a medical institution, the Tung Wah in the nineteenth century rendered many different kinds of services to Chinese in Hong Kong and overseas, services that were full of social and cultural meaning and that helped to establish the Hospital's Directors as community leaders. As the first highly organized merchant elite recognized by the colonial government, the Hospital Committee played a crucial political role in colonial Hong Kong, mediating between ordinary Chinese and the colonial administration and becoming indispensable to the latter's scheme of things as an instrument of social management and control. The Hospital's extra-territorial impact was equally significant. It established strong connections with Chinese officials on the Mainland who appreciated the value of its philanthropy, especially its contribution as a major fundraiser for disaster relief in China; but Chinese officials were also eager to exert their influence in Hong Kong through the Tung Wah Directors. The book shows how this picture was complicated by the desire of the Hong Kong merchant elite for social legitimacy, according to age-old Chinese principles, and for recognition within the Chinese Imperial order. Even as the merchants tried to establish their social and political status in Hong Kong vis-à-vis the colonial government, they were equally concerned with maintaining good relations with Chinese officials and gaining honours from the Chinese Emperor, interests that events often proved to be conflicting and a source of trouble.

The Tung Wah story thus illustrates perfectly the ambiguous nature of Hong Kong's position between two Empires.

By tracing carefully the immense volume of services the Hospital provided for Chinese overseas and on the Mainland, *Power and Charity* documents the vast networks that made such services possible, and emphasizes the fact that one of the Hospital's greatest assets was its ability to tap into these networks. In particular, by stressing the Hospital's strong connections with Chinese overseas, the book demonstrates for the first time the importance of Chinese emigration to Hong Kong on the one hand, and, on the other, the key role Hong Kong played in the Chinese diaspora.

Confrontation between Western and Chinese medicine is another principal theme of the book. The Hospital was founded in 1869 fundamentally as a result of the rejection of Western medicine by the Chinese population, and the great contribution of the Hospital was in providing medical care that Chinese believed in, and dispensing it within culturally meaningful ways. Yet, at the same time, Western doctors, full of the superiority of white Western men and faith in the infallibility of Western medical science, poured contempt on Chinese medicine, and backed by the coercive powers of the colonial regime, were able to force their will on the Hospital and make the practice of Western medicine there compulsory. In time, Western medicine became 'mainstream' in the Tung Wah, while Chinese medicine became circumscribed and marginalized. The Tung Wah story, therefore, is also a chapter in the greater drama of the encounter and clash of the world's cultures in the nineteenth century.

Power and Charity is based on the extensive use of primary sources, many of which had never been used before, or at least, not in the study of Hong Kong's social history. Archival records such as those in the Tung Wah Hospital Archives, the Po Leung Kuk Archives, the Hong Kong Public Records Office, the British Public Record Office and the US National Archives, along with contemporary English and Chinese newspapers, shed new light on individuals and events, policies and practices, ideas and desires. These materials enable the construction of new narratives as well as the reinterpretation of old ones. Pointing scholars to the richness of these sources constitutes another contribution of the book.

Many important events have occurred and many books have appeared since 1989, making it opportune to revisit *Power and*

Charity — to re-evaluate and recontextualize it. Some of these books were prompted by the return of Hong Kong to China in 1997; primarily concerned with the present and the future, they nevertheless refer, even if only in passing, to the past as prelude to the present. Many of these works are marred by distortions and over-generalizations and their tendency to be either crudely 'pro-colonial' or 'anti-colonial' further obscures rather than illuminates the complex social and political dynamics of Hong Kong.[2] Fortunately, recent years have also witnessed a countertrend of serious studies of Hong Kong's history, representing a cumulative process of intellectual evolution built on the use of new sources, greater sophistication of interpretation and originality of approach, and forming a new landscape in which to reposition the history of the Tung Wah Hospital.

One issue in the study of Hong Kong that has certainly demanded re-examination is the relationship between the Chinese population and the colonial government. In this respect, Christopher Munn's excellent book *Anglo-China: Chinese People and British Rule in Hong Kong, 1841–1880* is most edifying. Combining meticulous and minute study of source materials with bold interpretation, Munn questions such common assumptions as indirect rule, racial segregation and small government, which historians of Hong Kong have used unquestioningly as basic premises upon which to build their narratives. In particular, his work has prompted me to re-assess the first thirty years of colonial rule in Hong Kong, the period prior to the appearance of the Tung Wah Hospital Committee as the local Chinese social elite. Assuming indirect rule and small government as constants of British rule from the start, I overlooked the powerful apparatus that the colonial regime had erected to control the Chinese, with the courts, the police and the military as indispensable, and intrusive, accessories for domination. Munn shows that, far from relying on indirect rule, government interference was pervasive and exerted considerable impact on the daily lives of Chinese in Hong Kong. I had not realized that 'Hong Kong possessed one of the most top-heavy governments and one of the largest police forces in the British Empire. It had a military and naval presence that was roughly double the size of the civilian European population and was frequently called upon to aid the civil authorities.'[3] The courts, backed by the military and the police in the enforcement of the law, became a site for inter-racial encounter. By showing that the first three decades or so of British rule were more than 'only a kind of chaotic prelude to the political engagement and conflict later in the century'[4] and filling them with vivid details of colonial life, Munn recontextualizes the emergence of the Tung Wah Hospital and highlights its significance in a different way. In brief, direct and oppressive rule prevailed before the Tung Wah Hospital's establishment but later on, the Hospital's existence enabled the government to supplement its governing apparatus with the more persuasive social management and moral intervention of the Hospital, resulting in a combination of direct and indirect rule.

The court, as Munn shows convincingly, was a powerful instrument of colonial control, but it should be noted also that there was another side of the coin. My recent study shows that, whatever the original intention behind the legal and judicial system might have been, Chinese were quick to learn that the court could be used to their advantage as well. However ignorant they might have been initially of British law, suspicious of its effectiveness, frustrated by its modus operandi, and mystified by many of its judgments, they nevertheless resorted to it as a means to demand justice and seek compensation.[5] Long before the Tung Wah Hospital appealed to English law to prosecute kidnappers,[6] Chinese had used it to seek protection of their commercial and personal interests.

Munn's reservations toward the so-called 'abyss' separating the governors and governed, further alerts me to the fact that I have overstated the degree of segregation between the Chinese and foreign populations. The term 'abyss', so often referred to by governors and civil servants and used by me widely in the book, certainly needs refinement. Indeed, my recent study of the economic activities of the early years of the colony also leads me to redefine 'abyss' on other levels. It is commonly assumed that Chinese and European business networks were quite discrete, with compradors being the main bridge between them, but a closer examination of business records shows a more intricate picture. Apart from the fact that Europeans could not avoid relying on Chinese businesses to supply them with goods and services, the inter-dependence ran very deep. Their relations, moreover, were not confined to trade. Chinese were valued by European and American businessmen both as borrowers of their loans and depositors of funds long before formal banks were established. Chinese were, among other things, consumers of their goods, charterers of their ships, even shareholders in their companies. Chinese merchants depended no less on their European and American counterparts to survive and thrive. By as early as the 1860s, one can find close and complex long-term business associations between Chinese and foreign entrepreneurs which could only have been founded on trust and not just on opportunism or expediency.[7] Undoubtedly there were Chinese networks and European networks but the degree to which they overlapped and criss-crossed appears to be greater than previously assumed. Such relationships need much closer scrutiny for a better understanding of the social and economic dynamics of Hong Kong, and, in particular, for a more nuanced understanding of the meaning of 'segregation'.

Focusing on the Chinese merchant elite, *Power and Charity* necessarily pays attention to the European communities and the Chinese grassroots only where they became, from time to time, players in the Tung Wah story. Two books, happily, have appeared that by exploring Hong Kong society from different angles, help to draw a fuller picture of it. Chan Wai-kwan's *The Making of Hong Kong Society: Three Studies of Class Formation in Early Hong Kong*, looks at three 'classes' — a European merchant class, a Chinese labouring class and a Chinese merchant class. Exploring several important archives, including the Jardine, Matheson Archive which had never been examined for this purpose before, Chan reveals welcome new information about the first two groups. In addition, he analyses the intricate interplay among the three. One of his main arguments is that, ultimately, class divisions within Chinese society became more important than the racial cleavage between European and Chinese, as the common interests of the Chinese and European merchant elites increasingly distanced Chinese merchants from the politically marginalized Chinese labouring class. Chan provides a far sharper analysis of class relations than I did. I used the Seamen's Strike of 1922 to reflect the decline of the Chinese merchant elite's function as a cohesive agent bridging class differences. Chan, approaching it from another angle, uses the Strike to analyse how seamen and other trades successfully exploited class solidarity to extract concessions from a now entirely adversarial Chinese merchant elite. Combining these views, readers may construct a more comprehensive picture of this very significant historical event and gain greater insight into the multi-layered nature of class conflicts in Hong Kong.

Our understanding of the Chinese labouring class is further enhanced by Tsai Jung-fang's *Hong Kong in Chinese History: Community and Social Unrest in the British Colony, 1842–1913.* Tsai explains that he is interested not only in ' the wealthy Chinese merchants surrounded by their concubines in the magnificent residences overlooking Victoria harbor' but also in 'a sweating sedan chair coolie bitten by a dog owned by a European, the riotous Chinese crowd spitting on the British imperial troops patrolling the streets of Hong Kong, and a ricksha puller spitting blood at the end of a long hard journey.' Using a 'history from below' approach, he chooses to explore the social reality hidden behind the veneer of prosperity, stability and harmony so often portrayed by the colony's dominant groups and ruling elite.[8] In the process, he yields valuable information on the living conditions — wages, cost of living, housing situations — of several groups of manual workers, whom he describes as the most abused, exploited and neglected group in Hong Kong. While filling a gap in the social canvas I paint in *Power and Charity*, he throws new light on the dynamics of class relations by putting the labouring classes at centre stage.

Tsai's book also brings out the complex issue of nationalism. However, even though realizing that 'nationalism is Janus-faced' and that Chinese merchant and professional elites did have nationalist sentiments, he nevertheless seems to indicate that the nationalism of the labouring classes was somehow 'purer'. This is not the place to debate the problematics of nationalism,[9] especially why it should be treated as some kind of First Principle. What is relevant to our discussion here is the fact that the Chinese merchant elite in the late nineteenth and early twentieth centuries was deeply interested in Mainland politics: the Tung Wah Hospital elite showed their patriotism first toward the Qing government and later to various Republican Chinese regimes on the Mainland.

Those interested in further exploring the fascinating relationship between business and politics in China will welcome, as I do, Stephanie Chung Po-yin's work, *Chinese Business Groups in Hong Kong and Political Change in South China, 1900–25* (1998).[10] Chung demonstrates how members of the Hong Kong elite, including the commercial elite, were instrumental in Chinese nation-building from the late Qing onwards, taking part aggressively in such nationalistic activities as the 'rights recovery' movement and 'commercial war' against foreign economic intrusion. After the fall of the Qing government, Chinese elites in Hong Kong continued to work closely with the various Mainland regimes, with one group supporting the government in North China and a rival group the government in Guangdong. Of equal interest, Chung describes how the conflicts between North China and Guangdong mirrored conflicts among the different merchant groups in Hong Kong, thus further underlining the intricate configuration of Hong Kong society.

In Hong Kong, political sentiments and ambitions were as often as not oriented more toward China than Hong Kong itself, and conditions in China became a crucial factor affecting alignments within Hong Kong society. Thus, while race and class are easily recognizable factors for alignment, conflict and alienation, two other factors — the China factor and regional identity — further complicated the situation in Hong Kong.

Chung's work draws attention to an element fundamental to the internal differentiation of Hong Kong society — native-place affiliation — that is sorely underestimated in *Power and Charity*. Indeed, if I were to rewrite the book, the one statement that I would wish most to retract is this: that guilds rather than regional associations provided the main framework for social activities in Hong Kong![11] I realized almost immediately after completing the manuscript that the statement was invalid, and since then, in several of my publications I have emphasized the impact of regional sentiments on Hong Kong's development.[12] It is particularly useful here to point out the close co-operation between the many native-place organizations and the Tung Wah Hospital, with the raising of funds for famine relief and the repatriation of emigrants' bones from abroad being the two most outstanding collaborative activities.[13] In Hong Kong, native place organizations existed, and still do, at different levels of society, often straddling class divisions. In the nineteenth and early twentieth centuries, they contributed to social stability by providing welfare services to their less privileged members and, by emphasizing comradeship among the different classes, relieved some of the tensions of society and contained some of the contradictions. However, as might be expected, native-place consciousness could also be a factor for exclusion and disruption. Rivalry among different regional groups could manifest itself in manifold forms: from subtle jockeying for economic and political power among merchants to street brawls among 'coolies'. The

Hong Kong government did not hesitate to manipulate native-place divisions to ensure domination, the classic ploy of divide and rule. Though most members of the Tung Wah Committee were representatives of guilds, many of them were at the same time leaders of their own regional groups, a point that reminds us of the importance of multiple identity.

The reality of multiple identity and countless conflicting interests should call into question the overly homogeneous picture of the Tung Wah Committee presented in the book, and it is through a deeper understanding of how its members negotiated their many identities — sometimes as crosses they had to bear, and sometimes as social and political capital — that we can achieve a clearer vision of the dynamics that shaped the Hospital's policy, practice and course of development. A careful study of the interplay between the intricate and often conflicting identities of individual merchants and groups of merchants based on native-place origin, political affiliation, religious and cultural upbringing and intellectual inclination, to name just the obvious ones, will be a potent antidote to the too often overgeneralized views of Hong Kong society.[14]

One focus of *Power and Charity* is the Hospital's work with Chinese emigrants at different stages of their sojourn — when they left China, when they were in transit through Hong Kong, during their stay abroad and when they returned to the native village. Moreover, the Hospital played a vital role in the whole process of Chinese emigration by keeping Chinese in Hong Kong and China informed about the conditions of those overseas and in touch with them in a variety of ways. Though the book demonstrates the significance of Hong Kong as an emigration port as seen through the Hospital's operations, it is only from subsequent research that I have discovered the full impact of Chinese emigration on the development of Hong Kong, and, as importantly, how Hong Kong in turn shaped the Chinese diaspora. Chinese emigration touched almost every level of Hong Kong society. Many businesses were connected directly or indirectly with it, and the livelihood of people in many walks of life, from the most powerful merchant to the humblest transport labourer toiling on the waterfront, depended on it. Among the Hospital's Directors were so-called California Traders who exported goods to overseas Chinese consumer markets, mainly in North America, Australia and Hawaii, and imported goods from these places, often conducting business with their own overseas branches or with close associates among Chinese merchants abroad. Others were engaged in passenger shipping as compradors of shipping companies, ships' charterers and agents, passage brokers, provisioners and general contractors for repairing and other services. They were recruiters of migrant labourers and money changers who, with their expert knowledge of foreign exchange, handled emigrants' remittances. Whatever their business, they almost invariably had close links with Chinese overseas. Donations raised on ships carrying Chinese passengers were a major source of income for the Hospital. These intimate and pervasive economic and personal connections with Chinese emigration deepen our understanding of the Directors' concerns and the meaning of the Hospital's activities. Notably too, by facilitating the migration process, Hong Kong also directly contributed to the growing number of *qiaoxiang*, localities on the Mainland that sent their natives overseas and that became increasingly dependent for their wellbeing on migrants' remittances. Dealing with countless individuals, regional associations and other institutions in Hong Kong, China and abroad, the Hospital was in fact collectively and on a day-to-day basis, weaving, sustaining and consolidating global and multi-layered networks that bonded the Chinese emigrant to his native place. Taking these into consideration, we may appreciate even more its role in the Chinese Diaspora and its significance in modern Chinese history.

There is, indeed, no reason why we should confine the study of the Tung Wah Hospital within the boundaries of Hong Kong or China's history. There are at least two other arenas of enquiry it can engage in, one being comparative studies, the other, world history.

Many themes in *Power and Charity* can easily lend themselves to broader thematic and comparative studies. Take philanthropy, for instance. Philanthropy has in recent years grown into an enormous field of study — there are even degree programmes on it offered by universities. Numerous books, articles in academic journals and newspapers, newsletters and websites devote themselves to it. Topics range from practical matters such as fundraising and capacity building of non-profit organizations to pragmatic issues such as the relationship between business and philanthropy, especially between corporate image and good works, to philosophical questions such as the ethics of giving. Clearly, the Tung Wah's experience in all its various aspects can enrich these discourses, and contribute a useful historical perspective on contemporary concerns.

Other studies can, in turn, illuminate our understanding of the Tung Wah elite, its role in society and the environment in which it operated. The practice, rhetoric and motives of philanthropy naturally vary in different places and different times, and yet they can be remarkably similar. Recently, reading Andrew Herman's work, I was struck by the degree to which the Tung Wah Directors resembled the late twentieth century American philanthropists he studies. Herman describes philanthropy as an instrument that makes financial worth symbolically equivalent to moral worth, and claims that the dispensation of charity legitimizes the accumulation of wealth. This was exactly what philanthropy did for the Chinese merchant elite in nineteenth century Hong Kong. Herman also inspires one to look at the deeper psychological dimension of giving. His view that the identity of wealthy, philanthropic men 'comprises a mythical place of masculine desire in the social imagination of the "American Dream"' compels one to ask the same questions about the psychology of the Tung Wah Directors. We know that Chinese philanthropists were driven by a combination of the Confucian ideal of disseminating civilizing influence and the Buddhist ideal of mercy, but did this combined ideal function psychologically in the same way as the 'American Dream' in prompting men to do good? Indeed, how innovative it would be to analyse the behaviour and mindset of the Tung Wah Directors in terms of masculine desire!

Apart from the individual, it is equally instructive to compare the collective. While on the individual level, the effect of the interplay between wealth, philanthropy and self-image in the two above situations is largely similar, on a societal level, the effect differs dramatically. Philanthropy, Herman claims, is a social practice by which wealthy individuals in late twentieth century America are able to transform their individuality, expressed in personal desires, cultural interests and political-economic priorities, into a principality or a sovereign realm of autonomy, freedom, and control. Clearly this does not apply to nineteenth century Hong Kong where Chinese philanthropists laboured under a strictly authoritarian and watchful regime. But will it apply in the twenty-first century?

This is a particularly exciting time for reflecting on philanthropy in view of the fact that 'capitalistic welfare' is beginning to appear in socialist China, where an increasing number of wealthy entrepreneurs are coming on the scene, and where the gap between rich and poor is fast growing.[15] Bringing to bear the multifarious forms, justifications, rhetoric — and yes, even gendered desires — related to philanthropy, a host of interesting questions can be raised. For example, we may come closer to distinguishing which elements of philanthropy are universal and which are 'culturally determined'. Such comparative studies may indeed inform debates on whether there is even such a thing as 'culturally determined' phenomena, when the very notion of 'culture' being something immutable is being contested. Moreover, now that private philanthropy is being practised in a socialist state, new and compelling questions about class relations and about the political economy, even the moral economy, of giving will certainly arise — not only with regard to contemporary China or nineteenth century Hong Kong, but other societies in other times as well.

There is, in addition, a transnational dimension to philanthropy. One major recent concern in the field is private foreign aid.[16] It leads me to wonder whether what the Tung Wah Hospital practised was not a kind of foreign aid in reverse, as one of its major activities was to organize fundraising among overseas Chinese for relief in China. Can we not see this as a different paradigm of philanthropy, what we might tentatively call 'diasporic philanthropy'?

This and many other questions can be formulated on the subject of philanthropy from a comparative studies point of view, and I hope readers of *Power and Charity* will be stimulated and encouraged to raise and debate them in different arenas.

The other arena that the study of the Tung Wah Hospital may enter is world history. The Hospital's history reflected many phenomena that are now key issues in world history study, including migration, network societies, disease and medicine and colonial relations. Through becoming part of the British Empire, which was an immense global network in itself, and a growing hub for commercial and shipping links, for missionary movements and Chinese migrants, Hong Kong had become an integral and crucial part of world history at least since the 1850s. As a 'space of flow', its open and prompt access to information and the disproportionately immense energy it generated consolidated its central position in many different kinds of networks.

To claim for Hong Kong a place in world history is by no means an expression of my personal chauvinism. For many years, the Japanese economic historian, Takeshi Hamashita, has emphasized Hong Kong's central position in the Asia region.[17] Moreover, while Manuel Castells acknowledges Hong Kong as a megacity, he carefully points out that being a megacity is not necessarily an unmixed blessing, for megacities concentrate the worst as well as the best.[18] The history of the Tung Wah Hospital can be extrapolated more fully to demonstrate important global processes; at the same time, we can also gain new insights into its historical meaning by approaching it from a global perspective. It is as important to understand the internal dynamics of Hong Kong society as it is to appreciate how they interact with pervasive external forces that constantly influenced them, although the boundaries between 'internal' and 'external' factors are never clear-cut. Writing Hong Kong history from the perspective of Hong Kong's people, as suggested by Tsai Jung-fang, may be valid and meaningful, but it need not and should not be the only approach.[19] With Hong Kong's history being so rich, multifaceted and fascinating, only by studying it from as many perspectives as possible will we do it justice.

Let us return to Hong Kong where the Tung Wah story is still unfolding. Through its schools, hospitals, old people's homes and many other kinds of social services, Tung Wah continues to contribute vigorously to Hong Kong society today, and its enormous philanthropic operations keep growing in scale and diversity. Even though its Directors no longer play the high-level political role they did in the nineteenth century, there being now so many alternative routes to influence, fame and status in Hong Kong, a place on the Tung Wah Group of Hospital's Board is nonetheless still very much a feather in one's cap. But, in a way, it is the development of Chinese medicine that forms the most intriguing part of the Hospital's recent history.

The Hospital was, as earlier mentioned, founded to provide Chinese medicine for the Chinese population; indeed, its main mission in the nineteenth century was to protect Chinese patients from Western doctors and their practice. However, under pressure from Western doctors and the government, the Hospital was forced, step by step, to adopt Western medicine, until by mid-twentieth century, Western medicine had become its mainstream medical service. Up to the 1990s, most of the Hospital's resources had been invested in developments in Western medicine, and any progress that was made was made in that area. Even though it never ceased providing herbalist and bone-setting services, these had become marginal to the Hospital's overall operation. In the late 1970s, the Hospital demonstrated the headway it had made in Western medicine by becoming integrated with the training of the University of Hong Kong's medical students. It worked closely with the Queen Mary Hospital, the main government hospital and the University's teaching hospital, in both medicine and surgery, and when the University opened a Dental Faculty in the 1980s, its students also did their practical training at the Tung Wah. What a far cry from the days during the bubonic plague when Chinese patients were forcibly removed from the Tung Wah Hospital to government hospitals because it was considered harmful to patients! In fact, the Hospital became so enamoured with Western medicine that in 1982, its official historian took the liberty to rewrite its history. He notes that Western style medical methods were only introduced to the Hospital quite late, but instead of acknowledging the Directors' resistance to those methods as the cause of the delay, he writes, 'In spite of the promotional efforts made by the [Tung Wah] Group [of Hospitals], Western medical methods were not widely accepted until the early years of the twentieth century.'[20] Obviously it had become 'politically incorrect' to admit that the Hospital's leaders had, at one point in time, preferred Chinese medicine to Western medicine!

In general, the Chinese population in Hong Kong never quite lost its faith in Chinese medicine even though increasingly in the twentieth century, people also embraced Western medicine as more effective for some treatments and grew less fearful of some of the procedures. The colonial administration also helped to preserve the dominant position of Western medicine, by ostensibly leaving Chinese medicine unregulated, an extension of the segregation policy expounded by Captain Elliot in his 1841 Proclamation. Under a system where only Western medical practitioners could be registered, which meant in effect that only *their* letters of leave were recognized by employers, and insurance policies only covered Western medical services, it was unavoidable that Western doctors were privileged.

In the last decade or so, however, the status of Chinese medicine has risen dramatically, reflecting changed political and intellectual circumstances on many fronts.[21] At the local universities, which had long been the stronghold of Western medicine, Chinese medicine is now being taught, and is also an important topic of academic research. In 1999, after years of intense and bitter debating, the SAR government passed the Chinese Medicine Ordinance to regulate the practice, use, trading and manufacture of Chinese medicine. Accordingly, the Chinese Medical Council set up a registration system for Chinese medicine practitioners, and finally, in 2002, a list of such practitioners is available for the first time.[22] Although the main motive behind the ordinance had originally been to regulate the practice of Chinese medicine in order to eradicate abuses, the end result was to enhance the status of Chinese medicine. With the SAR government's recently declared ambition to make Hong Kong the world's Centre of Chinese Medicine, it seems highly likely that the position of Chinese medicine in Hong Kong will continue to rise.[23]

Naturally, these developments have affected the Tung Wah Group of Hospitals; indeed, the Group has played an important role contributing to the transformation. The first major sign of change occurred in 1995–96, when the Group turned to the First Affiliated Hospital of the Sun Yat-sen University of Medical Sciences of Guangzhou for advice on how to expand its Chinese medical service.[24] More positive steps in this new direction followed in the next few years. At first, they were only small steps. The Group added an acupuncture clinic in 1997, and set out to promote and educate the public on Chinese medicine by organizing herbs exhibition cabinets as well as distributing pamphlets and brochures introducing Chinese traditional medicine.[25] But soon, the steps became bigger and more purposeful. In December 1997, it organized the first Medical Symposium of Chinese Medicine for scholars from the Mainland and Hong Kong.[26] Perhaps even more significant are its collaborative efforts with the University of Hong Kong and the Chinese University, and later the Baptist University, in medical and health education, training and research on Chinese medicine.[27]

By the early 2000s, there is no doubt that Chinese medicine has become a main focus of the Tung Wah Group's overall strategic planning.[28] The scope of collaboration with local universities continues to expand, as does its connections with medical institutions on the Mainland. Research on Chinese medicine is as much emphasized as clinical practice and training, while the idea of integrating Western and Chinese medicine is quickly gaining ground. The outbreak of SARS (Severe Acute Respiratory

Syndrome) in 2003 has further prompted the medical authority and local clinicians to consider an integrated approach to treating SARS patients using a combination of Western and Chinese therapies, thus ensuring that the process of integration will intensify.[29] This surely represents another major development in the history of medicine in Hong Kong.

However, combining Western and Chinese therapies is one thing; reconciling the doctors of the two traditions is a very different matter. Not only is the gulf between the two systems based on radically disparate philosophies toward medicine and health, but in Hong Kong, the historical trajectories of the practice of Chinese and Western medicine in the last 150 years are bound to make reconciliation even more difficult. The widely divergent social and cultural backgrounds of practitioners of Western and Chinese medicine in general, not to mention vested interests, keep the two worlds apart, and it seems that any attempt at a 'forced marriage' — such as placing them in the same functional constituency — is as likely to widen the rift as to close it.[30] If one of the main lessons we learn in history is the limitations as well as the possibilities of any given place and time, the Tung Wah's own experience shows clearly that the encounters between Western and Chinese medicine do not happen in a social, political and economic vacuum. Such a realization should caution us against simple-minded and overly-optimistic expectations that real merging between practitioners of the two systems in Hong Kong could happen any time soon.

One final reason why I welcome the re-issue of *Power and Charity* is a personal one. When I submitted the manuscript to Oxford University Press in 1988, I had originally intended to dedicate the book to the memory of my father and to my mother, but when the events in Tiananmen in May and June of the following year rocked Hong Kong, I changed my mind. Instead, I dedicated the book to the people of Hong Kong as a way of expressing my solidarity with them during those days of hope, exhilaration, horror, despair and grief. Over fourteen years later, I seize this second opportunity to make a dedication, and it is comforting to know that, as long as I wish to express my gratitude and love to my parents, it is never too late.

ELIZABETH SINN
Hong Kong
June 2003

Notes

1. For example, in his review, Ian Scott writes, 'Dr Sinn's book will stand as the definitive study of the early history of the hospital and it is essential reading for anyone wishing to understand Hong Kong society and politics in the nineteenth century.' (Review by Ian Scott, *Journal of the Hong Kong Branch of the Royal Asiatic Society*, vol. 29 (1989) pp. 400–401).

2. See Carol Jones's review article of Albert H. Yee, ed. *Whither Hong Kong: China's Shadow or Visionary Gleam?* (Lanham: University Press of America, 1999).in which she also discusses the crop of not very good books that appeared just before and after 1997 (*China Review International* volume 8: no 2 (Fall, 2001), pp. 305–332.

3. Christopher Munn, *Anglo-China: Chinese People and British Rule in Hong Kong, 1841–1880* (Richmond, Surrey: Curzon, 2001), p. 3.

4. Christopher Munn, *Anglo-China: Chinese People and British Rule in Hong Kong, 1841–1880*, p. 11.

5. See the *Sultan* case in which Chinese passengers sued the ship's captain for refusing to allow them to board the ship even though they had bought tickets for their passage (*Friend of China*, 7 and 14 July, 1852); also the case of the *Libertad*, whose owner Chook Sing, having a quarrel with the ship's captain, prevented the ship from leaving the harbour by having the Vice Admiral seize the ship. (*Friend of China*, 1 April, 1854).

6. *Power and Charity*, p. 98, pp. 189–190.

7. One good example was the relationships between the American Charles Ryberg and his Chinese business partners in Hong Kong as revealed in his correspondence with Augustine Heard & Co., in the 1860s: Volume LV-1, Folder 52, Heard II at the Baker Library, Harvard Business School.

8. Tsai Jung-fang, *Hong Kong in Chinese History: Community and Social Unrest in the British Colony, 1843–1913* (New York: Columbia University Press, 1993), p. 6. It is interesting to observe that the labourers Tsai deals with in his book are all men. Granted that, by comparison, the number of women in nineteenth and early twentieth century urban Hong Kong was small, but they did exist. If anything, many of them, including the concubines of merchants living in magnificent residences overlooking the harbour, were abused and victimized. And yet, there was much social mobility within the labouring classes, even among women, and the high degree of social mobility was unquestionably one of Hong Kong's most outstanding characteristics. One channel of social land economic advance for working women was to become brothel keepers, who by Hong Kong law, could only be women. My work on women could fill some of the gaps in Tsai's book. See my article 'Chinese Patriachalism and the Protection of Women in nineteenth Century Hong Kong', in Maria Jaschok and Suzanne Miers, eds., *Chinese Women and Patriarchy: Submission, Servitude and Escape* (London & Hong Kong: ZED Books and Hong Kong University Press), pp. 141–167. In that work, I take a 'top-down' approach, and look at the way the (male) elite and the (male) colonial government dealt with the issue. However, the women's own voices are heard in a later work of mine — 'Her Sisters' Keepers: Brothel Keepers as Entrepreneurs in nineteenth century Hong Kong' which will appear in a volume edited by Helen Siu on women in South China.

9. One of the most stimulating discussions on Chinese nationalism is provided by Prasenjit Duara in *Rescuing History from the Nation: Questioning Narratives of Modern China* (Chicago: University of Chicago Press, 1995).

10. Stephanie Chung Po-yin, *Chinese Business Groups in Hong Kong and Political Change in South China, 1900–25* (London: Macmillan, New York: St Martin's Press, 1996).

11. *Power and Charity*, p. 56.

12. My works on regional associations are: 'A History of Regional Associations in

Pre-War Hong Kong', in Elizabeth Sinn, ed. *Between East and West: Aspects of Social and Political Development in Hong Kong* (Hong Kong: Centre of Asian Studies, University of Hong Kong, 1990) pp. 159–186; '*Xin xi guxiang*: A study of Regional Associations as a Bonding Mechanism in the Chinese Diaspora' *Modern Asian Studies* volume 31: no. 2 (1997), pp. 375–398; 'Cohesion and Fragmentation: A County-Level Perspective on Chinese Transnationalism in the 1940s' in Leo Douw, Cen Huang and Michael R. Godley, eds. *Qiaoxiang Ties: Interdisciplinary Approaches to 'Cultural Capitalism' in South China* (London and New York: Kegan Paul International in association with International Institute for Asian Studies, Leiden and Amsterdam) pp. 67 –87.

    13. See my paper 'In-between Places: The Key Role of Localities of Transit in Chinese Migration', presented at the AAS Annual Meeting, Washington D.C., 4–7 April 2002.

    14. The idea of multiple identity of the Hong Kong elite is also discussed in various chapters in Ngo Tak-wing, ed. *Hong Kong's History: State and Society under Colonial Rule* (London, New York: Routledge, 1999).

    15. Alex Kwan and Joseph Y.S. Cheng, *Capitalistic Welfare Development in Communist China : The Experience of Southern China* (Chicago: Imprint Publication, 1996) and Clara Li, 'Publicity Blitz turns Remote Charity Group into China Icon', *South China Morning Post*, 3 September 2002. The end of the cold war has also witnessed the rise of the non-profit sector in former socialist states, and as new forms of philanthropy are emerging all over the world, philanthropy becomes an even more exhilarating subject of research.

    16. David Sogge, Kees Bichart and John Saxby ed. *Compassion and Calculation. The Business of Private Foreign Aid* (London and Chicago: Pluto Press with Transnational Institute (TNI) 1996).

    17. Takeshi Hamashita 濱下武志, *Xianggang da shi ye: Yazhou wang luo zhongxin* 香港大視野: 亞洲網絡中心 (Hong Kong in Greater Perspective: The Centre of Asian Networks) (Hong Kong: Commercial Press, 1997).

    18. Manuel Castells, *The Information Age. Economy, Society and Culture* (Cambridge, Massachusetts and London: Blackwell, 1996) Volume I. *The Rise of Network Society*, p. 403.

    19. It is also important to remember that since 'Hong Kong people' are by no means homogenous there can be many Hong Kong people's Hong Kong histories. See Cai Rongfang 蔡榮芳 [Tsai Jung-fang], *Xianggang ren de Xianggang shi* 香港人的香港史 ('The Hong Kong People's History of Hong Kong')(Hong Kong: Oxford University Press, 2001).

    20. *Tung Wah Today* [Hong Kong: Tung Wah Group of Hospitals, [1982]].

    21. A number of reasons account for such radical change in direction. The return of Hong Kong to China in 1997 and the need to link different aspects of the Special Administrative Region with the Mainland more closely certainly was a major impetus. The phenomenal progress on the Mainland since 1949 in Chinese medical education, training, service and research — mainly through regulation, systemization and standardization and state support — was also critical. China's opening from the 1980s further made medical institutions in China more accessible to the outside world in terms of knowledge, training and research facilities and supply of medical products. In particular, the potency of Chinese medicine demonstrated through Western analytical methods helps to convince the medical fraternity, in Hong Kong and overseas, of the soundness of Chinese medicine, so long as quality control could be assured. But there are less obvious reasons too.

    One should not overlook the possibility that the acceptance and recognition of the merits of Chinese medicine in Hong Kong is partly due to the fact that Chinese medicine is increasingly being appreciated and promoted by the medical establishments in many Western countries as alternative/ complementary/ holistic medicine. In addition to the support of these mainstream establishments, in the West, the New Age enchantment with spiritual health and alternative health systems, further creates a thriving market for Chinese medical and health products. In Hong Kong, it is unfortunately true that often, even 'Chinese' things gain credibility only after they have received the stamp of approval in the West. Perhaps dependency, a key concept in the study of colonial relations and the colonial mentality, can yet serve as another frame of reference for our study of the development of Chinese medicine in Hong Kong!

22. http://www.info.gov.hk/info/tcm.htm.

23. Speech of the Secretary for Health and Welfare at the National Day Celebration of the Hong Kong Chinese Medicine Sector, 3 October, 2002: (http://www.hwfb.gov.hk/hw/english/archive/index.htm).

24. Tung Wah Group of Hospitals, *Annual Report,* 1995/96, p. 68.

25. Tung Wah Group of Hospitals, *Annual Report,* 1996/97, p. 49.

26. Tung Wah Group of Hospitals, *Annual Report,* 1997/98, p. 48.

27. One of the first joint research projects with the University of Hong Kong was a study of the effectiveness of using acupuncture in the treatment of acute facial nerve palsy conducted in 1998/99. (Tung Wah Group of Hospitals, *Annual Report,* 1998/99, p. 37). Another was a joint project with the Chinese University to explore the effectiveness of integrated practice of Western medicine and traditional Chinese medicine to the treatment of diabetic foot ulcer (Tung Wah Group of Hospitals, *Annual Report,* 1999/2000, p. 36).

28. 'Foreword', Tung Wah Group of Hospitals, *Annual Report,* 2001/2002.

29. 'Press Release' Hong Kong Economic and Trade Office Tokyo, 21 May 2003.

30. Chinese herbalists had demanded representation on the medical functional constituency but their demand was denied. See 'Doctors fear chaos from "forced marriage" of Profession in Legco', *SCMP,* 11 December 2002, and 'Herbalists miss out on a voice in next legco', *SCMP,* 21 February, 2003.

Preface to the Original Edition

THE Tung Wah Group of Hospitals is one of the oldest and best known charitable institutions in Hong Kong. The local community is familiar with the hospitals, schools, old people's homes, youth centres, and nurseries it runs, and its annual fund-raising show is one of the social and entertainment highlights of the year. Yet most people are ignorant of its history, its origin and, in particular, its social and political significance in the nineteenth and early twentieth centuries. Until eight years ago, I too shared this ignorance.

My blissful oblivion was shattered by the writings of Professor H. J. Lethbridge and the Reverend Carl Smith, which point out the central social and political role the Tung Wah Hospital Committee played as a local élite group.[1] Their pioneer works convinced me that here was a fascinating subject, a key to the understanding of Hong Kong history and society, begging for further attention. When I learnt of the existence of the Hospital's archives, the desire to pursue the subject became irresistible.

My aim is to put the Hospital in historical context. Though Hong Kong is much studied by the sociologist, anthropologist, economist, lawyer, and political scientist, historians have not given it equal attention, and the Chinese community is particularly neglected as a research topic. The Tung Wah is an ideal locus for exploring the many dimensions of Hong Kong's history. A historical study providing insights into one's own society requires no justification. At a time when the world is turning its eyes on Hong Kong and contemplating its future, a deeper knowledge and understanding of its past are even more timely.

This book has grown from my doctoral thesis. I wish to thank my supervisors, Dr Alan Birch, and Professors L. Y. Chiu and L. K. Young, for their encouragement and guidance. I am especially indebted to Dr Birch for introducing me to Hong Kong history. My colleagues at the History Department, University of Hong Kong, have given me unfailing support; in particular, Professor C. M. Turnbull was most sympathetic, and Dr Priscilla M. Roberts was good enough to read parts of the manuscript.

The work would have been impossible without the use of the

archives of the Tung Wah Group of Hospitals and the Po Leung Kuk, and I wish to thank their Directors for giving me access. My gratitude also goes to the staff of those two institutions, as well as to the Hong Kong University Library, the Public Records Office (Hong Kong), the National Diet Library (Tokyo), and the Meiji Bunka at the Tokyo University for their patience and assistance. Special acknowledgement is made to the Public Records Office and the Hong Kong Museum of History for permission to reproduce photographs in their holdings.

I wish also to thank the many individuals who have given me invaluable help: Professor Edgar Wickberg, who alerted me to the significance of the Tung Wah outside Hong Kong; Dr James Hayes, a constant source of information and inspiration; the late Sir Tang Shui-kin and Mr Leo Lee, former Tung Wah Chairmen, who provided information on the Hospital's workings in the past; Mr Peter Yeung of the Hong Kong University Library, and Mrs Robyn McLean, formerly of the Public Records Office (Hong Kong), who helped tirelessly in my search for materials; Mrs Gail Pirkis, formerly of Oxford University Press (Hong Kong), for her encouragement; and Miss Yan Woon-Yin, who helped to prepare the final draft.

To my friend and teacher, the Reverend Carl Smith, who has in countless ways supported me through the ordeal, I owe my deepest and most humble gratitude.

While the work owes so much to so many, any error in fact or interpretation is of course entirely my own.

ELIZABETH SINN

Abbreviations

BPP	*British Parliamentary Papers*
CM	*China Mail*
CO 129	Great Britain. Colonial Office. Original Correspondence: Hong Kong, 1841–1951. Series 129.
DP	*Hong Kong Daily Press*
FO 17	Great Britain. Foreign Office. General Correspondence: China. Series 17.
FO 228	Great Britain. Foreign Office. Embassy and Consular Archive: China. Series 228.
FO 233	Great Britain. Foreign Office. Miscellanea 1759–1935. Series 233.
JHKBRAS	*Journal of the Hong Kong Branch of the Royal Asiatic Society*
HKGG	*Hong Kong Government Gazette*
HKSP	*Hong Kong Sessional Papers*
HKT	*Hong Kong Telegraph*
HKWP	*Hong Kong Weekly Press*
LQJ	*Li Wenzhong Gong quanji (Complete Works of Li Hongzhang)*
LYJ	*Liu Kunyi yiji (Works of Liu Kunyi)*
MAS	*Modern Asian Studies*
TWR	*Report of the Commission appointed by H. E. Sir William Robinson...to enquire into the Working and Organization of the Tung Wa Hospital together with the Evidence taken before the Commission and other Appendices*
XH	*Xunhuan ribao (Universal Circulating Herald)*
ZQJ	*Zhang Wenxiang Gong quanji (Complete Works of Zhang Zhidong)*
ZW	*Zhongwai xinwen qiri bao (China and World News Weekly)*

Romanization

It is impossible to standardize the Romanization of Chinese words. Local names of persons, institutions, and places are Romanized in the way they most frequently appear in contemporary Western-language documents. Certain names are Romanized according to convention. The pinyin system is applied to the rest.

Introduction

FOR the Tung Wah Hospital, the years 1869 to 1896 were significant and dramatic. An inquest into the death of a Chinese emigrant in 1869 revealed the appalling lack of medical facilities for the Chinese community in Hong Kong, causing a scandal which rocked the colony and reverberated in London. In the wake of the scandal emerged the Tung Wah Hospital, which went on to carry out philanthropic work on a grand scale, winning wide acclaim, not least of which came from the Emperor of China himself. Its Committee, whose members wore Chinese Mandarin robes on formal occasions, soon grew so powerful among the local Chinese that it was feared as an alternative government challenging the colonial one. Officials in London, Canton, and Peking alike became involved with its activities, and more than once it became an issue in Sino-British diplomacy. Its work pervaded so many aspects of society that it became inevitably caught up in the most mundane as well as the most sensational matters — communal quarrels, kidnap cases, emigration fraud, riots, and epidemics among them.

But high drama aside, the Tung Wah story, so closely tied to the development of Hong Kong society itself, is an ideal vehicle for investigating some of its fundamental realities, and in particular three essential aspects: the relations between the government and the Chinese community, social organization in terms of the concept and function of Chinese community leadership, and the relations between China and the local Chinese.

Several factors affected relations between the colonial government and the Chinese community. Hong Kong's annexation was predominated by one aim — trade. It was Captain Charles Elliot's vision of Hong Kong as the 'chief seat of our commercial intercourse'[1] with the Chinese Empire and Sir Henry Pottinger's (Administered 1841–43; Governed 1843–44) conviction of the 'desirability and necessity' to possess Hong Kong as an 'Emporium of our trade'[2] which led them to insist upon its acquisition against the will of London. When London finally accepted this new addition to the British Empire for 'Diplomatic, Commercial and Military purposes'[3] trade was undoubtedly the major rationale. As the historian Stanley Lane-Poole commented, Hong Kong illustrated 'the commercial instinct which has so powerfully pervaded and strengthened the expansion of England'.[4] Britain's primary concern was to establish the necessary organs of law and order and administration to make trade possible.[5] Given this background, the management of the Chinese was not initially a problem in the sense that the problem did not at first exist independently in the minds of those administering the colony, except as part of the general concern to maintain conditions conducive to trade. In addition, for most of the nineteenth century, Hong Kong, from an administrative point of view, was in what Harold Ingrams calls the 'exploratory phase' of colonial history, when the government was minimal and primitive.[6] This helps to explain why many problems in the early years were dealt with casually and haphazardly.

A second factor dictating the government's attitude toward Chinese inhabitants was the individual Governors themselves. So much diversity characterized the British Empire that it was accepted that, apart from the broadest principles and structural outlines, each colony should be governed according to local conditions. While preventing the development of a uniform imperial 'native policy', it left large discretionary powers in the hands of the 'man on the spot'.[7] Individual Governors, with different backgrounds, personalities, attitudes, and styles, profoundly affected the course of events and the development of institutions in Hong Kong.

Colonial officers' general ignorance of Chinese customs, values, practices, and language was a third factor. To compound the difficulty, the high mobility of the Chinese population meant that Chinese prejudices and practices were constantly reinforced by newcomers from China. This made them more reluctant to give up old ways, and more resistant to government interference in any form. Government officers, in their ignorance, initially found it convenient to leave the Chinese to their own devices so long as public order and revenue were not threatened. In the early days, they simply resorted to *ad hoc* measures whenever crises arose.

The Chinese who came to Hong Kong after 1841 to take advantage of the new opportunities of a boom town also had their own fixed ideas of government and social organization in which the British had no part. The 'unbridged chasm' yawning in the midst of Hong Kong society, observed by Dr E. J. Eitel,[8] was indeed characteristic of the colony in those early days. But the rapid growth of the Chinese population, the increasing complexity of society, and changing concepts of government in Britain combined to make the management of the Chinese assume ever greater importance. It continued to be part of the larger framework of maintaining law and order and raising revenue, of course, but it attracted more official attention as time went by and developed from its crude beginnings to a more sophisticated, systematic, and skilled business. The Tung Wah Hospital played a significant part in stimulating this process. Ironically, though, a more coherent policy toward the Chinese made the government more intolerant of an independent native power group responsible only unto itself.

The creation of the 'Chinese Hospital' was a manifestation of the segregation between the government and the governed. Conflicting ideas about sickness and death and about specific medical treatment and medical organization had made the medical facilities which the government offered irrelevant to the Chinese. Chinese concepts determined the way the Tung Wah Hospital operated for the first 20 years of its history while European ideas of how a hospital should be run gradually took over and imposed changes thereafter. In the process, communal hostilities came to the fore, transforming medical issues into social and political ones. These offer us a chance to test the extent to which segregation could survive, and see how the medical reforms which were eventually forced upon the Hospital in 1896 symbolized the gradual 'de-segregation' of the Chinese community. As in Britain, public health became one of the first areas where direct government interference was introduced into society. But the acceptance of these reforms in Hong Kong was partly due to the emergence of a new Chinese élite whose comparative receptiveness to government proposals and Western ideas and practices was also a sign of the gradual de-segregation in society. Special circumstances in Hong Kong conditioned the Hospital's development from a medical institution to a more widely based charitable organization. Government did little in the way of welfare for the Chinese community, and there were many specific Chinese needs which it did not understand. This lack of understanding and interest created a vacuum and was a major factor affecting the development of Chinese community leadership, the second theme of this study.

The Chinese brought to Hong Kong, even after British occupation, their own ideas of social organization and leadership, and much of Hong Kong's history can be understood in terms of their adaptation to colonial rule and to the special geo-political circumstances of Hong Kong. With these elements in the background, certain tendencies can be detected. In time, in terms of scale, small localized groups representing particularistic, sectarian interests gave way to larger and more universalistic groupings. In terms of status, the Chinese merchants' increasing wealth and rate-paying ability transformed their self-image as well as their position *vis-à-vis* the government, the foreign communities, and the common people, and gradually led them to demand a greater voice in public affairs.

In 1869, a Chinese Hospital to be named the Tung Wah was planned and organized. Its Committee consisted of the wealthiest and most influential members of the Chinese community. It was the first permanent Chinese association which could justifiably claim to represent the whole Chinese community, and more importantly, to be recognized by the government as an élitist group. In many ways, the Committee resembled Chinese local élites in China itself. It arbitrated disputes, carried out a wide range of charitable works, supported education, upheld moral principles, and acted as the medium of communication between the local population and the government. These functions were all the more necessary since the Hong Kong government was for the most part unable or unwilling to perform them. Of course in Hong Kong, as in other Overseas Chinese communities, the Civil Service Examination degrees, such an important determinant of influence and authority in China, had only limited application. Instead, wealth was the main determinant, and the annual selection of the Tung Wah Hospital Committee, based primarily on guild nomination, had a built-in mechanism to call upon the most esteemed, and presumably the wealthiest and most powerful, Chinese business men in Hong Kong. We will see how this élite tried to perform its functions under a colonial government which neither understood nor appreciated sufficiently the social control exercised by informal Chinese power groups. Conflicts and confrontations were common, and the government's dissatisfaction with the Hospital Committee's influence over the local Chinese was finally instrumental in forcing it to reassess its own management strategy towards the Chinese community. Changes in the

Hospital Committee's status and function within the twenty-odd years under study are highlighted to reflect changes that took place within the Chinese community and in Hong Kong itself. This affected the Hospital both as a medical and charitable organization as well as a social and political one. The special circumstances of its foundation had led to the emergence of a Chinese community leadership in the form of the committee of a hospital — itself a novelty in Chinese society — and it was fated to labour under the anomaly of performing political and social functions while existing formally as a medical institution.

The third theme of this book is the presence of China, a factor which overwhelmingly affected the development of the local Chinese community. There were several dimensions. First, China was contiguous to Hong Kong and this physical closeness was a source of much discomfort. Secondly, there is the other fundamental reality of Hong Kong history, the peculiar circumstances of its cession, and the almost universal reluctance among Chinese officials and civilians alike to accept the fact that Hong Kong was foreign territory. To the ordinary Chinese, there was some confusion as to where Chinese jurisdiction ended and British jurisdiction began, and Chinese officials contributed to this confusion by being much less vigorous in observing Hong Kong's territorial sovereignty than their British counterparts. The question of nationality also added to the confusion. Chinese living outside China remained Chinese subjects, but even though in the late nineteenth century the Chinese court conceded that Chinese might be naturalized as foreign subjects, it was especially reluctant to recognize as foreigners Chinese residents in Hong Kong who had become British either by naturalization or by birth. To them, Hong Kong residents were still subject to Chinese law and Chinese jurisdiction. The very clear distinction made today between 'Overseas Chinese' and 'Compatriots of Hong Kong and Macao' is a legacy of the nineteenth century.[9]

The struggle between the Chinese and Hong Kong governments for sovereignty over the Chinese in Hong Kong was long and bitter. Close connections with China — economic, familial, demographic, and political — made Chinese residents in Hong Kong susceptible to the influence and control of Chinese authorities, especially Canton's. It meant that besides a natural inclination to pay allegiance to the Chinese Emperor, vested interests made it additionally expedient to obey Chinese official instructions. This situation produced ambiguity, trapping the Chinese resident in Hong Kong in an ambivalent position as both the Chinese and Hong Kong governments claimed his allegiance and loyalty. It also enabled him, at other times, to play one government against the other, appealing to the one that could protect his interests more effectively on any particular occasion. This reveals the ambivalence of the Chinese resident in Hong Kong, sometimes serving two masters, sometimes serving none. The Tung Wah Hospital's experience effectively revealed this interplay of political forces, and the extent to which China's presence affected the making of government policy and the nature of the Chinese community itself.

The Hospital's role as a link between Chinese at home and those overseas was another dimension of Hong Kong's connections with China. As Hong Kong developed into a major shipping and communications centre and emigration port, the Tung Wah Hospital extended a whole range of services to Chinese in transit in Hong Kong and Chinese living abroad, services especially indispensable in the absence of a Chinese Consul in Hong Kong. They illustrate not only the Tung Wah's importance in connecting Chinese everywhere with the motherland, but also Hong Kong's importance as a pivot in connecting China to the outside world.

These three aspects of Hong Kong history were intimately interwoven, and are separated here only for the purpose of academic analysis. In relating the story of the Tung Wah Hospital the interplay of these themes becomes apparent.

The Tung Wah story is as dramatic as it is significant. Taking us through the vicissitudes of Hong Kong's history, it also reveals fundamental realities. By tracing the fortunes of the Hospital as a medical, social, and political body, the story will provide insights not just into one institution but into the history and changing society of Hong Kong.

1

The Chinese Community before the Tung Wah Hospital

THE Tung Wah Hospital's emergence in 1869 was a turning point in the medical, social, and political history of Hong Kong, and one can fully appreciate its impact only by looking at the situation in Hong Kong before 1869.

Hong Kong's early history was one of segregation — segregation between the government and the Chinese community. Segregation was, for the most part, a tacitly agreed principle in their co-existence. When this was inexpedient and they were forced to meet on the same plane, they groped for ways to communicate.

It was an experiment. Though by 1841 the British had been governing foreign peoples for many years, this did not necessarily produce experienced and efficient government. Most of the Secretaries of State and Parliamentary Under-Secretaries at the Colonial Office were politicians with little detailed knowledge of the vast and diverse Empire they ruled. They relied on career civil servants who were better informed, but even these, preoccupied with 'process[ing] the torrent of papers' on their desks, left the running of the colonies to local officials.[1] Though theoretically more familiar with local conditions, local officials were moved from colony to colony so rapidly that they too often showed a 'dangerous ignorance' of the indigenous societies they controlled, and serious mistakes were made.[2]

Even if the Colonial Office had accumulated some kind of expertise, it was not possible to transfer it wholesale to Hong Kong, the first Crown Colony with a predominantly Chinese population.[3] Other factors also made it unique — the circumstances of its acquisition, the proximity to China, the absence of a 'host' population, or any established institution of authority except those in the small villages — demanding new arrangements. Learning to govern and manage the Chinese was, like all experiments, characterized by trial and error, disappointments and bitterness. The Tung Wah Hospital's emergence in 1869 was an important landmark in this process.

Jurisdiction and Chinese Customs

On 2 February 1841, a few days after formally occupying the island of Hong Kong, Captain Charles Elliot, the Chief Superintendent of Trade and Britain's Plenipotentiary to China, issued a proclamation announcing British sovereignty over the island. But the proclamation also pacified its inhabitants by reassuring them that although they were now British subjects, they would be governed according to 'the laws, customs and usages of China, every description of torture excepted',[4] so that despite the change of regime, life would remain largely the same. As a colonial power, Britain had learnt that apart from establishing its administration by force, it also had to cultivate native acquiescence by making as few changes in native life as possible.[5] Moreover, at the time, British sovereignty over Hong Kong had not been officially confirmed by treaty, and the home government gave no indication that the settlement would be permanent. With this underlying uncertainty, administrators clearly found it expedient to leave the Chinese to themselves as much as possible. Whether unwittingly or otherwise, Elliot set the pattern for the segregation of the Chinese in Hong Kong.

The Treaty of Nanking of 1842 formalized Hong Kong's cession but as jurisdiction over Chinese inhabitants on the island remained unresolved, negotiations continued. At first British officials considered letting them be governed by Chinese laws administered by a Chinese sub-magistrate[6] and Sir Henry Pottinger, the new Plenipotentiary, agreed. However, as London began to realize that Hong Kong was too small a place for two systems of criminal jurisdiction to co-exist, it instructed Pottinger to demand 'unqualified and complete' British jurisdiction.[7] The home government's insistence on full jurisdiction was based on the principle of British sovereignty over Hong Kong. The men on the spot were equally insistent, having learnt from experience that it was mandatory for maintaining law and order and effective control over the overwhelming Chinese majority in the population.

Throughout the negotiation, the Chinese proved unexpectedly intransigent in demanding continued jurisdiction over Chinese residents in Hong Kong. However, the British finally got their way. In December 1843 Pottinger announced that the Chinese had waived the right to try all Chinese persons residing on the island charged with serious crimes.[8] Finally, at the end of 1844, the new Governor, Sir John Davis (Governed 1844–48),[9] obtained from the Chinese Imperial Commissioner, Qiying,[10] a written acknowledgement of British sovereignty over the whole of the island and its people.[11]

Qiying's reluctance to concede jurisdiction surprised Pottinger; it is in fact an important point that both contemporaries and historians have underestimated. It grew not only from Qiying's fear that any further concession would compromise his own position, but also from a more deep-seated belief that all Chinese remained subjects of the Chinese Emperor wherever they went. The Western notion of 'nationality' based on territorial sovereignty took the Chinese a long time to understand and accept. Underlying Qiying's argument over who should try Chinese criminals was the principle that, regardless of where he lived and what new nationality he might *acquire,* a Chinese was always subject to Chinese jurisdiction.

This struggle for sovereignty over the Chinese in Hong Kong reveals a more fundamental problem. An almost inevitable outcome of a migrant population under a foreign government was dual allegiance. In Hong Kong, ties with China did not decline because of migration. Deep attachment to the homeland is natural among Overseas Chinese, but in the case of Hong Kong, China's proximity made the 'migration' an illusion. Residence in Hong Kong was often temporary, and both rich and poor travelled — one is tempted to use the word 'commuted' — back and forth frequently. In this sense, the movement of people had no regard for the political boundaries, and few Chinese regarded Hong Kong as their home. The Chinese kept their families on the Mainland, and for the wealthy, business interests tied them even more closely to China. With these connections they became vulnerable to the control of Chinese authorities, especially Canton's. This long, bitter struggle, with Chinese residents in Hong Kong caught in the middle, had far-reaching consequences.

The legal issue was finally decided in 1844 when the Supreme Court was set up by ordinance. The principle was laid that the law of England as at 5 April 1843 was to prevail in Hong Kong except where inapplicable; and the ordinance gave power to punish Chinese criminals according to Chinese law. As for Chinese customs, they were to be respected except where they conflicted with local ordinance.[12] Thus by 1844 Captain Elliot's promises were very much diluted; but the willingness to allow

Chinese to observe their own customs was sufficient to nurture a real sense of separateness.

As in other colonies where the British promised to observe native customs within the larger framework of British law, the tension was inherent. Natives invariably sought protection in the promise to respect customs while the government relied on statutory law and the courts for social control. In most cases, Hong Kong among them, the increasing centralization of government powers and functions led to the erosion of 'customs', and advocates justified this by calling it 'modernization'.

Control

Once the British had gained jurisdiction over Chinese residents they confronted the even more difficult business of governing them. This difficulty was partly due to the kind of Chinese who came to Hong Kong in the early 1840s. In 1841 there were about 2,000 Chinese scattered about the villages all over the island.[13] The population expanded quickly as builders, stone-cutters, craftsmen, domestic servants, coolies, prostitutes, small traders, and other hangers-on arrived on the heels of the British, and by 1844 the Chinese already numbered 19,000.[14] Besides outright pirates and outlaws,[15] it is safe to speculate that the early arrivals were mostly marginal to Chinese society, since those possessing either wealth or social position in China would not risk breaking the Imperial ban against emigration.[16] Moreover, during and after the Opium War, the Chinese government officially regarded those living under the British as traitors.[17]

Policing such a community was a formidable task, aggravated by the fact that Chinese were ignorant of British law and legal proceedings. Moreover, the early police force was composed mainly of Europeans and Indians, none of whom spoke any Chinese or understood Chinese ways.[18] Government interpreters were mostly Portuguese who had not mastered the written Chinese language. Various means were therefore devised to control the Chinese more effectively.

One method was to impose special restrictions on their movements. As early as October 1842, orders were given prohibiting the Chinese from being out of doors without a lantern from eight to ten o'clock at night, and from being out at all after ten.[19] From then onwards it was stipulated from time to time that Chinese must carry passes and/or lanterns when out at night, a practice formalized by ordinance in 1857. This was only one of the more blatant injustices.

Chinese criminals were also subject to harsher punishments, and caning with rattan, wearing the cangue, and cutting the queue were meted out only to them. The Governor, Sir John Davis, believed that more lenient English penalties would be ridiculed by the Chinese who were too poor to be fined, and whose standard of living was so low that it would be a boon for them to enjoy a spell in prison.[20] With experience in China dating back to the Amherst Mission (1816–17), he prided himself on his knowledge of the Chinese and their social behaviour. This obvious injustice was noted by Sir James Stephen, one of the few Under-Secretaries of State for the Colonies who actively tried to apply the principles of humanitarianism and racial equality to colonial administration.[21] Yet even he could do nothing to restrain Davis.

But Davis's policy must have looked even more unjust to the Chinese. However much he and other Governors pretended that Chinese in Hong Kong enjoyed the same legal privileges and protection as British subjects,[22] the fact remains that they suffered more restrictions and more brutal punishments than other ethnic groups.

The government also tried to control the Chinese with their own policing system. This segregationist approach was adopted in Ordinance 13 of 1844 which created Chinese officers entitled 'Paouchong' (baozhang) and 'Paoukea' (baojia), giving them the same power and authority as the regular police. This seems to be modelled upon the baojia system in China, a system of collective neighbourhood responsibility and mutual surveillance, under the leadership of a baozhang who was 'at once the peace officer and the Tribune of the people'.[23] Though only inheriting this ordinance from his predecessor, Davis was prepared to defend it, arguing rightly that the European police were unable to regulate or restrain the Chinese population and believing Chinese inhabitants would find it more congenial than the 'unnecessary importation into their villages of foreign regulations'.[24] Being gratis, the system had the added advantage of costing the government nothing. In early 1845, Davis was reporting its success. However, E. J. Eitel's opinion, expressed in his book Europe in China, was that the system was practically disregarded from the start and, indeed, very little was seen of these officers in the courts.[25] In the original Hong Kong villages, the *baozhang* had acted as spokesman and policeman, their traditional roles. In the new urban areas, by contrast, the system seems never to have worked. In 1853 the office was greatly modified by ordinance, showing that its success must have been limited.

Davis also hoped to control the population through registration. In August 1844 he proposed a poll tax on all inhabitants, who were to present themselves annually for registration at the Registrar General's office created for this purpose.[26] Reaction was violent. The European inhabitants protested against taxation without representation. As for the Chinese, a public meeting was called by a compradore, and placards were posted, extolling the need for solidarity — to 'enthusiastically share the same intent' (*yongyue tongxin*) — in beseeching the government to abandon the policy.[27]

In response, merchants closed their shops and workers, including cargo boatmen, coolies, and domestic servants, struck — an action known as *bashi*, the classic Chinese form of protest. Three thousand Chinese left Hong Kong, and business was at a standstill. The government yielded in face of stiff resistance. A new ordinance was passed in November 1844 exempting everyone except the lowest and poorest classes of Chinese from registration. Two years later this ordinance was repealed by one which gave the Registrar General the additional title of 'Protector of Chinese Inhabitants'. He was given new powers and the Paouchong and Paoukea became subordinate to him.[28] But this too bore little fruit.[29] The Registrar General's duties were actually confined to registration and the collection of 'Chinese revenues' and, from 1850,[30] the Superintendent of Police took these over. The functions of 'Protector of Chinese' were never carried out.

Chinese Social Organization in Early Hong Kong

In the meantime, the Chinese community in Hong Kong evolved. Though the early comers arrived on a so-called 'barren rock' with minimum urban development, they brought with them the concepts and experience of social organization.[31] Some of the organizations were temporary and informal — with people coming together to deal with a common problem and then disbanding.

One of the first examples of this occurred in 1844, when the government forced Chinese houseowners to move from the Central district to the Tai-ping-shan area. They were naturally reluctant to move, having been permitted to build houses there only two years before. In desperation, they jointly petitioned the government to let them mortgage their shops for money to move. In effect it was blackmail, and the government, which had sold the lots over their heads, eventually paid an average of $40 per shop as moving expenses,[32] showing that such combined action could pay off. Later in the year, Governor Davis's unpopular registration ordinance provided another occasion for the Chinese to demonstrate their ability to organize themselves.

Of course such drama did not occur too often, but day-to-day problems also required joint action. Participants of such action identified themselves variously by a list of persons' names or shop names, by neighbourhood, or by trade. In a few cases they even referred to themselves as 'merchants of all Hong Kong' (*he Gang hangshang*) or as 'shop keepers and inhabitants of the three districts' (Sanwan *zhong puhu zhumin*). It is inconceivable that they literally included every shop in Hong Kong or every inhabitant in the three districts, yet it is still significant that a consciousness of a community larger than the immediate neighbourhood or the craft and trade emerged fairly early.

There were also formal associations — transplanted replicas of those in China, including *huiguan* (regional associations), craft and trade guilds, temple committees, street/neighbourhood associations and, of course, the omnipresent secret societies. But secret or otherwise, Chinese associations tended to share these functions — they provided their members with protection and relief and, most important of all, a sense of identity. In an alien environment with incomprehensible concepts of law and order, these associations had a strong appeal to new immigrants.

Traditionally, Chinese secret societies[33] were formed to oppose the reigning dynasty, and in the nineteenth century they were dedicated to the overthrow of the Qing. The Tiandi hui (literally 'heaven and earth society') with the slogan 'Overthrow the Qing and restore the Ming', dominated the South China region. But, besides pursuing their political ideals, the Triad societies, as Westerners called them, often stooped to mundane criminal activities such as piracy, smuggling, robbery, and protection rackets. It is claimed that Triad members had existed among the indigenous inhabitants of Hong Kong even before the British came.[34] But as more Chinese migrated to the colony, the organization grew with the arrival of old members and the recruitment of new ones, attracting them with their high-sounding ideology and promise of protection.

Both Chinese and Hong Kong officials were convinced that the colony was the rallying point for secret society members.[35] Chinese officials were frustrated that they had no power to arrest them in Hong Kong; they were so near and yet so far. Hong Kong officials too, understandably, tried to eradicate Triad societies which drew members from all walks of life, their sinister influence pervading the whole colony. But despite Davis's efforts at passing stringent laws against them, the police were hampered by their ignorance of their *modus operandi*. Thus, the secret societies would remain a powerful force in Hong Kong into the 1980s.

Less justifiable was the government's hostility towards Chinese guilds, which began organizing in Hong Kong in the 1840s.[36] Unlike the Chinese government, the Hong Kong government refused to accord guild activities any legitimacy. In China, by contrast, the scope of law administered by the state was so narrow that many aspects of society fell beyond it. Consequently, large areas of human activities fell within the jurisdiction of non-official institutions such as the family, clan, and village.[37] Guilds in particular were recognized arbiters in deciding weights and measures, controlled quality and the professional ethics of their members, and protected the interests of their trade or craft. Moreover, they settled cases which might now be classified as commercial crimes and business disputes, and Chinese officials tolerated their right to do so. Europeans regarded all these activities as conspiracies to restrict free trade,[38] and in Hong Kong they constantly questioned the legitimacy of the guilds' powers. Given these conflicting views and practices, Chinese guilds often found themselves at loggerheads with the Hong Kong government, and conflicting concepts of jurisdiction and social regulation were a continuing source of irritation and controversy.

The Hong Kong government dealt with Chinese guilds chiefly by applying to them English labour legislation originally aimed at suppressing trade unionism, such as the Combination Acts of 1800 and 1825, which outlawed all combinations of workmen for the purpose of regulating conditions of work.[39] In 1857 it issued the following notification:

Whereas, according to law in England, every tradesman is at liberty to perform his work at whatever rate of remuneration it seems good to himself to accept, and all combinations for the control of such liberty are illegal: this is therefore to give notice that any persons found to be interfering as above with the freedom of trade will be prosecuted by Government.[40]

This new regulation led to several 'important arrests' and a large number of men being fined.[41] The Chinese guilds were resentful of the loss of long-established privileges and undue interference. It clearly shows the incompatibility between Chinese practices and English law, and the resulting anxiety only drove the Chinese to find security in their own kind.

Man Mo Temple and the Kaifong Committees

Another form of Chinese organization was the temple committee, a prominent feature of Chinese urban life, also active among Overseas Chinese.[42] In Hong Kong, the establishment of the Man Mo (Wen Wu) Temple Committee marked an important stage in its social development.

The Temple[43] was built in 1847 by Loo Aqui (Lu Agui) and Tam Achoy (Tan Acai). Loo, having made a fortune provisioning the British during the Opium War, settled down in Hong Kong. A powerful man controlling all the pirates around Hong Kong, his position was further enhanced by a sixth rank Chinese official title he obtained by trickery.[44] Apart from his alleged criminal connections, 'those who were in distress, in debt or discontented' resorted to him for relief and, in time, he gained respectability.[45]

Tam Achoy, a foreman in the government dockyard at Singapore, came to Hong Kong in 1841, became a contractor, and built some of the most prestigious early buildings in the colony. His business ventures included property and a market and, later, when Hong Kong became an embarkation port for thousands of emigrants, he made a fortune in the emigration business. His wealth and influence among the Chinese earned him the title of 'Nabob of Hong Kong'.[46]

Loo and Tam became leaders of the Chinese community and

'judged the people in public assembly' at the Temple.[47] This should not be surprising, as Chinese people often submitted themselves to the jurisdiction of persons other than representatives of the state, such as village elders, clan leaders, guild masters, and the local gentry. In early colonial Hong Kong, apart from the original villages where such authority existed, newcomers had to build a structure of social power anew. With their wealth and public spirit, and possibly their underground connections, men like Tam and Loo managed to emerge as community leaders.

In 1851 the Man Mo Temple was repaired and enlarged. Though the *China Review* reported that it was repaired by the shopkeepers of Sheung-wan (Shanghuan),[48] it seems to have been a colony-wide project, and was known as the '*He Gang Wenwu Miao*' ('the Man Mo Temple of the whole Hong Kong').[49] Support for it cut across regional and dialect group divisions, and came from various guilds.[50] The enlarged Temple, costing nearly a thousand pounds to erect, testified to the Chinese community's growing wealth.[51] Tam, regarded as 'the most creditable Chinese in the colony',[52] managed its accounts, which he later handed over to Ho Asik (He Axi)[53] of the Kinan (Jiannan) firm, who would attain even greater prominence. Very early on, the Temple acquired property, grew extemely rich, and later became an important benefactor of both the Tung Wah Hospital and the Po Leung Kuk (Bao liang ju).[54]

The Temple Committee inherited and expanded Tam and Loo's influence. In 1851 the shopkeepers of Sheung-wan elected the Committee, and 'therein afterwards decided all cases of any public interest'. But in time the base of the Committee was extended to include other districts, and by 1874 the kaifongs of the five main administrative districts were represented.[55]

Kaifong (*jiefang*) is a term used variously to denote the residents of a neighbourhood and their leaders. Kaifongs had existed under one name or another in South China for a long time, and in parts of Hong Kong throughout the colony's history.[56] Their leaders were self-appointed; as Lethbridge writes, they were 'civic minded, status seeking and paternalistic citizens in a particular area of the city who set themselves up [and] voted themselves into a public body'.[57] The neighbourhood association varied in size and importance, encompassing a single street or an entire district. Though today kaifongs are relatively low-level social leaders, in early Hong Kong they included leading merchants such as Ho Asik and Li Sing (Li Sheng).[58]

By 1857 the kaifongs of four districts had organized the Yulan Procession Committee,[59] whose duty was to make preparations for the important Yulan festival, or ghost festival, which included processions, religious ceremonies, theatrical performances, and street decorations, as well as the giving of alms. The Committee, composed of the kaifongs of different districts, might have helped to weld them into one community.

The kaifongs settled community matters at the kung-so (gong-suo) next to the Man Mo Temple. The kung-so was traditionally a community meeting-place found in both Chinese villages and cities for discussing public matters. The couplet at the entrance of the Hong Kong kung-so, exhorting those who entered to abandon their selfish interests and prejudices, and to be upright, just, and clear-headed,[60] leaves little doubt that judicial decisions were made there. As the *Daily Press* reported, 'There is some kind of organization among the native residents and it is commonly understood that the arrangements of joint action are made at the kung-suh [*sic*], a Public Meeting Hall next to the Temple in Hollywood Road.'[61] Evidently, the Chinese community had already developed an apparatus for discussing community matters and arbitrating disputes. The kung-so symbolized the Chinese need and desire to take care of their own affairs beyond government interference and according to principles familiar to themselves.

The Man Mo Temple also marked the emergence of a fairly high-powered leadership group. According to Eitel, the Temple Committee

...rose into eminence as a sort of unrecognized and unofficial local government board (principally made up of Nam Pak Hong or export merchants). This Committee secretly controlled native affairs, acted as commercial arbitrators, arrranged for the due reception of Mandarins passing through the colony, negotiated for the sale of official titles, and formed an informal link between the Chinese residents of Hong Kong and Canton authorities.[62]

These functions were taken over by the Tung Wah Hospital once it was established.

The I-ts'z and Medical Care

The Chinese community also organized itself in other ways. In 1851 a group including Tam Achoy petitioned for a grant of land to build 'a temple for the reception of tablets of deceased persons'. This was necessary because when Chinese workmen, servants, and the like died in Hong Kong, there was nowhere for their death tablets to be placed or await transfer back to their native villages. The government granted the land in the crowded Tai-ping-shan area on condition that it was used only as a 'temple'.[63] Funds were raised, two persons were entrusted with carrying out the operation, and the Kwong Fook (Guangfu; literally 'wide benevolence') I-ts'z (yici), a common ancestral hall, was erected.

This concern for the dead was typically Chinese, and Chinese associations of every kind tried to service the dead. Among Overseas Chinese, the problem became paramount, making the ability and willingness to arrange for Chinese burials, together with exhumation, re-interment, and repatriation of bones to the native village, a keystone of community leadership and influence.[64] Thus this common ancestral hall, built only 10 years after the colony was established, reflects not only a growing sense of community consciousness but also the emergence of community leadership as well.

But the I-ts'z was to house not only death tablets. Soon, there were coffins awaiting shipment and, more interestingly, sick people awaiting death. This latter phenomenon was directly related to the founding of the Tung Wah Hospital.

The truth was that soon after the colony was founded Chinese in Hong Kong began disposing of dying people on the hills. The problem became so serious that the government tried to prevent it by tracking down the offenders. The community was alarmed, and as a result the leading Chinese petitioned for the I-ts'z. It is not difficult to see that they had in mind not just a repository for death tablets but a death house as well.[65] Though this was not stated explicitly in the petition, government officials at the time seem to understand that the 'temple' would also serve this purpose.

In the course of time six or eight small rooms at the back of the I-ts'z were let out to dying people. No regular doctor attended the place, but doctors were sometimes called in to visit individual patients. Facilities were limited to the I-ts'z keeper giving tea and food to those who could take them;[66] but there was nothing designed to relieve suffering.

Underlying this phenomenon was the peculiar Chinese attitude toward sickness and death. It was considered unclean to have someone die in the house. If it was a family member the death of course had to be tolerated. Otherwise, the dying person would be removed either to an open space or to a matshed erected for this purpose. Apparently places similar to the I-ts'z existed in China too.[67] In Hong Kong, where the population was primarily migratory and living mainly in tenement houses, there was perhaps a special need for it. Naturally landlords were anxious to avoid the 'uncleanness' on their property, and some gladly paid the I-ts'z to have their sick tenants admitted.[68] Others took their friends and relatives to 'avoid the troublous rites and ceremonies connected with death'.[69]

As Hong Kong grew into a major embarkation port, would-be emigrants swelled the numbers at the I-ts'z. Sick men, unwanted on board, were taken there while the ships sailed off without them. Suspected victims of infectious diseases were instantly removed there to prevent infection at the emigration depot. A more or less regular account was even kept between the emigration agencies and the I-ts'z keeper who also arranged for the coffin and burial.[70]

Some of the I-ts'z's inmates did survive, but its main purpose was to house the dying. In fact patients who were considered not ill enough were sometimes turned away. But the I-ts'z served a purpose, and was well know and regularly used among the Chinese community. In 1869 some 200 patients went there.[71] By that time, too, the place had become filthy, but apparently the Chinese themselves never complained about it.[72]

The I-ts'z also shows that the Chinese had their own concepts and practices regarding sickness and death. The segregation so apparent in social and political affairs was just as apparent in medical matters. Not until 1866 did the government admit the need for a separate hospital for the Chinese.

The government's medical set-up, like everything else in those days, was skeletal. In 1843 a Colonial Surgeon was appointed to oversee the health of the civil establishment and prisoners.[73] In 1850 a Civil Hospital was established catering mainly to the police force, and to destitutes and injured persons the police picked up. Around 1864 it became accessible to private paying patients as well. Statistics show that in 1868, admissions to the Civil Hospital of Europeans and Indians were 934 as against 228 Chinese, though the Chinese population was between 15 to 18 times greater than that of all other nationals.[74]

Admittedly the Chinese demand for hospital facilities was limited. The idea of a hospital as a place for cure was a novel one among Chinese. In the course of their long history they had had institutions which resembled hospitals as we know them, though it is doubtful whether they were ever very widespread.[75] By Qing times, however, these seem to have disappeared completely. Chinese operated institutions for the blind, the aged, lepers, and otherwise disabled people, not to cure them but to provide relief. The same was true of foundling 'hospitals', which were really orphanages.[76] Dispensaries where doctors consulted out-patients, sometimes called *yiyuan* (hospitals), existed, but unlike modern hospitals with wards for in-patients,[77] they were more akin to today's clinics or dispensaries. The idea of a hospital as a specialized and permanent place where sick people went to reside for care and cure seems to have been introduced in the nineteenth century by Western doctors who operated a number of them in China.[78]

The Civil Hospital in Hong Kong might have led the Chinese to see the merits of a hospital, but they responded negatively to it. Very few Chinese went there voluntarily. The one dollar charge was of course a deterrent, but there were more profound reasons for their reluctance.

The Chinese had their own unique holistic medical system.[79] The average Chinese in the late Qing period might not be versed in the philosophy of medical theories based on man's relations with the whole cosmos, but he would have some idea of the properties of *yin* and *yang* and the five elements which governed the working of his body. When unwell, he would go for treatment, whether herbal, acupuncture, bone setting, or even magical. He might consult one doctor after another until he got well, or move from one form of treatment to another, but basically he would remain faithful to the system without suspecting the existence of a viable alternative. It was accepted that Chinese, having a different constitution from foreigners, should only receive Chinese medical treatment, and any attempt to impose Western treatment was seen as an intrusion.[80] Thus, the medical aspect, like other aspects of the Chinese world, was self-sufficient.

The Chinese repulsion for the Civil Hospital also stemmed from a deep-seated aversion to Western medical practice. Although by the 1840s some Western medical practices had made inroads in South China, notably the treatment of eye diseases and smallpox vaccination,[81] on the whole Western medicine and surgery were viewed with suspicion. In part this was due to a general distrust of Westerners and belief in their extreme evil. The Chinese also found specific practices disgusting. *Post mortem* examinations and amputations, anathema to the Chinese who believed in the inviolability of the human body but performed regularly at the Civil Hospital, were major reasons keeping them away.[82] As Eitel put it, 'Nearly all Chinese in the colony would rather die like dogs than enter the Government Civil Hospital.'[83] Moreover, mid-nineteenth-century Western medicine did not inspire faith. Remedies against specific diseases were few, hospitals were badly administered, and ignorance of hygiene was general. Though ether and chloroform had been invented, the non-prevention of infection limited the success of surgery.[84] The Chinese, who made little use of surgery, found their own treatment less final.

In Hong Kong there were other efforts to provide medical care for the Chinese. From 1843 the London Missionary Society ran a hospital at Wanchai under Dr Benjamin Hobson's supervision.[85] According to the missionaries' own reports it was very popular with the Chinese. In a three-month period from 1 May 1844 there were as many as 168 in-patients.[86] However, it seems that they were attracted not so much by the medical care as by the allowances given to the poor to buy rice.[87] Still, the hospital could not have been as successful as the reports claimed. In 1848 the popular Hobson was sent away to Canton; his successor was sent to Amoy in 1853, and the hospital closed down after that — according to one report because it had 'lost its hold over public sympathy'.[88] It was some twenty years before the London Missionary Society attempted another hospital in Hong Kong.

The Catholics also ran a couple of 'small hospitals' at Wanchai, but the hospitals, being small and constantly short of funds, made only a limited contribution.[89]

However well intentioned, the missionary efforts did not adequately meet Chinese needs. The I-ts'z showed that they needed a different kind of hospital, a place to house the poor and homeless sick, where there was no imposition of either Western medical practices or religious propaganda, and which would attend to their burial after death. It was a Chinese problem that needed a Chinese solution.

Management of the Chinese: Tepo and Registrar General

The limited documentation on the Chinese community in this period gives the impression that it kept very much to itself, looking inwards for security, relief, and justice, apparently very successfully. A telling piece of evidence is that in the six years after 1848, significantly the year after the Man Mo Temple was built, not one civil case in which both parties were Chinese went to the Supreme Court.[90] The government appeared pleased with this situation, which was in line with its principle of governing the Chinese with the least effort and the greatest economy.

Thus, in 1853, when certain Chinese petitioned for permission to settle civil suits affecting only Chinese, the Officer Administering the Government, Major-General William Jervois,[91] readily complied. In fact for some time he had been pointing out that the Supreme Court in Hong Kong was ill adapted for settling Chinese cases. Seeing that the Chinese had so far settled their own disputes according to their own customs, he felt it would be advisable to legalize 'an arrangement so convenient'.[92]

To do so, the government repealed the ordinance which had created the Paouchong, and passed Ordinance 3 of 1853 to introduce the Tepo (*dibao*). In China, the *dibao* was an agent of social control very similar in function to the *baozhang*. By this ordinance, the Hong Kong Tepo's main function was to arbitrate civil disputes among Chinese. He was to be chosen by the rate-payers of each district. Anyone with a complaint against a Chinese might apply to him for redress. He was in effect an arbiter, but instead of a man of stature and prominence, he was to be a salaried officer, paid for from rates.[93]

The Tepo system did not work either, and one can only guess why. Jervois might have been right in thinking that the Chinese wished to settle their own disputes, but he was wrong in assuming that they would submit to the arbitration of a salaried civil servant. Men like Tam Achoy and Loo Aqui had previously 'judged the people'; it was unlikely that the Tepo could command the same respect or even inspire the same terror. Jervois perhaps did not realize the fact that the arbitrator the Chinese sought was one who had social position and moral authority, not a glorified yamen runner.

Even though the government had realized for some time that the Chinese were able to manage themselves, it did not officially authorize any Chinese or group of Chinese, other than the Tepo, to administer justice. It must also have known that certain influential individuals and associations, by carrying out that function, were contributing substantially to the colony's stability, and yet, while not actively interfering with them, it gave them no formal recognition.

In the 1850s both the Chinese community and its élite continued to grow, partly as a result of developments in China. From the early 1850s onwards the disturbances caused by the Taipings and other rebel groups in South China forced many Chinese merchants to flee to Hong Kong, bringing with them their capital, business experience, and organizing powers. As a contemporary observed:

It has always seemed to me that this was the turning point in the progress of Hong Kong. As Canton was threatened the families of means hastened to leave it, and many of them flocked to this colony. Houses were in demand; rents rose; the streets that had been comparatively deserted assumed a crowded appearance; new commerical Chinese firms were found.[94]

The number of large Chinese merchant establishments — 'hongs' — grew. They formed a new category in the Census of 1858, numbering 35 in that year and 65 in the following.[95] Some of the capital brought into Hong Kong in the 1850s was invested in real estate, and a group of large land-owners emerged.

The colony's political structure, however, took no account of these social and economic realities despite an attempt by Sir John Bowring (Governed 1854–59) to change things.[96] Seeing the growing economic power of the Chinese, he proposed associating them more closely with the government's work. Among other constitutional changes, he suggested giving the vote to leaseholders, who included a number of Chinese.[97] The idea was unpopular with the European community in Hong Kong, and in London, the Secretary of State for the Colonies, Henry Labouchere, was hesitant. Rather than question the principle of sharing power with the natives, he queried the moral quality of the Chinese, doubting if they had 'acquired a respect for the main principles on which social order rests'.[98] Thus, in order to avoid having to leave out the Chinese leaseholders from the electoral body, the idea of elections was abandoned altogether. Another important consideration for Labouchere's objections was China's proximity. The fear of the Chinese population and their close ties with China was a major impediment to admitting them to political participation in Hong Kong. Though an additional unofficial member was added to the Legislative Council in 1857, none of the three members was Chinese.[99] In fact not until 1880, when the dynamic John Pope Hennessy (Governed 1877–82)[100] forced his way through in a rather unorthodox manner, was the first Chinese Legislative Councillor finally appointed.

Labouchere, however, did advise that the colony's affairs be conducted with consideration to the Chinese community's feelings and interests but this was easier said than done. The Chinese remained a separate community with whom the government had little means of communication. This became dangerously apparent in a crisis.

This came in October 1856, when the *Arrow* Incident led to the outbreak of hostilities between China and Britain. In Hong Kong tension heightened as placards issued by Canton officials called upon Chinese residents there to make war against all Europeans, who naturally lived in constant terror. The government's lack of communication with the Chinese became obvious in the crudest way when it failed in November to deal with disturbances because of the absence of an efficient interpreter![101] The ridiculous situation prompted Bowring to take action. He hastily appointed D. R. Caldwell,[102] a former police interpreter, Registrar General with the function of Protector of Chinese.[103] This dependence on one man, who alone seemed capable of facilitating communications between the Chinese and the government, is a sorry comment on the paucity of either institutionalized liaison or understanding between rulers and ruled.

The Registrar General's new duties were first announced by notification on 4 December 1856. Any Chinese who had difficulty in understanding the law or had wrongs to be redressed were to call at Caldwell's office, or in cases of emergency even at his home.[104] Moreover, it announced that registration was designed to protect good citizens from vagrancy and asked respectable inhabitants to send a deputation to call on Caldwell to suggest a system which might work more effectively.[105] This notice was a rather remarkable document, representing the first occasion when the Hong Kong government officially asked the Chinese for advice regarding administration. But it was more a desperate attempt to pacify the Chinese at a difficult time than part of a coherent policy towards them. It is not known what came of these early efforts at consultation and communication.

The Hong Kong government survived the *Arrow* War. In early 1857 there was much alarm over the Esing poisoning case, a rather horrendous attempt to poison the entire European population.[106] The government responded to the general feeling of insecurity by tightening control over the Chinese population, giving general powers of arrest and deportation, and introducing Night Passes for Chinese.[107] It also depended on the Registrar General to conciliate them.

'Thoroughly conversant with Chinese customs',[108] Caldwell was apparently a fairly effective Protector of Chinese. In 1858 the Registrar General's establishment was enlarged with clerks, minor staff, and 16 Tepos.[109] Unfortunately, Caldwell did not devote all his energies to managing the Chinese. While using his special knowledge of the Chinese to manage them on the Crown's behalf, he seems also to have used it to enrich himself. Charged with owning brothels and associating with outlaws and pirates, and even of being a member of a secret society, he resigned in 1861.[110] This severed the only effective link between the government and the Chinese community, showing how precarious the arrangement had been.

Governor Hercules Robinson (Governed 1859–65)[111] was appalled by the state of affairs. Complaining to the Colonial Office, he wrote that no civil servant, except interpreters, understood Chinese. The interpreterships at the Supreme Court and the Registrar Generalship were vacant, but no qualified gentlemen could be found to accept these positions. There were nine or ten interpreters, Chinese and Portuguese, but they had no education and their knowledge of English was insufficient to qualify them for higher duties. On the other hand, English officers were not keen to learn Chinese. The only solution was to introduce cadetship to Hong Kong. Cadets — graduates of English universities with a knowledge of Chinese — would first serve as interpreters at courts for three years and, if competent, would then be considered for other appointments in the civil service, including the Registrar General's office.[112]

The first cadet to fill this office was Cecil Clementi Smith,[113] appointed at the age of 24 before finishing his Chinese studies, when the original holder died at sea.[114] In fact, the first cadets were in such demand that they were all appointed to fairly senior posts without first becoming interpreters as planned. Smith turned out to be quite capable, but the strange ways of the civil service reduced his effectiveness. Between 1865 and 1869 he moved from office to office, either acting in other offices or was away on leave, frequently leaving the Registrar Generalship to acting officers.[115] On the whole, the arrangement was unsatisfactory. Many felt that for such an important office Chinese scholarship alone was insufficient. A young and inexperienced Registrar General might intimidate the lower classes, but would be unable to exert authority over the 'better class' Chinese.[116]

The communication gap remained. Governor Robinson was painfully aware that of the 120,000 Chinese in Hong Kong, no more than 500 had any idea of the general nature of the institutions and laws under which they lived.[117] Despite their general quiescence regarding government policies, he did not think this conducive to progress. There was no means for the government to communicate with them except through the Protector of Chinese, but he only did so verbally, and only with persons immediately interested in a specific issue. With the Chinese susceptible to rumours, misrepresentations, and false reports in newspapers, the situation was particularly serious. Robinson decided to publish a Chinese *Gazette* to let the Chinese know the government's decisions and wishes.[118] The first issue appeared on 1 March 1862, but it soon fizzled out, and it was not reintroduced until 1880 by Hennessy.[119]

Robinson deserves admiration for attempting to reach the Chinese, and he was right in seeing the language barrier as a major impediment. He did not appear, though, to notice that language was only one factor. The government had made very little attempt to understand Chinese society and its principles, or how the Chinese acted, thought, and felt; this was perhaps a greater obstacle. At the same time he seemed oblivious to the existence of organizations among them which managed their own affairs. Or, if he had realized this, he chose not to recognize them as channels of communication. Not until 1866 did the Chinese seek the government's recognition as managers of their own community.

District Watchmen and the Nam Pak Hong

One of the most obvious causes for the gulf between the Chinese and the government was the police force, established on a permanent basis in 1845 with 168 men — 71 Europeans, 46 Indians, and 51 Chinese.[120] None of the European or Indian policemen spoke Chinese, and the Chinese were especially contemptuous of the Indians. The Chinese policemen, like the rest, were of dubious character.[121] The force was so ineffective that many trading houses and residences employed their own watchmen; watchmen were also employed by neighbourhoods. This practice was especially common in the Chinese quarters, partly because it was traditional for neighbourhoods in Chinese towns to provide their own security, and partly because they felt the police force was not equipped to detect Chinese crimes.

On 1 February 1866 the Chinese community held a meeting to discuss the formation of a District Watch Force.[122] This was a scheme to centralize the watchmen employed in the many different neighbourhoods and, more importantly, to seek government sanction for it. A petition was sent asking the Governor for permission to set up such a force, and the Victoria Registration Ordinance, no. 7 of 1866, was passed authorizing a body of Chinese district watchmen 'with all the powers and authorities as constables'. Supported entirely by subscriptions from the Chinese community, they were to be appointed by the government on the recommendation of the district's inhabitants and to be under the Registrar General's control.

The Chinese were dissatisfied with this arrangement, in which they paid for the services of the watchmen but had no control over them. The set-up differed significantly from the original plans for an officially recognized managing committee. There had been some disagreement among the Chinese themselves regarding details. Some preferred a central committee while others preferred a separate committee for each district.[123] Whatever the details, it was apparent that the promoters of the original plans envisaged a fairly powerful committee/s with Chinese members controlling an instrument of law enforcement, almost a municipal council. The squabble reflects that the stakes were high, and Registrar General Smith commented on the jealousy displayed regarding the powers which would be exercised.[124]

As it turned out, power went to the Registrar General, and for many years the District Watch Committees responsible for recommending watchmen seem to have been rather low-level neighbourhood organizations, with little weight in community matters. It was only in 1891 that the committees were reorganized and upgraded. Thus this early attempt by the Chinese community to win government recognition for its right to control Chinese affairs failed.

Despite this, government officials saw it as a sign that 'substantial and intelligent Chinese were prepared to deal with public matters'.[125] It indicated that social organization among Chinese in Hong Kong had reached a certain maturity. The small traders, contractors, and shopkeepers were joined, if not outflanked, by merchants of a different calibre, who not only made money on a grand scale, but could also conceive of social organization on a grand scale.

Hong Kong being a free port, trade statistics are unreliable, but the list of rate-payers and leases indicate that by the 1850s Chinese rate-payers outnumbered non-Chinese many times over, with several being major property owners.[126] Among the wealthiest merchants were Nam Pak (*Nan bei*, literally 'South-North') Hong (*hang*, literally 'a trade') merchants engaged in the North-South trade between China and Nanyang. They dealt in a large variety of commodities, making full use of Hong Kong's favourable geographical position and free port status.

In 1868 the Nam Pak Hong Guild was formed, signalling the trade's coming of age. Besides carrying out traditional guild functions, it also arranged for services such as a fire brigade, a watch force, and religious and other celebrations.[127] Its establishment marked a turning point not only in the colony's commercial history but also in its social history. Though there had been earlier guilds, it was by far the most important in terms of wealth, influence, and sophistication of organization. And because the Nam Pak trade was so closely related to other trades and crafts, it could exert considerable influence over them too. It was the closest thing to a Chinese Chamber of Commerce Hong Kong was to have for many years to come. In time, the government would find it a useful body to consult on commercial matters, and would exploit its connections with other guilds to maintain law and order.

Conclusion

By 1868, after 30 years of colony-building, the Hong Kong government remained isolated from the Chinese community which it nominally governed. From 1850, unofficial members had been appointed to the Legislative Council but none was Chinese. It is perhaps not surprising that in a colony no 'native' representative participated in the law-making process, but this lack of contact was not compensated in other ways. The officers empowered to deal with the Chinese either lacked personal integrity, knowledge, or time to fulfil their function adequately. Though several Chinese community organizations existed, the government neither officially recognized their authority nor actively sought their support. There was in reality indirect rule of the Chinese, but it was not acknowledged.[128]

The hospital situation illustrates a more fundamental reality — the government's failure to understand and provide, and the Chinese determination to do things their own way. In practising non-intervention, the government found it convenient to ignore the Chinese community, spending taxes the Chinese paid on public facilities irrelevant to them. The Chinese in turn, distrustful of Europeans and obstinate in their own prejudices, looked to their own kind to solve problems in their own preferred way.

Under these circumstances, Chinese community leaders and organizations, though unrecognized by the government, managed the various aspects of Chinese life and tended to the community's needs. They enabled the Chinese community to exist, as it were, on a different plane and made segregation possible.

2
The Origin of the Tung Wah Hospital

THERE is a tendency to write about social institutions in terms of patterns and models as though they were inevitable and merely stereotypes. To the historian this approach has only limited value. Generalizations based on a flat time-dimension only answer questions about certain abstracted factors of behaviour without enhancing historical understanding. Society is not static and human affairs happen in time. To understand them, we need to look at them in historical context. Though we may classify institutions, no two institutions are identical. Each exists in a particular place and time and, in that sense, each is a unique historical event. One needs to look at the 'objective factors' — social, economic, political, and cultural developments — as well as the subjective. The decisions and actions of individuals are often catalysts which, given the necessary objective conditions, make things happen, and make them happen in a certain way. What matters is not just the circumstances but the particular combination of circumstances, the unpredictable interaction of objective and subjective conditions, the necessary and the incidental. By looking at all the variables and contingencies, one arrives at a more complex but truer picture of the historical reality.

In the Tung Wah Hospital's case it is particularly important to scrutinize the circumstances of its emergence. For one thing, the story itself was full of drama, a vignette capturing the essence of Hong Kong society at the time. For another, these circumstances conditioned its development for many years to come, developments which were to have a great impact on the history of Hong Kong itself.

In 1869 the Tung Wah Hospital was conceived and planned. The hospital situation as far as the Chinese were concerned had remained substantially unchanged since 1851, when the I-ts'z opened. A chance did arise in 1866 for providing better hospital facilities for the Chinese, but it was an aborted effort.

An Earlier Proposal for a Hospital

In May that year, Fan A-wye (Fan Awei), a government interpreter, and four other Chinese government clerks and school teachers planned a Chinese hospital to provide quarters and medical attendance for the sick, and act as a soup kitchen. After forming a committee to raise a subscription they petitioned the government for a grant of land in the city. The site they requested was behind the new chapel at Tai-ping-shan,[1] and since the acting Registrar General, M. S. Tonnochy,[2] knew some of them personally and believed them to be sincere, he endorsed the petition.[3] Governor Richard MacDonnell (Governed 1866–72),[4] newly arrived in Hong Kong a month before, was also sympathetic. By nature energetic and reformist, he was to rule the colony 'without fear or favour of the Colonial Office or of local opinion'.[5] He went along with the idea and consulted the Surveyor General, W. Wilson, regarding the expediency of granting the land.

Wilson was discouraging. He valued the proposed site at $10,000, and because it was adjacent to the night soil depot, he considered it unsuitable for a hospital.[6] Accepting this opinion without asking how such a site could be worth so much, the Governor ruled that it was too valuable to be given up for such a purpose.[7] This was on 26 May.

Fan and his friends soon found another site, this time directly opposite the Man Mo Temple. Again Wilson objected. Though the site had no value, the soil, he said, being of the nature of quicksand, was not safe for construction.[8] But MacDonnell thought otherwise. On 29 June he wrote, 'On the understanding that the intended hospital will be used for relief and cure of sick and destitute Chinese, I am unwilling to withold my sanctions for a project which is creditable in its objects', and announced that he would grant their land if something could be done to make it safe.[9]

It seems that the Governor, amenable to the idea of a Chinese hospital in May, had become positively enthusiastic about it by June. What had happened in the meantime to transform him? To answer the question, let us return to the Kwong Fook I-ts'z, the common ancestral hall.

As we have seen, besides ancestral tablets, the I-ts'z also

housed coffins and dying persons, and European officers familiar with Chinese ways were complacent about it. To the uninitiated, however, the practice could be horrifying. In June 1866 an Inspector of Nuisance, responsible for overseeing the colony's general cleanliness and orderliness, was stunned to discover there coffins containing bodies, and a report was made to the acting Colonial Secretary.[10] In the course of enquiry, the Colonial Surgeon, Dr I. Murray, discovered a 'greater nuisance' — poor people being sent there to die — and he minuted accordingly on that report.[11]

Murray's discovery on 9 June might have made the Governor more appreciative of the proposal for a Chinese hospital, for it was apparent that sick Chinese needed a place to receive them. This was perhaps the cause of his unwillingness to refuse Fan's second request for a site as well. True, the land had no value but had the Governor been less accommodating, he could have sent them away to look for yet another site. Apparently, the second site was agreed upon, and in the following February Fan A-wye and company were proposed as trustees for the property.[12] Pleased that the project had not fallen through, MacDonnell expressed his readiness to help in every way.[13] The project, however, *did* eventually fall through and all that came of it was a dispensary in Wanchai and not a hospital for in-patients in Taiping-shan, the centre of Chinese activities, as originally planned.

We can only guess why the plan failed. It was possible that being mere government clerks and schoolteachers, Fan's group lacked the social standing to rally support and failed to raise the necessary funds. Some of the influential Chinese also obstructed their efforts,[14] perhaps thinking that if ever such a project were undertaken, they would like to control it. The circumstances of this early effort contrasted sharply with those of the founding of the Tung Wah Hospital a few years later.

The I-ts'z Scandal, 1869

The little stir the I-ts'z created in 1866 soon died down. No positive action was taken on the reports and, with the hospital project aborted, things reverted to their old ways. In 1869 the I-ts'z attracted attention again, but this time the matter developed into a full-scale scandal that threw the government into disarray, and out of this drama rose the Tung Wah Hospital.

A man from an emigration depot died at the I-ts'z in April 1869. In the course of investigation, Alfred Lister,[15] the acting Registrar General, stumbled across the appalling conditions there. It was not just small, dark, and filthy; there was a complete lack of any care for the inmates. He wrote:

At my first visit there were, dead and alive, about nine or ten patients in the so-called hospital. One, apparently dying from emaciation and diarrhea [sic], was barricaded into a place just large enough to hold the board on which he lay, and not high enough to stand up in, another room contained a boarding on which lay two poor creatures half-dead, and one corpse, while the floor, which was of earth, was covered with pools of urine. The next room contained what the attendants asserted to be two corpses, but on examination one of them was found to be alive.... and other rooms contained miserable and emaciatied creations, unable to speak or move, whose rags had apparently never been changed since their admission, and whom the necessities of nature had reduced to an inexpressibly sickening condition.[16]

The testimonies of Lister and others at the Inquest so publicized the horrors of the I-ts'z that it was impossible to suppress the scandal. In Hong Kong, the press, provocatively highlighting the question of official responsibility for this state of affairs, added pressure on the Governor.[17] When the news reached London, the National Association for the Promotion of Social Science saw the opportunity to hit at the abuses of the so-called 'coolie trade' from Hong Kong and immediately created an uproar.[18]

When MacDonnell first learnt of the I-ts'z's conditions he seems genuinely disturbed that 'such heartless cruelty and filth could be found in any building in this city'.[19] Though Dr Murray had mentioned sick people there in 1866, he had not described the place in detail. But it would have been difficult for anyone to be unaffected by Lister's graphic description. However, as the episode gained publicity, MacDonnell became increasingly concerned with pinning the responsibility on someone, not just to meet the accusations of the local press, but also in anticipation of the Colonial Office's censure.

He first blamed the acting Registrar General, Alfred Lister. MacDonnell referred to Ordinance 8 of 1858 which authorized this officer to look after the interests of the Chinese. It was his responsibility to visit houses and tenements of every description where Chinese coolies, emigrants, and others lived, and to ensure that they were in good order.[20] Lister objected, reminding the Governor that as far as supervising emigrants was concerned, there were 'depots' for them under the Harbour Master's control. He admitted that the problem of sick emigrants was a serious one; in Chapter 4 we shall look at the important problem of emigration in greater detail. Lister gave the example of a batch of 600 intending emigrants from Fujian of whom only 290 were taken on board, and he was sure that almost all the rest would be buried within a few weeks at public expense.[21] But this was not his business, he claimed; it was the Harbour Master's duty to oversee the medical requirements of intending emigrants and their well-being both before their departure and during their voyage.[22] The buck was passed in the best bureaucratic tradition.

The Governor then turned his wrath on H. G. Thomsett, the Harbour Master, who was also Emigration Officer. In defence, Thomsett sketched out his duties as Emigration Officer as laid down both by Act of Parliament and local ordinance — seeing that emigrants were not fraudulently obtained, that they understood the nature of their contracts, that the provisions for the voyage were fit and sufficient and, with the assistance of a medical man, to see that none but healthy persons embarked. It was mainly to carry out these duties that he visited the depots. He denied ever seeing any sick persons on these visits, adding that he would be surprised to find any since the recruiting agents knew very well that only the strong and healthy would be accepted. There was no special connection between the I-ts'z and emigration, he asserted, and dismissed Lister's allegation about sick emigrants as nonsense.[23]

The witch-hunt continued. The Colonial Surgeon, Dr I. Murray, was the next target, and MacDonnell expected that he too would 'claim similar immunity'.[24] And of course Murray did. 'No one could have been more surprised and shocked at the frightful revelations' than he, who had never seen a 'living sick person' there, he claimed.[25] He had conveniently forgotten his own minutes of 1866; the Governor, however, had not, and could see the doctor lying through his teeth.[26]

This inquisition yielded very little, except perhaps a fairly good picture of how bureaucracies work. It showed that despite the plethora of rules and regulations concerning emigration, health, and 'protection' of the Chinese, in reality there was only confusion, callousness, and neglect. Unable to single out any officer on whom to lay the blame, MacDonnell told the Colonial Secretary that the Secretary of State would surely find all three responsible. Still, it would be difficult for him to avoid implicating himself. After all, he had done nothing about the I-ts'z in 1866 and, as chief executive, he would be compromised by the incompetence of his subordinates. Anticipating displeasure from London, he went about setting things right at the I-ts'z and then reported on the affair in the least damaging way he could.

The Idea of a Chinese Hospital

While conducting his inquisition and striking terror into his officers' hearts, MacDonnell had the I-ts'z set right. On his instructions Lister, Murray, and the Superintendent of Police cleared out the building and sent the inmates to the Government Civil Hospital. The government resumed control of the place on the grounds that the original purpose of a temple had been violated, and forbade all further admission.[27]

However, closing the I-ts'z did not solve the problem — it only resurrected an old one. Immediately, dead bodies and dying persons began appearing on the streets,[28] making apparent the impracticality of suppressing the I-ts'z altogether. The episode did not have the quick, short ending that everyone must have hoped for. Instead, it was only the beginning of another long story. It was in these circumstances that the idea of a Chinese hospital was revived.

Apparently Fan A-wye had not abandoned his plans for a hospital and Lister, impressed with the cleanliness and order of his dispensary at Wanchai, was ready to support him. After closing the I-ts'z, he took the idea to MacDonnell,[29] who was now even more zealous about a Chinese hospital than he had been in 1866, for reasons which will be analysed, and proceeded to realize it with gusto. In early May, he appointed a Commission of Inquiry composed of Murray, Lister, and the Coroner to find out the Chinese community's views on a Chinese hospital and to recommend a Committee of Management for setting one up.[30] As it turned out, the Chinese who were eventually to establish the hospital were entirely different from Fan's group.

On 5 May MacDonnell wrote to the Colonial Secretary officially proposing the establishment of a Chinese hospital on condition that 'its regulations and general superintendence be subject to

Government control'.[31] He assumed that funds could come from the Chinese. For one thing, he believed that the 'better class of Chinese' were ashamed of the exposé of such questionable Chinese usage connected with the I-ts'z,[32] which was probably true. For another, he felt sure that they could afford it. He referred to their 'great wealth' and the large sums of money they spent on 'their puerile national processions and "shows" every year', and was confident that an appeal to them to forego some of that expenditure for a well-conducted hospital for the relief of their countrymen would probably succeed.[33] There should be no trouble raising $12,000 to $15,000 from them, while he was prepared to have the government contribute either through a fund or a grant of land. His observations of the Chinese show his perceptiveness and shrewdness, and how quickly he exploited the situation.

He put forward some preliminary ideas. The hospital was to accommodate at least 100 Chinese, 'of whom 20 might be regarded as the moribund class for whose accommodation Chinese prejudice and superstitution require apparently some place like the notorious I-ts'z'. He also envisaged it as a residence for a Chinese doctor and a dispensary for native and European medicines, to be visited by a European medical man almost daily.[34] It is interesting to compare these initial ideas with what would actually come into being.

MacDonnell then formally presented the proposal to Lord Granville, the Secretary of State for the Colonies. In a series of dispatches, he argued its necessity; no matter how well maintained the Civil Hospital might be, 'Chinese customs and prejudices' made it impossible to meet Chinese needs.[35] A Chinese hospital was the only way to prevent the suffering which had prevailed at the I-ts'z. He had pin-pointed the problem. However, one might well ask why he had not pursued the idea of a Chinese hospital more vigorously before the I-ts'z scandal erupted. MacDonnell's proposal for a Chinese hospital was truly a departure from the government's tradition of non-interference, and his extraordinary concern for the Chinese community cannot but arouse our suspicion.

It was all very well to be visionary and speak positively of reforms to come. Unfortunately for the Governor, he could not avoid having to explain the I-ts'z issue to the Colonial Office and this he did with considerable skill. One could almost sense that he had brought the subject up in anticipation of inevitable questions coming upon the heels of such a grand scandal. In one of the dispatches he gave a brief history of the I-ts'z and went to great lengths to show that given Chinese objections to people dying in a house, such a repository was indispensable, implying that so long as it was kept clean — and until April there had been no indication that it was otherwise — there was no reason for government to intervene. He concluded by congratulating himself that considering reforms since introduced and reforms soon to be introduced, 'the incidents had resulted in good' [my italics].[36] Thus, in one clever stroke, he side-stepped the issue of government responsibility for the abuses at the I-ts'z, and focused attention on his grand project.

Planning the Hospital

Even as MacDonnell was persuading Granville of the absolute necessity for a Chinese hospital, he informed him that he had already committed the government in funds and a land grant, and that as far as funds were concerned, there was no better source than the Special Fund raised from the Gambling Licence.[37] To understand this Fund, we need to look briefly at its origin.

Gambling among Chinese was an endemic problem in Hong Kong. It offended Victorian evangelical sensibilities as well as being a cause of social disorder. When illegal it was a source of police corruption. The situation had led Governors John Bowring and Hercules Robinson to apply for permission to license gambling, the logic being that doing so was the only means of controlling the vice.[38] But their applications were turned down. Faced with the same problem, MacDonnell cunningly slipped it in through the back door, as it were, and before the Colonial Office realized what had happened, a gambling licencing system had been established in Hong Kong in 1867. Later it was changed to a monopoly bringing in huge revenue for the government,[39] but this soon proved to be so 'embarrassingly large' that the question of what to do with it became urgent.

The Colonial Office, inveigled by MacDonnell into accepting the system in the first place, opposed the idea of government endorsing vice. Accepting it only on a temporary basis, it insisted that at some future date the system would be abolished and gambling again banned. Consequently, the Secretary of State instructed MacDonnell categorically to keep the Gambling Fund as a separate exchequer with its own expenditure and receipts, and not to integrate it with the regular revenue of the colony.[40] It was even hoped that the Fund could be eventually used, somehow, to suppress gambling altogether.

MacDonnell did not anticipate much success in suppressing gambling, but he was eager to spend the 'embarrassingly large' Fund.[41] Finding loopholes in London's instructions, he proceeded to spend it on building police stations, roads, and telegraph lines, and on police launches, which he claimed to be indispensable in fighting crime, arguing that to suppress gambling one must first eradicate criminal elements from Hong Kong. Unfortunately these measures were disallowed in 1869, just before the I-ts'z scandal erupted, and he was told to pay the Fund back from regular revenue.[42] The Gambling Fund remained as large as ever.

The I-ts'z incident showed MacDonnell an opportunity to spend the Fund which had become such a source of conflict between himself and the Colonial Office. This time he reasoned that since the Chinese were the sole contributors to the Fund, it should be spent on their physical and moral improvement. Thus on 2 June he proposed expending $8,500 of it on the new hospital, and a further $3,000 to prepare the site to be granted.[43] Three weeks later he increased the grant to $10,000, to be paid upon the Chinese completing and paying into the bank a subscription of $15,000.[44]

MacDonnell tried to shame the Colonial Office into agreement by reporting that Chinese subscription lists for the hospital amounted to over $30,000, and he predicted that despite the current depressed state of trade, at least $15,000 would be forthcoming.[45] But the fact remained that he had committed the government to support the hospital, and if the Colonial Office disapproved of his using the Special Fund, the grant would have to come from regular revenue. In his usual unorthodox way he had bulldozed the Colonial Office into an awkward position. His 'determination not to obey the Secretary of State' was noted with some resentment by Lord Granville himself.[46]

Before the Governor's explanations and rationalizations could reach London, the Colonial Office had already read about the I-ts'z incident in the *London and China Telegraph*. The National Association for the Promotion of Social Science, concerned not only with the horrible conditions at the I-ts'z but also with the abuses of the emigration trade from Hong Kong which it compared to slavery, protested to the Colonial Office.[47] As a result, the latter wrote to MacDonnell demanding answers to a series of questions: how the I-ts'z could have been unnoticed by the police, whether other such places existed, what was being done to remove the evils, whether any investigations were being carried out, and whether the emigration conducted by D. R. Caldwell, now the major emigration agent in Hong Kong, was accompanied by abuses.[48]

MacDonnell had anticipated these questions and had already dealt with the I-ts'z and the new Chinese hospital in dispatches which had crossed with Granville's. To a large extent, he satisfied Granville, mainly, it seems, by his argument that whatever the abuses might have been, they were now being put right. He was able to convince Granville of the need and desirability of a properly constituted Chinese hospital as a remedy.

With the customary respect for the man on the spot, and also perhaps because he saw the genuine benefit of a Chinese hospital, Lord Granville approved of the hospital, and sanctioned both the grant of land and the sum for preparing the site.[49] But, in line with the principle that the Special Fund was only temporary, he told MacDonnell not to commit the government to the hospital's annual maintenance.[50] The Governor must have been relieved that his manipulations had succeeded, as the question of maladministration regarding the I-ts'z was not pursued. Obviously his strategy of using the proposal of a Chinese hospital as a remedy — even as a smoke-screen — had worked.

The Chinese and the Hospital

Meanwhile, the Commission MacDonnell had appointed to ascertain the Chinese community's views on a hospital and to recommend a Chinese Committee of Management set to work. By 1 June a Hospital Committee had been formed. It was composed of some 20 influential residents with Ho Asik,[51] a leading kaifong, as its chairman. Its other leader was another leading kaifong, Leung On (Liang An),[52] compradore of Gibb, Livingston & Co. It was obviously due to the existing kaifong organization, which had managed Chinese community affairs for several decades, that the new Hospital Committee could be established and function so quickly and efficiently. It is not known whether the official Commission had approached the kaifongs or the other way around, but in any case it was this group which was officially accepted as the Committee for planning the hospital. The number soon grew to 125, and from it emerged the first Tung Wah Board of Directors.

Though the Tung Wah Hospital was rooted in an older association, the kaifongs, the difference between them was profound. The Tung Wah Committee was the first Chinese group in Hong Kong to be recognized by the government as representatives of the Chinese community. The Hospital Ordinance of 1870 gave legal sanction and official status to its existence and further enhanced its social status. This first official recognition of a group of influential Chinese community leaders made the founding of the Tung Wah Hospital a turning point in Hong Kong's history.

From the start, the earnestness of the Chinese was manifest. According to the *China Mail*, all sections of the community saw the need for a Chinese hospital, but even then, the willingness of 'influential residents' to devote their money and energy to such a project must have been beyond all expectations. Some of them had obstructed Fan A-wye's plans in 1866 and their enthusiasm now revealed their ambitions both to operate the hospital themselves and, perhaps more importantly, to form themselves into a public body to run a community project with the government's approval. They also showed their effectiveness. Almost as soon as the Committee was formed, $10,000 to $15,000 was promised towards the Hospital, and by early 1870 the final paid-up subscription was over $47,000.[53] This ability to raise funds was an important reflection of the economic capacity, community spirit, and organizational powers of the Chinese in Hong Kong. The Tung Wah Hospital's capacity to do so would soon become legendary and internationally known.

While planning the new Hospital, the Committee also operated the I-ts'z as a temporary hospital. When it had become clear that closing the I-ts'z was impractical, MacDonnell allowed the Committee to renovate it to admit a small number of patients for the time being.[54] Two thousand dollars was spent on its renovation, and soon patients started arriving.

Just as things appeared to be going well, trouble erupted. The Colonial Surgeon discovered that a dying patient at the I-ts'z had been removed to a room where a corpse had been deposited.[55] When Lister, the Registrar General, heard about it, he put up a stinging notice at the I-ts'z, warning that in future on no account was a dying patient to be removed from his room. Anyone who did so or who gave such an order would be punishable for manslaughter according to English law.[56]

The new Hospital Committee, which supervised the I-ts'z, protested strongly to the Governor. The members, led by Leung On, explained in a petition that it was Chinese practice to remove a dying man from his room. There was nothing cruel about it, and it was certainly not intended to hasten his death. They pleaded that they had no wish to risk disobeying the notice, and complained that after spending so much money and energy in giving relief to the poor, they did not deserve such treatment. They reminded MacDonnell that they had undertaken to operate the present hospital and establish the new one on the understanding that 'the general conduct of the affairs and the framing of regulations will devolve on the Chinese, in whose hands the management will be'.[57] According to their understanding, Chinese customs would provide the operating principle. They put forward a telling point: if the Hospital was to be run on English principles, there was really no need for them to take the trouble of building a new hospital when the Civil Hospital already existed.[58]

The message was clear. They were threatening to call the whole thing off unless the Governor would rescind Lister's instruction and give the Committee a free hand in the Hospital's management. They had acted so boldly only because they knew they held the trump card. They were shrewd enough to see the Governor's eagerness for a Chinese hospital and this could not be built without either *their* money or *their* participation. Besides, they were determined that the ground rules concerning the control of the future Hospital should be clarified once and for all.

MacDonnell's reaction was unexpectedly accommodating. Instead of being offended by their impertinance, he thought the petitioners reasonable; rather, it was Lister's blunder which annoyed him. Sympathetic with the Chinese prejudice against allowing a person to die in a room where there were living persons, he thought it permissible to remove him so long as it was done carefully.[59] He was ready to compromise his officer and yield to Chinese pressure because, as he admitted, to refuse their 'reasonable request' 'would have completely checked the movement for building a new Hospital'.[60] It was a small price to pay.

MacDonnell instructed Lister to publish his decision among the

Chinese. For Lister, the gesture was nothing short of a public apology. In response, the Hospital Committee thanked the Governor for his permission to conduct the Hospital on Chinese principles, and stated their intention to engrave the proclamation on stone together with an account of the proceedings connected with the Hospital as a permanent reminder of MacDonnell's and Lister's goodness.[61] This was obviously also designed to prevent the government from going back on its word and to pre-empt future dispute.

The Committee had reason to be pleased. Having won the first round with the government, it was disinclined to let the victory go without due fanfare. It had gambled, banking on the assumption that the Governor would go a long way to safeguard the Hospital project, and had won. The Governor's earnestness was unmistakable. Though enthusiatic about the idea of a Chinese hospital in 1866, then he had played a passive role, and when the plans were eventually dropped, he did nothing to salvage them. The site which the present Committee had received was exactly the one Fan's group had originally asked for in 1866. Not only was the Governor undeterred by its high value, now he was even prepared to pay for the site formation. His zeal became even more obvious when he compromised his own subordinate and gave in to the Chinese Committee's demand in order to preserve the Hospital project.

MacDonnell and the Hospital

Why was MacDonnell so keen to bring about the Chinese hospital?

First of all, the need to atone for the abuses at the I-ts'z was obvious. By helping to bring about a new Chinese hospital, he could at least argue that some 'permanent good' was coming out of the whole fiasco and use the smoke-screen to divert attention from the real issue. He even tried to turn the situation to his advantage by claiming credit for taking 'so leading a part in extracting finally so much good from the original abuse'.[62]

The Chinese hospital would also provide an opportunity to reduce the 'embarrassingly large' Special Fund. This Fund, born of such unsavoury circumstances, had put MacDonnell in a most awkward position. Spending part of it, at least, would relieve some of the pressure on him, and spending it on a good cause would reduce some of the stigma. The Fund certainly allowed him to be magnanimous.

His intention to involve the Chinese in this scheme was another consideration, though perhaps a minor one. He had been impressed with the District Watchmen's work, which showed the value of letting the Chinese co-operate with the government. It would be a 'politic' as well as a charitable move.[63] This reference to the political need to solicit Chinese co-operation is significant. Up to 1869 the government's management of the Chinese had not been particularly successful. Despite the Registrar General's office, it was oblivious to much that was going on among the Chinese. The I-ts'z episode was an excellent illustration. There were government policies which alarmed and repelled the Chinese community. MacDonnell must have remembered, for instance, that when he introduced the Registration Ordinance in 1866, 10,000 Chinese left the colony in protest.[64] The lack of communication was obvious. If the acting Registrar General, whose business was the Chinese community, did not know its customs, how much more ignorant the other government officers must be of them. At the same time, there were prominent Chinese residents who exerted influence on the community and MacDonnell might have seen them as a possible medium through which he could manage the rest. This could partly explain why he gave so much more countenance to Leung On's Committee than to Fan A-wye and his humble friends.

Throughout, MacDonnell was emphatic about the wealth of the Chinese. By the end of the 1860s, Chinese merchants in Hong Kong had indeed accumulated great wealth, and this was clearly manifested in the ease with which the Hospital subscriptions were raised — not only in 1869 but also in all the years to come. Apart from the Special Fund, which was a windfall, the government was constantly threatened by deficits. The sources of revenue of a free port were limited, and it was forced to practise very strict economy. MacDonnell saw the situation presenting an excellent opportunity for the Chinese, who he believed were embarrassed by the whole scandal, to use some of *their* money for a good cause. It would be a feather in his cap at someone else's expense.

His expectations were well founded. Initially, he had hoped that the Chinese would raise $12,000 to $15,000. By August the subscriptions had already exceeded $30,000.[65] Eight months later the fund had grown to over $47,000. This confirmed his observations. This is also an important indicator of the type of Chinese involved in the founding of the Tung Wah Hospital.

The Chinese Hospital Ordinance

An ordinance 'for establishing a Chinese Hospital to be supported by voluntary contributions, and for erecting the same into an eleemosynary Corporation' — Ordinance 3 of 1870 — was passed. The full Ordinance is reproduced in Appendix I, but a few significant points should be noted.

According to the Ordinance, the Chinese Hospital would be a corporation, and its legal rights and liabilities as such were specified. The Schedule named the Founding Board of Directors. From the beginning, the Chineseness of the Hospital was established, for it was stipulated that all its members were to be of Chinese origin. However, this also became one of the first rules to be broken, since subsequently the register did contain, even if nominally, foreign members.[66]

This emphasis on Chineseness was made again when the Hospital's aim was spelt out. It was erected 'for the purpose of establishing and maintaining a public free hospital for the treatment of the indigent sick among the Chinese population'. Provisions were also made for fee-paying patients, for it was expected that emigrants returning from abroad, especially from California, would patronize it and provide a regular source of income.[67]

For the first two years there would be a 'Preliminary Board of Directors', which the Chinese called *Chuang jian zongli* (literally 'Founding Board of Directors'). Afterwards, a permanent Board of Directors would be formed, consisting of not less than six and not more than twelve members of the Corporation, to be elected from time to time by the members, each having one vote. The Directors would appoint a President (the term 'Chairman' was later more commonly used) among themselves and each Director would hold office for one year only, though he would be eligible for re-election. Questions arising in Board meetings would be decided by majority vote, and in case of a draw, the President had the casting vote.

Great powers were given to the Directors during their term of office. The Board had 'full power and authority generally to govern, direct and decide all matters whatsoever connected with the administration of the affairs of the Corporation and the accomplishment of the object and purposes thereof'. For the immediate supervision and management of the Hospital, the Board of Directors could also appoint a Board of Management. To check the Board's power, the Ordinance provided for government intervention. In important matters such as the change in the term of the Directors' office, or the qualification of membership, the consent of the Governor-in-Council was required. The Board had the right to frame regulations relating to the Hospital's administration and discipline provided that copies of them were furnished to the Colonial Secretary, subject to the disallowance of the Governor-in-Council. He also had the final say over the interpretation of the Ordinance.

The Ordinance also provided for a government role in the day-to-day running of the Hospital. The Registrar General, the Colonial Surgeon, and any other person appointed by the Governor, were authorized to inspect the premises at any reasonable time. In addition, an annual statement of accounts was to be presented.

Final powers were vested in the Governor-in-Council. Section 16 provided that 'in case it shall at any time be shown to the satisfaction of the Governor-in-Council that the Corporation have ceased or neglected or failed to fulfil the conditions thereof, or that sufficient funds cannot be obtained by voluntary contributions to defray the necessary expenses of maintaining the said Hospital or that the Corporation is unable for any reason to pay its debts', the Governor would have power to repeal the ordinance and declare the incorporation void. In such an event, the Hospital's property would revert to the Crown. This particular provision was made at the Governor's request,[68] and may be interpreted as a sign of his caution, perhaps even his fundamental distrust, of the Chinese.

While preparing this Ordinance, the Attorney General, Julian Pauncefote,[69] was in constant communication with the Chinese through Lister, the Registrar General, who worked hard to meet the Committee's wishes. It appeared satisfied; the only point of disagreement which seems to have arisen was over membership fee. The Committee had originally proposed 50 cents but the government demured. This small sum would have enabled 'grass-root' participation which the government would not encourage. As a result membership was restricted to those contributing at least $10, making it much more exclusive.[70]

Otherwise, the terms were satisfactory. It provided the Corporation with ample autonomy and the Board with vast powers of governance. So long as things went smoothly, the Chinese could run the Hospital as they wished. Although nowhere was it specified that it would be run according to Chinese customs and principles, implicitly the Board could apply these principles so long as the Governor did not find them objectionable and overrule them. Pauncefote himself believed that the intention was to interfere as little as possible[71] and it is likely that the Chinese had been informally reassured of this. Certainly the general vagueness of the Ordinance gave the Board much leeway.

Should any extraordinary circumstances or abuses arise, however, or should any changes be desired, the government was empowered to intervene. More importantly, in the event of a débâcle, it would be in a position to declare the Hospital's abolition. One could say that the interests of both sides were fairly well taken care of, the Ordinance vesting ample power in the government to control and supervise, but at the same time avoiding 'vexatious interference with an institution so purely Chinese'.[72]

Initially, a trusteeship rather than an incorporation had been proposed for the Hospital, but the Attorney General, Pauncefote, much preferred the latter. He claimed the Chinese, being ignorant of the English language and laws, would never comprehend a deed and most probably disputes would arise among the Hospital's supporters. Another reason he gave — a more convincing one — was that land was invariably granted for a Crown Lease of 999 years, but the population was so transient that it would be necessary constantly to reappoint new trustees, and each new appointment involved much technical complication. The present Ordinance gave the land to the corporation and its successors and allowed government to control its management.[73] The I-ts'z had been managed by trustees and the terms of the land grant had not provided for any government control so long as it was used as a 'temple'. Thus when its original trustees lost interest in its operation, no one could be held responsible, and short of resuming the land, government could not intervene. Clearly, the Hospital Ordinance was designed to avoid a repetition of the I-ts'z fiasco.

This Ordinance is an interesting framework within which to see the Hospital's development and relationship with the government in the years to come. In normal times, armed with the autonomy it provided, the Committee would run the Hospital as it saw fit, but when the government detected things getting out of hand, it would invoke the Ordinance to remind the Hospital authorities of the limits to its powers. The tension was inherent. Even when their relationship appeared harmonious on the surface, there was always an undercurrent of conflict. At times the undercurrent turned into a tempest and open confrontation took place. In 1896, for example, the Governor forced the Hospital Committee to toe the line by threatening to abolish the Hospital. Thus the Ordinance which gave the Hospital Committee legal status and great administrative powers also circumscribed its powers.

The Chinese Hospital Committee

The 20 member Committee soon grew to 125. Out of these, the 12 most active in promoting the establishment of the Hospital and the greatest donors were elected as the Founding Board of Directors.[74] They included the most powerful and wealthy Chinese business men of Hong Kong, and the mechanism they soon developed for selecting the Board, which we shall see in the next chapter, ensured that this tradition should be upheld. As kaifongs, they were familiar with managing the Chinese community. As merchants and compradores,[75] of whom there were five on this Board, their knowledge of the international business world gave them a measure of worldliness and confidence when dealing with government. The First Chairman, Leung On, who had led the protest against Lister, was a perfect illustration of the assertive Chinese representative, ready to demand rights for the Chinese. A number of Directors had also received an English education, which might have opened their minds to an intellectual world beyond the strictly Chinese one. Many of them held Chinese official titles,[76] an important subject to be discussed more fully in Chapter 4. The Board not only represented wealth, dynamism, and astuteness, but also knowledge and experience in managing business and community affairs. These were important and formidable qualities and, to a large extent, they became a part of the Tung Wah tradition.

Conclusion

This chapter reveals the origin of the Tung Wah Hospital, re-creating a historical situation where incidental factors played a large part. Objectively, political, social, cultural, and economic developments provided the necessary conditions. Primarily, the Chinese community had reached a stage where its leaders had the economic and organizational powers to bring a hospital into effect and, at the same time, were ambitious for government recognition of their social and political status. There were also cultural gaps which made the medical facilities offered by the government irrelevant to the Chinese, and Hong Kong's function as an emigrant port created extra medical and welfare problems. There was little communication between the government and the Chinese community, and the Registrar General's office did little to remedy the situation. Added to these objective factors were a series of incidental ones, catalysts which produced a dynamic situation.

If the death at the I-ts'z in 1869 had gone unreported, like so many others before it; if the Governor had decided to expand the Civil Hospital with special provisions for the Chinese; if he had put the Hospital project in the hands of Fan A-wye; if the Colonial Office had allowed the Governor to include the Special Fund as regular revenue; if the Hospital Committee had succumbed to Lister's interference; if Pauncefote had considered a trusteeship sufficient safeguard... Any of these variables would have affected the outcome, perhaps quite radically. But what *did* happen led to the establishment of the Tung Wah Hospital and to a large extent determined its character. The story shows that in studying history, even the history of a social institution, one must make allowances for contingencies.

The Tung Wah Hospital became the first hospital in Hong Kong operated by Chinese and offering Chinese medical treatment. The special circumstances not only resulted in the Hong Kong government according official recognition for the first time to a group of Chinese community leaders but, more significantly, dictated that it took the rather unusual form of a hospital committee.

The site of the new Hospital was on the west of the Tai-ping-shan district, across the street from the I-ts'z. The street originally bore the morbid name of Cemetery Street, Fan Mo (*fenmo*, literally 'grave') Street in Chinese, because to the south of the site was a burial ground where Chinese had been burying their dead rather haphazardly for many years.[77] After the land grant was made in 1869, it was renamed Po Yan (*puren*, 'universal benevolence') Steet,[78] signifying the optimism of those involved with the Hospital's foundation, and it had turned out to be an accurate prophecy. From Fan Mo Street to Po Yan Street... The birth of the Tung Wah Hospital indeed marked a new page in Hong Kong's history.

3

Management, Organization, and Development, 1869–1894

THE Tung Wah Hospital building was opened on 14 February 1872 with great fanfare. All the newspapers reported on the 'greatest ever witnessed' ceremony in Hong Kong.[1] It began at an early hour. Between 70 and 80 Hospital Committee members assembled at the kung-so next to the Man Mo Temple. They were all dressed in ceremonial robes, some even with peacock feathers attached to their headwear, showing off their official titles. A little before eight o'clock, accompanied by a band of Chinese musicians, they proceeded from Hollywood Road down to Bonham Strand, the Chinese business centre, and back again toward the Tung Wah Hospital on Po Yan Street. Throughout, Leung On, Chairman of the Founding Board, played the most prominent role. Arriving at the great hall of the Hospital, he placed three incense sticks before an altar dedicated to Shennong,[2] the legendary Sage-Emperor, traditionally believed to be the inventor of medicine and the patron saint of medical practitioners. (This offering is still made daily at the Kwong Wah Hospital, one of the Tung Wah Group of Hospitals.) The morning's ceremony was rounded off with fireworks, the booming of guns, and a theatrical performance. The spectacle drew such a great crowd that the police and district watchmen were called out to keep order.

The ceremony continued into the afternoon. Governer Mac-Donnell was received by about 30 Committee members all dressed in official robes, and shown around the premises. This rare appearance by a Governor at a Chinese function must have added moment to the occasion. Speaking to the meeting, Mac-Donnell referred to the I-ts'z and the circumstances in which the Hospital was conceived, and he praised the Committee's excellent work in raising funds and in building a very commendable hospital. However, he did not omit to mention his own contribution.

He reported on the greatly increased subsidy — from $15,000 to $115,000 — which he had managed to obtain for the Hospital.[3] The home government had approved of the increase — to be taken from the Special Fund, of course — because, he explained, he had convinced it of the cordial co-operation from the respectable members of the Chinese community and the growing mutual understanding which existed between the government and the Chinese. He concluded the speech by handing a cheque to the Hospital.

The Hospital which the Governor opened had taken two years and cost about $45,000 to build.[4] It consisted of several two-storeyed buildings of granite with large windows on each side. The complex was surrounded by a garden and bounded by a very high wall. (See Appendix II for the Ground Plan.) A central building contained the Directors' hall, the doctors' accommodation, and the business offices. The hall was 'lofty and very handsome', the roof supported by massive pillars. It had a 'superb' ebony table in the middle with a chair 'massive enough for a throne' for the Chairman and six carved ebony chairs on each side.[5] The grandeur was later enhanced by the many plaques and couplets, some very elaboratedly carved, presented over the years by grateful people all over the world, including the Emperor of China and many high Qing officials.[6] One may recapture some of this grandeur today by visiting the Tung Wah Group of Hospitals' Museum.

The Hospital had a capacity of 80 to 100 patients. The lower wards were intended for poorer *gratis* patients while the upper storey, better lighted and ventilated, was reserved for paying ones.[7] The wards were divided into wooden stalls, each containing two beds — matted wooden platforms with white wadded quilts as bedding. Above each bed was a shelf, and over each patient hung a ticket with his name and the hours he was to take his medicine written on it. There was also a women's ward, strictly out of bounds to men.[8]

Medicine was prepared in a large kitchen. There were 150 earthen furnaces for 150 pots, for each patient had his own. Preparing Chinese medicine was generally a time-consuming and complicated process and was undertaken by attendants with special training. There was also a dispensary where the doctors saw out-patients, an apothecary, and a mortuary.[9]

According to Dr John Kerr,[10] the Tung Wah Hospital was 'the first establishment by natives of a permanent institution for the treatment of the sick'.[11] Kerr, an American medical missionary who had run the Canton Missionary Hospital since 1855, should know. The hospital as a specialized and permanent place where sick people went for care and cure was an alien concept in Qing China, having been introduced, it seems, by Westerners in the mid-nineteenth century. Even the Tung Wah's founders acknowledged that the establishment of a hospital by private contribution was quite a novel idea in China.[12] In fact the concept of a hospital itself was novel. This explains why when Guo Songdao, the Chinese Minister to London, passed through Hong Kong on his way home from England in 1879, he commented that the Tung Wah was run 'entirely according to Western ways' (*yi yi Xi fa wei zhi*).[13] This shows that, in Chinese eyes, the hospital as we know it was something Western.

The paradox is that while in concept the Hospital was 'Western', in practice the Tung Wah was extremely Chinese. The Chinese hospital started by Dr William Lockhart in Shanghai in 1844 was Chinese only in the sense that it catered for Chinese patients, but it was operated by Westerners and used Western medicine.[14] The Chinese hospital in Hong Kong, however, was Chinese in a much more profound sense. It was managed by Chinese for Chinese patients, employing only Chinese doctors using Chinese treatment. If the modern concept of a hospital was a Western one, then we must say that the Tung Wah, as a 'Chinese hospital' was in fact a hybrid, a Western form with a Chinese content, a classic expression of the East–West cultural exchange which Hong Kong was a most likely place to produce. In this sense, the Tung Wah was a landmark in the medical history of both China and Hong Kong.

It was also an experiment. While Chinese might be experienced in organizing institutions such as guilds, *huiguan*, temples, schools, kaifong associations, and so forth, running a hospital was a new experience.[15] Despite Guo Songdao's observation, the Tung Wah was operated quite differently from contemporary Western hospitals. The situation was anomalous. On the one hand, there was a management committee very similar in structure and *modus operandi* to that of conventional Chinese associations. On the other, there was a hospital, an unfamiliar institution as far as the Chinese were concerned. The impression is that one was rather artificially grafted on to the other. Often they were out of gear, sometimes with serious consequences. From a Westerner's point of view, the Chinese hospital was a curiosity, even a disaster, and conflicting views as to how a hospital should be run eventually led to controversy and conflict. As the Hospital Committee's other social commitments increased it appeared that the institution's medical work had become a minor concern, and the Hospital's role and function inevitably became suspect and subject to scrutiny. A look at the Hospital's organization and work shows not only how the Hospital worked but also reveals interesting features of Hong Kong society itself.

The Management

From the start the founders demonstrated that they intended the Hospital to endure. In their Regulations, they expressed their eagerness to distinguish themselves from the run-of-the-mill temple committees which lacked continuity and discipline[16] — possibly a reference to the failure of the I-ts'z's trustees — and it is perhaps due to this spirit that the Hospital they started, in spite of changes over the years, still exists today. They realized that one way to ensure permanence was to establish a rigid system under a strict set of rules. As a result, they compiled a code of Regulations setting out the basic constitution and rules of operation. The degree of detail is evidence of the amount of thought which had gone into its compilation. In one way, the Regulations supplemented the broad outlines of the 1870 Ordinance. In others, however, they differed from it, though the Regulations were not disapproved by the Governor.[17] In practice, both the Ordinance and the Regulations were contravened on occasions. Both are worth attention for revealing the original intentions of the people involved, but we need also to look at what actually happened to understand the Hospital's work.

The Hospital's operation was regulated by page upon page of rules, bearing upon every activity and every level of administration. These are too many to deal with in full, but several are particularly interesting. The rules were more like declarations of principle. There was great emphasis on honesty. Money, medicine, coffins, and other items were to be meticulously accounted for so that there would be no fraud or even room for suspicion. All Committee members and staff members were required to take an oath each year to show their consciences were clear.[18]

There was a detailed prescription for every job to be done to prevent sloppiness and disorder. Emphasis was on cleanliness, punctuality, discipline, temperance, and the strict segregation of the sexes. It is obvious that the founders aimed not only at a well run hospital but also at a respectable and dedicated institution. There was a complex arrangement of checks and balances to ensure that the system would not be wrecked by the selfishness and dishonesty of individuals.[19]

The Board of Directors and the Guild Connection

The management system was clearly laid down in the Regulations. Central to it was the Board of Directors (*zongli*) which, according to the Ordinance, was to be elected by members of the Hospital. The Founding Board comprised five compradores, two Nam Pak Hong merchants, and one merchant each from the Rice, Piecegoods, Opium, and California Trade businesses. This was the basic pattern for subsequent Boards, which also consisted of representatives from these guilds. For the rest of the nineteenth century, these six guilds were represented each year, and in roughly the same ratio. By 1896 the Yarn Dealers' and Pawn Brokers' Guilds also regularly sent representatives. (See Appendix III.)

The so-called election process may be reconstructed from later accounts. Each year, when the current Board's term of office was about to expire, the Hospital would send notices to the guilds mentioned, which, according to the Regulations, were to nominate a few of its members for the kaifongs (the leaders as well as the people of the neighbourhood) and Hospital members to vote on.[20] In practice each guild only made one nomination, or as in the case of the Compradore and Nam Pak Hong Guilds, two or three according to the quota allotted them that year. Once the nominations were returned the Hospital would send letters inviting the nominees to serve. It was customary for the nominee to refuse on the grounds of poor health or incompetence, but after a second or third letter extolling his virtues, he usually complied.

Besides the guild representatives, for most years in the nineteenth century there was also one *yinhu*, or *yinshang* (wealthy merchant) representative on the Board. *Yinshang* were members of the Hospital who had made subscriptions of over $50 from year to year, and this entitled them to nominate someone among their own ranks as a Director.

When the nominations were completed, the names would be posted in the great hall of the Hospital and an election day would be announced. On that day, kaifongs and subscribers gathered at the Hospital for the election. As all the nominees were invariably elected,[21] the contest that really mattered had already taken place within the guilds and among the *yinhu*. However, the kaifongs and subscribers elected the Chairman and the two other Principal Directors.[22]

Such an annual election was both symbolically and practically significant. As a communal occasion focused upon the Tung Wah Hospital it inspired a sense of community, commitment, and participation. Each year the Board was presented as elected by the *He Gang jiefang tongren* ('all the residents of Hong Kong and members of the Hospital') thus legitimizing the Directors' claim to being the Chinese community's representatives. It also marked the continuity of the kaifong connection.

The guild-based structure deserves attention. Lethbridge has noted the merchant element of the Tung Wah executive[23] but he has not discovered the significant structural connection between the guilds and the Board. This structure was in fact a most lucid expression of the commercial nature of Hong Kong society. It was significant because the 'election' mechanism ensured that the most respected and successful members of the major businesses in Hong Kong would become the Hospital's Directors. It guaranteed the continuity of the concentration of power and wealth which had happened almost by accident in the first Board. No wonder contemporaries considered the Tung Wah Board as a kind of 'roll call' of Hong Kong's Chinese élite.[24] Its role as the local élite will be examined in the next chapter.

In addition, the mechanism was a means of translating commercial power into social influence. In Chinese cities guilds were an important social and economic factor, and increasingly in the late Qing, a political factor as well. In this respect, the prominent role guilds played in Hong Kong shows how closely this city resembled Chinese cities. But the influence of merchants was greater in Hong Kong than in China because, in the absence of a scholar-gentry class, they assumed the status and role of a local élite without competition. As most of the guilds included employers as well as employees, masters as well as apprentices, this guild-based structure was one way of allowing the Hospital Committee to influence, and find support from, the 'grass roots' of the Chinese community. In addition, the guilds provided one of the most constant sources of revenue, as we shall see.

This predominance of the guild element in Hong Kong contrasted with the comparatively low profile of the *huiguan*. A small number of *huiguan* existed in Hong Kong in the mid-nineteenth century, but they played a much less conspicuous part here than in other Overseas Chinese communities, where community-wide activities and organizations were often based on regional representation.[25] Guilds of course could be regionally based too, and there were *huiguan* which doubled as guilds.[26] In Hong Kong some occupations were dominated by people from certain regions in China. For example, the Nam Pak Hong merchants were largely Chaozhou people, and many compradores came from Xiangshan. But the situation was never exclusive. Though the subject is still very much under-researched, there is sufficient evidence to show that those guilds represented on the Tung Wah Hospital Board at least were cross-regional organizations.[27] It was the guilds rather than the *huiguan* which provided the main framework for social activities in Hong Kong. Thus the structure of the Tung Wah Hospital management system illustrates a fundamental but little known aspect of Hong Kong society.

However, the guild-based structure had its limitations. The early Committee members included some prominent local figures who were not merchants. There was Wu Tingfang, known in Hong Kong as Ng Choy (Wu Cai), who became its first Chinese barrister and first Chinese representative on the Legislative Council; later he rose in officialdom in China.[28] There was Wang Tao, one of the most progressive thinkers in modern Chinese history, a pioneer in Chinese journalism and the founder-editor of the influential *Xunhuan ribao* (*Universal Circulating Herald*).[29] Another noteworthy journalist on the Committee was Chen Aiting, known locally as Chan Ayin (Chen Axian), editor of the *Huazi ribao* (*Chinese Mail*) who eventually became Chinese Consul-General in Havana.[30] There was also Ho Fuk Tong,[31] (He Futang), a Chinese pastor of the London Missionary Society with immense personal wealth. He was the father of Ho Kai,[32] one of the colony's most illustrious sons. But they never became

Directors, perhaps because they were not guild representatives. The non-merchant element found it difficult to play a really leading role in the Hospital as Directors. The Hospital Committee's guild-based structure might also account for its failure to accommodate the Chinese professional classes emerging in the late nineteenth and early twentieth centuries. It was only in the 1920s that structural adjustments in the Board were made.

The General Committee

Besides the Board of Directors, the Management consisted also of the Assistant Directors (*xieli*) and Ordinary Committee (*zhili*). Collectively they formed the General Committee.[33] The executive was a three-tiered one, a form quite common among Chinese associations. Before 1878 the Assistant Directors were composed of the out-going Directors and others, but there is no indication of how the latter were selected. After 1878 they consisted exclusively of the out-going Directors and were rather like elder statesmen. As for the Ordinary Committee, there is simply no way of guessing how the members were chosen. Some individuals first served as Directors and then became Ordinary Committee members; others served in the reverse order. There was no discernible pattern. At first the Ordinary Committee included both individuals and firms; it is quite common for firms or other corporate bodies to be listed as members of Chinese associations, or even as members of their executive. From 1920 the Ordinary Committee consisted exclusively of firms.

The Ordinance had vested powers in the Board of Directors, but according to the Regulations, many of the powers and duties were shared by the entire General Committee. The Regulations provided guidelines for every activity. One special duty was the management of funds placed upon the three Principal Directors. Each year two Directors were chosen to be chairman and secretary of the meeting hall, and one was also appointed to audit the accounts.[34] But apart from these there was no further specialization, and no division of duties, giving the impression of much overlapping of functions. The Directors and other Committee members worked on a monthly rotation basis so that the division of labour was based on time rather than on the kind of duty. While on duty, they tended to every aspect of the administration, from checking accounts to inspecting patients' diets, from seeing to the general cleanliness and order of the place, to the hiring and firing of doctors. This was partly because the concept of specialized management was still new. But more significantly, there was a conscious effort to let the duties overlap. The Regulations explained that a strict compartmentalization of duties would induce one to become unconcerned and callous about the duties of others.[35] Making the duties and powers fairly general and diffused would more likely create a sense of shared responsibility and co-operation. In other words, everything should be everybody's business.

The diffusion of executive power was also a prominent feature in the management of Chinese associations, but the Tung Wah carried it out to an exceptional degree. Not only was power diffused within the current Committee, but members of past Committees also exercised certain authorities, often playing an important part in the decision-making process. Much depended on the personalities involved. In the period under study, Leung On and Ho Amei (He Amei)[36], who were exceptionally dynamic and aggressive, were able to exert influence on the Hospital long after their official retirement from the Board. This convention adopted by the Hospital meant that power was much more diffused than either the Ordinance or the Regulations had intended. It was institutionalized in 1906 by the establishment of the Advisory Board composed largely of past Directors.[37]

Ordinary Members

Another vital component of the Hospital was the body of ordinary members. The Hospital Ordinance provided that 'persons being of Chinese origin as shall from time to time become donors of any sum not under ten dollars to the funds' would be registered as members and, if in the colony, be entitled to vote for the Board of Directors. There were in fact a number of non-Chinese on the membership list, which was headed by Governor MacDonnell himself. The list also included John Pope Hennessy, several Parsees, taipans of European firms, a few Japanese, and others.[38] This is only one blatant example of the contravention of the letter of the Ordinance. Also among the listed members were a large number of associations — charitable organizations, *huiguan* and guilds, many of which were located in Macao, China, and other parts of the world. In this respect, the membership list is a noteworthy document showing the early connections between the Tung Wah and other Chinese societies and the network they formed; this will be discussed again.

Theoretically, the ordinary members could play an active part in the Hospital's operations too, and this was connected to the constant reference to the ballot box. Not only were Directors elected by ballot to office but, at least theoretically, they could also be voted out of office if they failed their duty. The vote would also be used to decide on the hiring and firing of doctors and every member of staff.[39] In fact, it was stipulated that any matter concerning the Hospital would be decided by the majority vote. Considering that each member was entitled to vote on all issues one must conclude that the Hospital was, in intention at least, run by consensus.

The Hospital's base was widened when the members' rights were extended in practice to 'the members of the kaifongs'. This means that anyone who was interested in public affairs, regardless of whether or not he had made a $10 donation, could participate in the Hospital's activities. There is evidence that the rights of the members and kaifongs were respected, and they did participate actively on many occasions where decisions about the Hospital were made.[40] Their influence was also felt because the Directors, however élitist they were themselves, were extremely responsive to public opinion. They never ceased to claim that they represented the Chinese community, which was their source of legitimacy. Indeed the Tung Wah Hospital was very much a 'people's hospital' and decision by consensus was generally maintained.

From the beginning, the Hospital authorities were not content with running a mere medical establishment. The Hospital's meeting hall was one of its central features, the place where matters relating to the Hospital as well as to the Chinese community as a whole were discussed. Any member who had a matter to raise could take it to the Directors, and if they thought it justifiable, a meeting would be called for that purpose. The agenda for meetings was posted beforehand to ensure that all interested persons would attend.[41] All office bearers were expected to attend all meetings, and a quorum of four Directors and 12 other Committee members was required.[42] Strict regulations governed the proceedings and minutes were meticulously kept. In the event that an unscheduled matter was brought up at a meeting and voted upon, absent members could call another meeting, give due notice that the same matter would be discussed again, and re-vote on it. This provision was designed specifically to prevent 'packing'.[43] By providing the mechanism for discussion and com-promise, the system aimed at safeguarding decision by consensus and, more specifically, it was designed to prevent disharmony and jealousy from destroying the institution.[44]

In the course of time, a wide variety of subjects came to be discussed at the Hospital, making it in reality a centre of com-munity affairs. 'He Gang jiefang tongren' became a familiar expression denoting an entity which the Hospital purported to represent. It emphasized the popular participation in Hospital affairs, however theoretical it might be. But above all, in social and political terms, it was a formidable entity implying unity and purpose within the Chinese community and legitimizing the Hos-pital Committee's role as the local élite.

The Tung Wah Hospital's management structure was typical of Chinese voluntary associations. Their principles of operation were also similar. Anthropologists claim that the management of Chinese voluntary associations shared certain characteristics — diffusion of executive powers, rotation of duties, decision by consensus — which served the purpose of mitigating the 'hierar-chical features of formal bureaucratic and descent ideologies'[45] and these were obvious in the Tung Wah Hospital. More impor-tantly, behind the structure and the principles, there were also the attitudes and modes of thought associated with traditional voluntary associations which would become manifest. One may argue that this was no surprise because the Tung Wah was Chinese. Yet it should be remembered that it was also a hospital, an essentially new institution among the Chinese. A study of the Tung Wah is therefore interesting to show how a group of Chinese managers familiar with running traditional voluntary associations would apply their experience to an institution of a different genre, and how they affected its work and course of development.

Hospital Work

Another factor that conditioned the direction of the Hospital's development was of course the application of Chinese medical practice — Chinese wine in a Western bottle.

The story of the I-ts'z reveals Chinese aversion to Western medical practice. The very basic antipathy between the two cultures with respect to medicine and the concepts of sickness and death had made a Chinese hospital necessary. It was laid down emphatically in the Regulations that all patients would be treated by Chinese doctors 'because Chinese customs were so different from those of Westerners'.[46] The earlier confrontation between Alfred Lister and the Chinese Hospital Committee over the removal of a dying patient at the I-ts'z demonstrated the Chinese community's determination to claim the right to abide by Chinese customs. They had argued convincingly that it was the basic *raison d'être* of the new Hospital, and the Directors jealously held to this principle which would be challenged many times and upheld many times. An examination of the Tung Wah Hospital affords a glimpse into Hong Kong as a stage where the conflicts of cultural attitudes were played out.

The Chinese Hospital Committee organized a temporary hospital as early as June 1869 by renovating the I-ts'z. The Chinese immediately recognized its value and by December a total of 211 patients had been taken there, compared to 302 Chinese admitted at the Civil Hospital for the whole of 1869.[47] These figures show how much such an institution had been needed and, by the same token, how little the Chinese saw the Civil Hospital as a viable alternative.

In 1872, when the new Hospital building was completed, it was staffed by three doctors, one of whom was a vaccinator.[48] The Hospital was designed to receive two grades of patients, destitute patients and private paying ones. It was recognized that special provisions were needed for visiting merchants and respectable persons, and reserved for them were the *qiao'an* (literally 'comfort for the sojourner') rooms, which were to be kept especially clean and comfortable — not, the Regulations explained, because the patients were richer, but in order to show hospitality to those from afar.[49] One of the Hospital Committee's greatest fears was to have the poor and sick of the surrounding region descend *en masse* upon it. Patients were not admitted unless the doctors thought them sufficiently ill, and it was stipulated that a security from a shop or one of the Directors was required.[50] The idea was that when the patients recovered, they would be taken away by someone and not left destitute at the Hospital. But the Regulations were not foolproof, and as the Hospital found itself saddled with many sick and destitute persons, repatriating them became a major undertaking.

In line with the Hospital's principles, only Chinese doctors were employed. Though formal medical education, like hospitals, may have existed in some distant past in China, in modern times it did not. There was no medical school or any board or college which conferred diplomas on doctors. Doctors who had been trained by others, or who had trained themselves by studying medical books, were accepted as long as they proved themselves effective.[51] When a doctor was recommended to the Tung Wah Hospital, he was required to write a medical treatise, which was judged by the doctors of the Hospital.[52] If he passed, he would be put on trial without pay for a month, and if he showed himself effective, he would be hired on a regular basis. The monthly salary was 20 taels of silver (approximately $27.60)[53] with food and board, and outside practice was permitted. These conditions remained largely unchanged up to 1896. Doctors were hired for only three months at a time to keep them on their toes.[54] The turn-over of doctors was fairly high: it could be that since it was prestigious to work at the Tung Wah, doctors were tempted to leave once they had served long enough to earn sufficient repute.[55] The number of doctors on the establishment varied from three to eight.[56] At times, there was also a house dentist.[57]

For a while the Hospital even trained doctors — the first institution in modern times to train Chinese medical practitioners.[58] The experiment was the brainchild of Governor John Pope Hennessy, whose close involvement with the Tung Wah will be discussed later. Eager to promote Chinese interests as well as introduce the benefits of Western knowledge, he advocated a scheme in early 1878 to train young Chinese in Western medicine, with clinical teaching to be done at the Tung Wah and 'a little instruction in physiology' at the Central School.[59] Promising funds, he suggested that Frederick Stewart,[60] Inspector of Schools, discuss it with his medical friends and the Hospital Committee.

By April 1879 the scheme was in operation,[61] with one medical tutor and ten students.[62] The course would take five years. According to Regulations drafted for the programme, priority would be given to candidates who knew both English and Chinese because, after two years, the better students would be sent to the Government Civil Hospital to learn Western medicine. Thus it was a joint effort between the Hospital and the government. The Regulations also expressed the hope that these prospective doctors, having integrated Chinese and Western medicine, might one day serve China.[63]

It seems the scheme, apparently very popular at the beginning, only lasted one or two years, and only seven trainee doctors in all were produced.[64] Ostensibly, it ended when the buildings used to house the students were taken over by the Po Leung Kuk,[65] but this could not have been the entire explanation. It is more likely that this method of training Chinese doctors was so radically different from traditional ways that it was found unacceptable. In China, medical knowledge was jealously guarded by the family or by the Master, and the idea of propagating it openly to a class must have appeared very odd. Moreover, combining Western and Chinese medicine might have sounded a good idea, but it could be difficult in practice. Even so, this brief attempt by an institution to train Chinese medical practitioners is another factor which makes the Tung Wah Hospital a landmark in Chinese medical history. The idea of combining Chinese and Western medical knowledge, though miscarried, was bold and progressive, an indication that Hong Kong was a potentially ideal place for cultural exchange.

Treatment at the Hospital was based mainly on herbs. Very little surgery was performed; though never using ether or chloroform, Chinese doctors had drugs to induce sleep.[66] Amputation, which horrified Chinese, was never performed. In 1872 the Hospital Committee even made a special request to the Governor that victims of accidents discovered by police be spared the Civil Hospital where amputations were so freely performed.[67]

The death rate at the Hospital was high compared to that of the Civil Hospital. From February till December 1872, 922 patients were admitted of whom 287 died, producing a death rate of 31 per cent against the Civil Hospital's 12.93 per cent.[68] In fact the 1872 death rate at the Tung Wah turned out to be low compared to later years. Up to 1894, it ranged between 42 to 54 per cent, with the exception of 1888, when it reached 62 per cent.[69] This did not seem to have alarmed the Chinese, who viewed the Hospital mainly as a place for stowing away the sick with no one to care for them and the dying with no home in which to die. In a place with a more stable population than Hong Kong, there would have been less demand for a Chinese hospital;

the circumstances which had turned the I-ts'z into a death house had the same effect on the Tung Wah. The high mortality rate was actually caused by people *wanting* to die there. The fact that in 1893, 1,231 out of 1,375 deaths in Hong Kong took place at the Hospital clearly confirms this tendency.[70] One attraction was that by dying at the Tung Wah, people hoped to avoid *post mortem* examinations. The Hospital's founders had declared their aversion to this practice as a matter of basic principle. The Regulations, asserting that there was no greater anathema among the Chinese than having the corpse 'punished' [by autopsy],[71] pledged to claim exemption from it as far as possible. Relatives requiring such examinations were warned not to take their patients there.

In 1873 the Committee went so far as to ask the Governor that *post mortem* examinations be avoided except when absolutely necessary.[72] It argued that if a patient died after treatment at the Hospital, it was obvious that he had died of illness. If the deceased had been poisoned before being taken to the Hospital again it was obvious that he had died from poison. Since doctors at the Tung Wah could tell the difference, they concluded that *post mortem* examinations were unnecessary.[73] The argument was of course superficial and simplistic, making no allowance for pathological considerations. But it reflects the Chinese mode of thought and prejudices. Above all, it reflected the Tung Wah's willingness to defend these prejudices, even to institutionalize them, as it were.

Another attraction was the provision of free coffins and a free burial service. For instance, in 1893, 869 patients who had died at the Hospital were given free burial.[74] In addition, the Hospital regularly exhumed the remains five years later for re-interment. At such times, notices would be posted for relatives to come forward to reclaim the remains and take them back to their native village. The relatives were subsidized by the Hospital whenever necessary. Where they did not come forward, the Hospital undertook the re-interment and, even then, records were carefully kept for future identification.[75] As James Stewart Lockhart,[76] one of the most energetic Registrars General, so rightly observed, to the Chinese, 'the dead are almost of greater moment than the living'.[77] The Hospital's ability to meet these special Chinese needs accounted for the community's respect and gratitude.

The Hospital's work cannot be dismissed simply because the death rate among in-patients was so high. Among out-patients, it was reasonably low. In 1877, for instance, among 54,974 out-patients, the death rate was only 1.105 per cent.[78] We can also see evidence of its popularity in the fact that neither the Alice Memorial Hospital[79] nor the Nethersole Hospital,[80] both founded for Chinese but using Western medicine, significantly diverted patients from it. Unlike the Tung Wah, they were never over-crowded.[81] In 1892, for instance, when the Alice Memorial Hospital treated 848 in-patients, the Tung Wah treated 2,455. There was never any serious rival to the Tung Wah's popularity.

Vaccination

One major contribution of the Tung Wah Hospital was vaccination. In a way this was an anomaly. For all its insistence that only Chinese medicine be used, Jennerian vaccination (*Yangdou*, 'Western vaccination') was one of the Hospital's most constantly and widely provided services, and also one of the most distinguished. The Chinese had inoculated against smallpox since the Song dynasty, but the method of obtaining lymph from an infected person was dangerously unsatisfactory.[82] Edward Jenner's method of inducing cowpox was introduced into China in the early nineteenth century through Macao.[83] Although the Chinese first resisted the idea of vaccination, as they did all foreign things, it gradually gained acceptance in the Canton area. As early as 1852 the Colonial Surgeon noted that the Chinese in Hong Kong were beginning to prefer vaccination to inoculation.[84] Even so, the Hospital Committee's enthusiasm for it was remarkable. From 1869 all vaccinations it gave were free. In fact it offered 100 cash (approximately 13.4 cents) to well-selected healthy infants whose families were willing to let lymph be obtained.[85] Ironically, the Colonial Surgeon and other Western doctors, who received their lymph from London free, performed a minimal number of vaccinations. In 1880, when the Tung Wah was vaccinating thousands, the medical officers altogether did only 76.[86] The supply of vaccine presented a problem for the Hospital until 1892, when a Vaccine Institute was established in Hong Kong and calf lymph was supplied free by the government.[87]

Hennessy praised the Hospital's vaccination work profusely. He pointed out that Hong Kong, being a major shipping and

emigration port, was particularly susceptible to an influx of smallpox, and yet, due to the Tung Wah's efforts, no full scale
epidemic had broken out. [88] Dr P. B. C. Ayres,[89] the Colonial
Surgeon, praised it too. Perhaps, seeing how well the Chinese
received vaccination from the Tung Wah doctors, he hesitated to
promote it at the Civil Hospital. Even in 1874, while he was
condemning other aspects of the Tung Wah's work, Ayres wrote,
'The one great good this Hospital does is vaccination, which it
has greatly assisted in spreading, 1,246 were vaccinated this
year.'[90] He even complimented the Hospital on being far-sighted
enough to see the benefit of vaccination when educated people in
Europe were sceptical of its efficacy.[91]

From 1876, Tung Wah vaccinators started going to various
places in Guangdong and, in 1878 alone, they performed 5,641
successful vaccinations there.[92] In sending these missions to
China, the Hospital not only saved lives, but also helped to
spread Western medical knowledge to China. Governor George
Bowen (Governed 1883–85)[93] wrote smugly that vaccination by
the Tung Wah 'is another of the many instances of the general
progress and extension of the practices of modern civilization
over the great neighbouring Empire from this British colony'.[94] It
was another way in which the Tung Wah contributed to China's
modernization.

The Hospital also ran a smallpox ward. In early 1871 a mild
epidemic of smallpox broke out. The medical authorities converted part of Stone Cutters' Island prison into a smallpox hospital for Europeans,[95] but not for the Chinese, whom the
Colonial Surgeon knew were suffering considerably. It was then
suggested that the I-ts'z should be converted into a smallpox
ward, and with Governor Arthur Kennedy's (Governed 1872–77)
approval,[96] it was accordingly cleaned and fitted out.[97] New Regulations for the new ward were added. Again, there was great
emphasis on cleanliness and ventilation, and all attendants had
either to be vaccinated or to have had smallpox. As with the
general ward, mortality was high, as many of the victims were
very young children. From a medical point of view keeping
patients with a contagious disease in the crowded urban areas was
of course inadvisable. Its one advantage was that the parents and
guardians of the young victims at least had the consolation of
attending to them until death.

Ironically, while the Tung Wah Hospital was so energetically giving vaccination, it was equally energetic in resisting government attempts to make vaccination compulsory. When Governor Bowen suggested this to the Directors in 1884 they astutely replied that it might be better 'to trust to the influence of reason and experience to combat prejudice'[98] than make it compulsory. It may seem paradoxical that the Chinese, who readily submitted to certain forms of authority — guild regulations and parental authority, for instance — could be stubborn in resisting other forms of imposition. With things foreign in particular, their resistance could be eroded only by long periods of observation and proof of effectiveness. To force anything on them was likely to destroy all inclination even to experiment. In this instance we see the Hospital Committee showing the Governor some home truths about the people he governed.

For better and for worse, the Governor took the Hospital Committee's advice, and the Colonial Office agreed to leave things as they were.[99] For better, because the Hospital Committee proved its ability to reflect Chinese attitudes and be an effective channel of communication between the Chinese community and the government. For worse, because a smallpox epidemic erupted three years later, claiming 374 lives.[100] Consequently, a Vaccination Ordinance making infant vaccination compulsory was passed in 1888.[101]

The Tung Wah's vaccination work not only demonstrates the value of its medical work in terms of saving lives but also its contribution to the dissemination of medical knowledge to China. The extension of its work to the Canton area is only one manifestation of its close connections with China. Its insistence on using only 'Chinese' methods was neither absolute nor inflexible. Yet Chinese preference for Tung Wah doctors to Europeans even for vaccination reveals their prejudice, and shows how much they needed the Hospital, if only to cater to those prejudices.

In Western Eyes

Contrary to Guo Songdao's observation that the Hospital used all Western methods, a Western visitor's opinion was that 'in it nothing European, either in the way of drugs or treatment, is tried'.[102] Dr Patrick Manson,[103] one of the founders of the College of Medicine for Chinese,[104] commented that 'by its constitution and the spirit of many of its directors and supporters, [the Tung

Wah Hospital is] closed to European methods of cure and administration'.[105]

To generous Westerners, the Tung Wah was a curiosity; to the critical, a disaster. Every medical officer in the colony doubted its value as a medical institution. Great medical development took place in Europe after 1870. Antiseptics had revolutionized surgery, and new ideas of sanitation, public health, and patient care contributed to the progress of Western medicine. Diseases such as typhus, typhoid, smallpox, cholera, and scarlet fever were being contained by the 1880s; there was increasing professionalization among medical workers, while medical knowledge was becoming more solidly based on scientific research.[106] Using Western medical development as a yardstick, Western doctors sneered at anything different. Hospitals as well were judged only according to the Western paradigm.[107]

Not surprisingly the acting Colonial Surgeon, Dr G. Dods, found the medical treatment of the new Chinese Hospital unsatisfactory. In his Report for 1872, he suggested that since the government had endowed it with such a large sum of money, the Directors should set apart one ward for treatment by foreign doctors or open a dispensary in another part of town where foreign advice and medicine might be given free.[108] Needless to say, the Hospital Committee ignored him.

Western doctors, generally keen on surgery, questioned the adequacy of treating medically cases they regarded as surgical ones.[109] The Chinese faith in herbal treatment contrasted starkly with the Westerners' contempt for it. They also found the Chinese way of dressing wounds dirty and conducive to infection, and wondered why they never used lint, cotton rags, cotton wool, or water dressing, so essential to the European doctor, and used paper for all purposes instead. Dods was particularly distressed by the way patients at the Tung Wah were allowed to dress their own wounds, 'perpetually meddling with the dressings and applying ointments or lotions'.[110]

No one was more dismayed by the Hospital than Dr Ayres. Shortly after arriving in Hong Kong in 1873 as Colonial Surgeon, he was instructed by the Registrar General to see that the Hospital was kept clean and in good order, that the patients were properly treated according to Chinese customs, that they were properly clothed and kept clean, and received enough food and drink; nothing more. Significantly he was instructed not to interfere with the medical and surgical treatment.[111] Thus began his relationship with the Hospital that was to last 24 years.

The young doctor who fought so vigorously to improve the Civil Hospital and the colony's sanitary conditions could not be silent about the Tung Wah's defects. In his Report for 1873, he dismissed it curtly. 'This institution at present hardly deserves the name of Hospital, in the ordinary accepted sense of the word', he reviled.[112] His next Report was even harsher. In fact he was so blunt in his indictment that parts of it remained unpublished and were not forwarded to London. Citing the mortality rate of over 50 per cent for 1874, he concluded that the Tung Wah had taken the place of 'dying houses'. He complained that the treatment at the Hospital amounted to nothing, except in surgical cases, and then, 'what is done is more harm than good'.[113] To him, Chinese medicine had no value since most prescriptions were composed of 'simples' — that is, uncompounded ingredients — which might be eaten in any quantity.[114]

In his zeal, he reported the Hospital's many defects to the Registrar General and the Governor but was told not to interfere. When he realized the government's reluctance to impose Western medicine, he gave up trying to convince the Chinese of its superiority. He soon came to terms with the limits of his power and the Committee's determination to uphold the principle that 'the general conduct of affairs and the framing of regulations will devolve on the Chinese in whose hands the management will be'. Gradually he accepted the basic need for a separate, Chinese, hospital. Absurd though Chinese doctors appeared to him, he recognized that as long as the Chinese did not go to Western doctors voluntarily, Chinese doctors had some value.[115] As years went by, his reports on the Tung Wah became more terse, giving only the barest statistics. The ferocious fight was abandoned and he mellowed. It was not until 1894 that a new generation of Western doctors again attempted to topple this citadel of Chinese medical practice.

Non-Medical Work

The Tung Wah Hospital's work was never strictly medical. The circumstances demanding a hospital for the Chinese also demanded a wide range of other social services. Hong Kong's development into a major shipping centre in South China coincided with increased Chinese migration both inside and outside China. Internal migration was stimulated by the opening of treaty ports and the Cantonese, with their long experience in dealing with foreigners, frequently travelled through Hong Kong as they moved up and down the China Coast. Shanghai in particular attracted a large contingent of Cantonese compradores, merchants, clerks, and prostitutes. Hong Kong's own growth was both a cause and a symptom of this movement. It also became a main embarkation port when Chinese emigration increased. Chinese migration, both internal and external, increasing the number of persons in transit in Hong Kong, created a variety of problems besides sickness and death.

Many transients were destitute and homeless; some were lunatic. Foreign destitutes and lunatics were cared for by their consuls. Portuguese born in Hong Kong and Macao could turn to their churches, and the Society of St Vincent de Paul catered to their needs.[116] The Chinese were less fortunate. There was no Chinese Consul in Hong Kong. The Hong Kong government did little for the poor. Though it had control of a Charitable Allowance Fund, given mainly to the missionaries' charitable organizations, its efforts amounted to little. It operated no poor house, no dispensary, no lunatic asylum for the Chinese.[117]

There was also pressing need for repatriation arrangements as large numbers were stranded penniless in Hong Kong — people kidnapped or decoyed as 'coolies', women sold as prostitutes, would-be emigrants failing medical examinations, victims of shipwrecks and mutinies. Many of these services — housing the poor and sick, providing free burials and coffins, repatriating persons and human remains — were traditionally carried out by various types of charitable institutions in China; in particular, *huiguan* provided these services for their members. In a way these services were inter-related and, in the Chinese mind, an integral part of community service. From this perspective, it seemed logical for the Tung Wah, which provided medical services, to provide the others as well. And yet, when it assumed these other functions, it created an unusual situation.

First, it was not a *huiguan* but a hospital incorporated for 'the care and treatment of the indigent sick', so that strictly speaking the other functions were extra-legal. Secondly, it carried them out on a grand scale, covering a much wider geographical area than the average *huiguan*. As emigration increased, it became a major contact point between Overseas Chinese all over the world and their native villages in China.

Much of its non-medical work dealt with the dead. Bodies were often taken there for free burials; in 1893 there were as many as 665 such cases.[118] In addition, its coffin home housed coffins and exhumed bones awaiting shipment to China. In time these came from all over the world, and the Hospital undertook to bury those which were unclaimed.[119] Its coffin home, initially situated near Kennedy Town and now at Sandy Bay, has always been an important arm of its operation. There was such constant traffic in coffins and bones that later the Hospital had to obtain an annual permit from the Canton authorities for exemption from import duties and, presumably, from customs inspection.[120] When major disasters such as typhoons or fires struck, the Hospital not only cared for the survivors but also buried the dead. In 1874, for instance, it buried 399 people drowned during a typhoon.[121] It is not known when the practice began but, by the end of the nineteenth century, the government, exploiting its expertise in dealing with matters related to Chinese deaths, was recruiting the Hospital's services wherever Chinese burials were concerned.[122] The exhumation of 4,000 bodies buried in its cemeteries in 1895 testifies to the scale of its work.[123]

Repatriation

The Hospital had feared that large numbers of the poor and destitute in the surrounding area would descend upon it and, despite precautions, this did happen. The only way to avoid becoming a regular poor house was to repatriate them. As with the burial service, the more successful its repatriation arrangements proved, the greater became the demand for it. Soon, the Harbour Master, the police, the courts, and the Registrar General were sending along all sorts of persons stranded in the colony. Initially, Chinese destitutes were repatriated via the British Consul in Canton, but it was a cumbersome bureaucratic process, and the Tung Wah had connections which bypassed this. In 1873 it repatriated 42 destitutes, of whom seven had been forwarded by the Registrar General and two from the Police Magistrates. At the same time, Overseas Chinese communities sent along persons for a safe passage home. In 1893, 159 patients and 1,287 destitutes were repatriated, including those from abroad. They were sent to 14 different destinations, including Penang, Haikou, and Shanghai.[124]

In fact, as well as persons, human remains, money, letters, and other personal effects were also sent to the Tung Wah Hospital for distribution. In 1882, when Chen Lanbin, former Chinese Minister to the United States, Spain, and Peru, set up a bureau in Canton to help people establish contact with members of their family abroad — particularly the kidnapped — the Tung Wah was appointed to transmit letters to major foreign cities where *huiguan* and Chinese Consuls would distribute them.[125] Hong Kong's position as a shipping centre enabled it to act as a pivot in the network of communication. It was also aided by its Chinese newspapers which circulated in the region.[126] With every case of repatriation, detailed information would be advertised in the papers to notify interested parties. The frequent appearance of its name not only showed the large volume of work it undertook, but boosted its image and transformed Tung Wah into a household word.

Other factors, however, also accounted for its active role. Repatriation was no simple matter. In the case of persons in particular, much was at stake. Every effort was made to secure a safe passage. Detailed instructions were sent ahead to ensure that the persons or objects would be collected only by legitimate parties. Security was regularly demanded from any addressee and acknowledgements of receipt were meticulously kept. For places up-country, the process involved a complicated relay through a series of associations.

Obviously the Tung Wah Hospital could provide such valuable service only by maintaining good relations with various organizations in China — gentry organizations, benevolent societies, militia groups, clan associations, temple committees, *huiguan*, even business houses and banks. These connections, indispensable for safe delivery, were one of its greatest achievements and assets. They were based on mutual trust and respect, cultivated over a long time. Every transaction enhanced the prestige of the organizations concerned, and the high esteem accorded to the Tung Wah by Chinese at home and abroad was the fruit of a long record of care, efficiency, and dedication which confirmed the élite status of its Committee.

The Hospital's membership list helps us appreciate the scale of its work. It consisted, on the one hand, of a whole range of associations in China located as far apart as Yantai in Shandong and Beihai in Southwest Guangdong and, on the other, Overseas Chinese organizations all over the world, predominated by those in Annam, Japan, Australia, and California. Putting these two groups side by side we see a clearer picture. There was a network of associations which linked the two worlds of the Chinese, the native village and the Overseas community, with the Tung Wah as its pivot. Its services to Overseas Chinese explain why they supported it so generously and subscribed so readily to fund-raising campaigns it organized.

Poor House and Lunatic Asylum

However, there were always people who could not be sent away — those with no family, or whose only family was the brothel from which they had been rescued in the first place. Accommodation therefore had to be provided for them, often at the expense of real patients. Even when the Po Leung Kuk was formally established in 1882, the women and girls it rescued were kept at the hospital premises.[127] Dr Ayres appropriately compared this situation to workhouses in England.[128]

The Tung Wah was in fact operating both a hospital and a poor house, and the priority was not always clear. The destitutes were a burden on its administration. Young girls and boys had to be put out for adoption and young women for marriage; boys were also offered as apprentices.[129] From a sanitary point of view, using the Hospital as a poor house was objectionable and the Po Leung Kuk inmates were often too noisy. But from a humanitarian point of view, there was little choice. If the Hospital was exceeding its legitimate scope of work, government was abetting it. As one official admitted, if government prevented the Tung Wah from providing those services, it would be forced to do so itself, and there was no reason for this when the Tung Wah could do it both cheaper and better.[130]

Yet another category of unfortunates swelling the number of inmates was lunatics. In 1877 a small building on Hollywood Road was used to house European lunatics awaiting repatriation by their consuls, but not Chinese.[131] In 1879 a lunatic ward was built at the back of the Hospital.[132] When the Colonial Office learnt about the situation in 1880, its staff were quite concerned, but it took 10 years before a special lunatic asylum for Chinese was finally built. Only in November 1891 was the Tung Wah Hospital able to transfer its lunatic inmates there. And yet, as late as 1894, lunatics were still kept at the Tung Wah, and their horrifying conditions became the subject of a sensational article in an English-language newspaper.[133]

Funds

To do all this, medical work and otherwise, funding was essential. In fact, raising funds had always been one of the Hospital's main concerns. Since the Colonial Office had decided against contributing to its recurrent expenses, the estimated annual expenditure of about $7,000 had to come from other sources. But the Hospital found it well within its means to raise this. For the next 30 years or so its income came mainly from subscriptions, both annual and occasional; from guilds, shops, passenger ships, and individuals; from bank interest and rent; and from donations in the form of cash, medicine, coffins, and clothing.[134]

The government remained its main benefactor with the donation of $115,000. After an advance of $15,000 for the building and $3,000–4,000 toward sundry matters connected with the site, the remainder of $96,760 was presented to the Hospital at the official opening in 1872. From this, expenses of furniture and other contingencies were defrayed, leaving a balance of $9,000 which was deposited in the name of the Colonial Secretary in the bank at a fixed rate of about 5½ per cent.[135]

The guilds were also important benefactors. In 1873, 25 guilds made a total contribution of $9,040.[136] (See Appendix IV.) Of these, 22 continued to subscribe at a fixed rate until after 1900. Others were less consistent. Between 1873 and 1900 a number of guilds appeared on the subscription list and then disappeared. The number of subscribing guilds fluctuated but it never exceeded 35 for any one year before 1900; after that, it declined. In terms of amount, the Nam Pak Hong Guild headed the list with $1,500, followed by the Compradores with $1,000. At the other end of the scale, some guilds only paid a few tens of dollars.

What made the guilds subscribe so loyally? It is difficult to ascertain how exactly the Hospital arranged the contributions with them. The European community in any case was inclined to believe the worst. In 1872, when it learnt about the subscriptions, there was an outcry. In particular, a rumour circulated that the Piecegoods Dealers' Guild had agreed not to employ any agent who refused to pay a third of their commission to the Chinese hospital.[137] The matter came up at the European-dominated General Chamber of Commerce meeting , and though some members dismissed it as a matter among the Chinese themselves, Phineas Ryrie,[138] the Chairman, thought otherwise. The 'fine' as he called it, coming indirectly from the goods, would hurt trade by jacking up the cost. With the current trade depression, he did not look upon such interference kindly, and believed this form of 'squeeze' needed investigation.[139]

The *Daily Press*, never slow to pursue a good scandal, took the matter up immediately. It questioned the Hospital's right to demand such subscription and insinuated at some secret arrangement for it to impose squeezes on trade.[140] In China, guilds frequently collected dues for the government. At the time, the Chinese government was fighting a running battle with smugglers from Hong Kong, mainly by stationing cruisers around Hong Kong waters to ensure that all the necessary customs dues were paid. This was known as the 'customs blockade'.[141] Rumours that Chinese officials had set up offices in Hong Kong itself to collect revenue further raised the question of infringement of territorial sovereignty. Thus Chinese taxation was a sensitive issue causing animosity between Hong Kong merchants and Chinese officials. It was the background to the *Daily Press*'s insinuation that subscriptions for the Tung Wah might be a disguised form of customs dues collected on China's behalf.

The Tung Wah's Chairman denied the charges, asserting that the Piecegoods Dealers' Guild had donated the $700 voluntarily; it was not the Hospital's business to know how the money was raised.[142] The *Daily Press*, however, persisted: it was not easy to distinquish between voluntary and forced contributions.[143] Besides, if only $700 were given to the Hospital, was the Piecegoods Dealers' Guild using the Hospital as an excuse to extract money for other purposes? As far as the *Daily Press* was concerned, whichever way one looked at it, it was bad business.

The *North China Daily News* of Shanghai chimed in,[144] demonstrating the foreigners' ingrained distrust of Chinese associations. Whatever the arrangement, it felt that a powerful native organization was lurking behind the Hospital, and asked 'how a hospital, an institution merely for the relief of the sick, could have so much influence'. Perhaps, it continued, there were other motives than benevolence?[145]

The foreigners' hostility towards the Tung Wah was obvious from the start — the method of fund-raising was only one of the issues attracting criticism. At the bottom of the controversy was the Europeans' ignorance of how Chinese guilds worked combined with the general paranoia of living in the midst of, in their view, a weird and barbaric people. At best they saw the guilds as dangerous combinations designed to strangle free trade; at worst, secret societies engaged in sinister activities. The discovery of the connection between the Hospital and guilds created so much fuss because to them it was proof of evil doings.

It is difficult to ascertain if the subscriptions or other forms of contribution were voluntary and we can only infer from the figures. There is sufficient consistency to indicate that certain guilds did feel a strong obligation to subscribe. It was common for Chinese guilds to subscribe to various religious and charitable causes.[146] Once the guild made the decision, it was binding on all its members. If compulsion existed, it was an internal matter among members. It was this willingness to submit to the guild's authority which foreigners found so incomprehensible.

The Hospital had no real means of penalizing guilds which ceased to subscribe and, over the years, a number of them did. Perhaps it was not fear of a formal penalty which prompted payment. It could be a strong sense of social obligation toward a worthwhile charity. The ultimate penalty was a loss of face. The subscription list appeared every year in the Hospital's *Zhengxinlu* (annual report) and in the local newspapers, so that any payment or non-payment was publicized. Any guild concerned about its reputation must have made all efforts to pay up.

An added incentive was that the Directors came from guilds paying the most subscriptions. There is evidence that guilds were keen to meet the obligation. In many cases, when a guild failed to pay for one year, it would try to make up for it the following year instead of dropping out from the list altogether. That some guilds did discontinue shows that they were free to do so.

Another important means of raising funds was the *yuanbu* (subscription lists) given to individuals, shops, and guilds to pass around. With every donation, the donor's name and the amount would be entered into it. Frequently, unsolicited donations were made by grateful people, challenging the theory that there was always compulsion.[147]

Yuanbu placed on passenger ships became a major source of income. In 1873 ships to California and Australia collected $9,802; in 1887, 76 ships going to California, Australia, as well as to the Philippines, Singapore, Honolulu, Siam, Haiphong, and the treaty ports in China, collected $2,498.[148] The Hospital's connections with emigration are also reflected in the donations Overseas Chinese organizations made periodically. In 1877, for instance, Chinese merchants in Cholon and Saigon gave the handsome sum of $4,513.[149] The Chinese in Peru and California, especially closely connected to the Tung Wah, were regular donors. In 1895 associations from as far afield as Peru, Panama, British Columbia, Burma, Siam, and Annam donated a total of Tl. 5,175 (approximately $7,089).[150] These expressions of gratitude confirm the Tung Wah's respected position in the China–Overseas Chinese network.

Other sources of income were bank interest and house rent. In 1873 the Hospital invested in property, and the first piece of property it acquired was in Wing Lok Street; it cost Tl. 3,240 (approximately $4,500) and yielded an annual rent of Tl. 324 (approximately $450).[151] It continued to increase its real estate holdings, and by 1896 these holdings, for which it had paid $86,300, were estimated to be worth $215,265, yielding $12,915 in annual rent.[152] While profitable, the investments added greatly to the Hospital's administrative burdens.

In 1875, when notices were put up concerning the renting of its property, the *Daily Press* commented that the Hospital had turned into a housing agency.[153] It was not far wrong. It fact this statement became increasingly pertinent as its housing properties grew. Its correspondence of a slightly later period gives some idea of how problems of collecting rent, making repairs, insurance, legal actions, sanitary facilities, and so on demanded much administrative attention.[154]

In fact, by the end of the century, the Hospital had became a major business operation. In 1894, for instance, it handled Tl. 34,676 (approximately $47,506) in income, including rents from 55 tenants.[155] In addition, a number of institutions had accounts with it for defraying various expenses. There was money paid into one charity fund or the other. It naturally became more powerful as its wealth grew. The creation of the Tung Wah

Hospital had resulted in an unprecedented concentration of the power and influence of the Chinese in Hong Kong. Its wealth added to this already formidable combination. And yet, this could be a great temptation to those needing money, and on more than one occasion the possession of such wealth had embroiled the Hospital in trouble, as we shall see.

Even the Hong Kong government was quite overwhelmed by the Tung Wah's financial success. Though occasionally dissatisfied with its mode of operation, and sceptical of its medical efficacy, it did little to interfere. It was after all doing *some* good, officials conceded. More importantly, it cost the government nothing. Without it, the government would have had to perform many of the functions, and pay for them. The Tung Wah was shouldering much of the burden because it could afford to. Thus its independent income to a large extent ensured its autonomy and survival. By the same token, the administrative machinery was stretched to keep pace with the growing accounts and assets.

The Direction of Development

It became apparent at a very early stage that the Hospital's many non-medical functions were outpacing the strictly medical ones for which it was originally founded. These non-medical functions created heavy demands on its administration, draining the Directors' time and energy which might have been spent on the supervision and planning of medical work. It may be said that up to 1894 medical work was the least dynamic of its activities.[156] This was partly because of the management structure; there was not one doctor on the Hospital's Committee. Neither was there a special person responsible for overseeing and supervising medical administration. At the executive level there was a complete lack of professional expertise, with the result that sanitary conditions and discipline among doctors, attendants, and so on fell short of the standard originally set.[157] All these shortcomings would be exposed during the plague in 1894.

Changes, when made, were *ad hoc*. Though the Hospital was overcrowded,[158] there was no long-term plan for expansion. In 1893, a year before the bubonic plague broke out, admissions had increased to 2,857 in-patients and 135,608 out-patients, and yet there were only four doctors, and the premises had been only slightly enlarged since 1872.[159]

It can be argued that the Hospital's medical operation developed slowly because Chinese requirements were minimal. Without the conception of better things there was no demand for improvement. Moreover, there had been no great breakthrough in the development of Chinese medical science in this period to stimulate new activities at the Tung Wah. Another reason is that the hospital as an institution solely for the care and treatment of the sick was still an novel concept, too novel for the Chinese to conceive of development on such a basis. But the ultimate reason was a gradual loss of interest.[160] With so many other problems faced by the Chinese community, the Hospital Committee's ambition to deal with them took priority over the mere running of a hospital.

The Chinese Hospital

And yet a Chinese hospital, however inadequate by modern standards, was not without its value. The oldest plaque at the Tung Wah dates from 1871, when the Chinese Hospital Committee was still only operating the renovated I-ts'z. It was presented by the Aiyutang, a charitable organization in Canton known to Westerners as the Hall of Sustaining Love.[161] The large characters on it, '*huizhou haiwai*', literally mean 'benevolence prevailing beyond the seas'. The small characters further point out that Hong Kong, a lone island several hundred *li* beyond Canton, had become a flourishing trading port where many merchants gathered. When sickness struck, they were desperate. Now, with the foundation of the Tung Wah Hospital by benevolent people, benevolent acts one after another had been performed and, it added, this was due to the prevailing benevolence of the imperial court.

This shows that from a very early stage the Chinese hospital's work had gained recognition beyond the colony. Many later plaques praising its medical work followed. The vaccinations it performed saved lives as well as helped to propagate Western medical knowledge. It had succeeded in training Chinese doctors, though the number was small. In addition, its other charitable works had benefitted thousands upon thousands, both the living and the dead, in Hong Kong, China, and other parts of the world.

The Chinese hospital made its impact in other ways too. The

hospital as a place for the care and treatment of the sick, as we have noted, was a novelty in late Qing China, and the Tung Wah was the first 'Chinese hospital' — employing Chinese doctors and Chinese treatment to cater for Chinese patients. It was, as we have said, a hybrid, a Western form with Chinese content. Yet after it was founded a number of such hospitals began to appear. In 1871 Chinese merchants in Macao founded the Jinghu Hospital.[162] In Canton, the Guangji (1893) and Fangbian (1901) hospitals were founded.[163] Overseas, the Thong Chai Medical Institution (Tongji yiyuan) of Singapore was proposed in 1885,[164] the Donghua Hospital of San Francisco was proposed in 1888,[165] the Fushan and the Guangzhao Hospitals were founded in Cholon in 1901 and 1907, and the Tianhua Hospital of Bangkok was established in 1907.[166] Clearly, by the early twentieth century, Chinese hospitals had become quite common among Chinese both in China and overseas.[167]

Some of them, including the San Francisco Donghua Hospital and the Thong Chai Medical Institution, were consciously modelled after the Tung Wah of Hong Kong. In 1886 there was another specific attempt — though an abortive one — to build a hospital like it in Hawaii.[168] Recognized for its experience, the Tung Wah's regulations and constitution were frequently copied by new institutions, and it was common for them to ask for its help in recruiting and recommending doctors.[169] No doubt it was looked upon as the senior institution. And no doubt too it had contributed much in popularizing the concept of a 'Chinese hospital' through its success, if not in creating it.

On another level, the 'Hospital' was also a façade, in the sense that behind the medical institution many other kinds of social and charitable work were carried out, so that in this respect the Tung Wah might also be considered the prototype of a new genre of Chinese voluntary society. Like the Tung Wah Hospital, these other hospitals were organized by merchants, and as its Committee assumed the role of a local élite group, so frequently did theirs.

The sociologist Lawrence Crissman has identified hospital committees as a community leadership organization common among Overseas Chinese;[170] however, he has not attempted to trace their origins. May we conclude that the Tung Wah's Committee was the first such hospital committee and had inspired others? The connections between these institutions need further research, but the hypothesis that the Tung Wah might be the origin of a new genre of Chinese voluntary association/medical and charitable institution is worth exploring.

A study of the Tung Wah Hospital involves more than just looking at its work, or assessing its shortcomings and contributions. It also demonstrates the relationship between the Hong Kong government and the Chinese community and highlights its position in the Chinese world, both in and beyond China. The hypothesis that it could be the first of a new type of medical, social, and political institution in China provides yet another exciting dimension to the study.

4
The Tung Wah Hospital Committee as the Local Élite

IN traditional Chinese society it was the local élite rather than the official administration which largely managed local affairs.[1] It acted as the bridge between the magistrate and the local community, settled disputes, conducted fund-raising campaigns, commanded local defence, and provided education and welfare of all kinds. It also professed to spread a moralizing influence on the locality by upholding Confucian principles.[2]

Until recently, scholars assumed that these functions were carried out exclusively by the *shen* (gentry), defined as degree-holders.[3] However, some scholars are now showing that in many regions groups other than degree-holders had performed those functions,[4] and even propose that the term 'gentry' could be more broadly defined as 'local people who controlled wealth, power and influence',[5] not necessarily degree-holders. Together, their works provide a more comprehensive picture of local organization in late Qing China. They also provide important reference for this chapter on the Tung Wah Hospital Committee's role as a local élite, that is, a group controlling local affairs by means of informal power,[6] and on how it attempted to fulfil that role in a colonial situation.

The Hospital's opening heralded a bright new era and the fanfare was of immense symbolic significance. Its grand scale of operation, manifesting both dynamism and philanthropy, was a source of pride to the Chinese community and signified its coming of age.[7]

The Committee members themselves saw the opening as a fitting occasion to show off their superior status by donning official robes. It was a display of the power, and the wealth to purchase it, that the Committee represented.[8] Its self-consciousness as the local élite is apparent. The Governor's presence was equally significant in endorsing its position as the community's representatives. It was the contact point between the Chinese

community and the government, which until now had largely
existed on different planes; from now on, the Committee would
act as the go-between. Thus the pomp and splendour of that
spring day celebrated not only the Hospital's opening but also the
initiation of a new local élite.

In a way it was also celebrating its achievements since mid-
1869. Much of its work, even then, was conspicuously non-
medical. Its role as community leader was so extensive that as
early as October 1871 the *Daily Press* charged that it had constituted itself the governing body in the colony of all Chinese
matters, as that newspaper had predicted.[9] The Chinese community thought very differently. It saw the Hospital as a great
benefactor not only in providing charitable services but also as a
moralizing influence rectifying society's decadence and eradicat-
ing its evils.[10] By helping the government rule more effectively
and wisely, it deserved the community's gratitude and praise.
These contrasting views on the Hospital Committee's role as the
local élite were based on different concepts of community leadership. They also stemmed from sharply conflicting communal
interests. Europeans looked upon the Committee's community
activities as attempts to usurp the government's powers while the
Chinese saw the committee as the champion of their cause. These
divergent views underlined the Hospital's history throughout the
nineteenth century; as it became the centre of communal controversy, its history also revealed the basic nature of Hong Kong
society.

The Makings of a Local Élite

The group forming the 'Chinese Hospital Committee' was an
unprecedented combination in several respects. First, it had
community-wide support. Unlike many of the Chinese associations in Hong Kong — guilds, kaifongs, *huiguan* — which were
particularistic in nature, the Hospital's membership was 'non-
segmentary' and the public in practice enjoyed all the rights and
privileges of formal members; in other words, it had a very
widely-based 'constituency'. Of course other bodies claiming to
represent 'the whole of the Chinese community of Hong Kong'
had existed, but they were either ineffective or ephemeral.

Second, the government recognized it as being representative.
Despite the dominant position of the Man Mo Temple Commit-

tee, the government had never given it countenance. The Chinese had an opportunity to form a committee controlling municipal matters when the District Watch Force was established in 1866, but the government frustrated the attempt. In short, until the formation of the Hospital Committee, there was a vacuum of social and political power.

The Committee could fill the vacuum for other reasons too. The mechanism for selecting it guaranteed that year after year it would include the most successful men in each major trade, and it even became a means for identifying the most influential Chinese. The Committee was composed of influential individuals, but the sum of their influence was greater than the parts; the process of calling forth these individuals became itself a recognized means of confirming élite status.

Traditionally, the Chinese local élite, both degree-holding and non-degree-holding, performed important and well-defined functions. With actual or potential connections with the state apparatus, the former were of course more influential and prestigious. Among Overseas Chinese, however, wealth was the operative word,[11] and likewise, in Hong Kong, since the earliest days, its local leaders were invariably the wealthiest merchants.

Their position was further strengthened from the late 1860s as both their number and wealth grew. In 1869 Governor MacDonnell noted this, and the ease with which they raised the Hospital funds proved this beyond doubt. They were active in making Hong Kong a shipping and trading centre, their connections with Overseas Chinese in Australia, Southeast Asia, and North and South America making them the main suppliers of Chinese goods to these markets. By 1869 all the British consuls in China agreed that the distribution of British and foreign goods was passing into Chinese hands.[12] The Chinese boasted that they could sell more Chinese goods on English markets cheaper than their English competitors and, at the same time, sell English goods cheaper to the Chinese in Hong Kong and in China than other traders. By the mid-1870s much of Hong Kong's entrepot trade was theirs.[13] By 1881 they were the largest owners of real estate, contributing over 90 percent of the colony's revenue and holding 90 percent of the note circulation. Since 1876, Nam Pak Hong firms had increased from 215 to 395, the number of Chinese traders from 287 to 2,377, and Chinese bullion dealers, who first appeared in 1876, now numbered 34. More remarkable still, of the 20 largest rate

payers, 17 were Chinese. The best indication of both their absolute and relative wealth was the $1,710,000-worth of property
they bought from European owners between January 1880 and
May 1881,[14] leaving no doubt that they were the predominant
economic force in the colony. Such wealth naturally inflated their
self-importance, prompting them to seek social and political recognition; in 1869 they did so by founding the Tung Wah Hospital
and in 1880 they petitioned the Governor to appoint a Chinese
representative on the Legislative Council.[15]

Third, many Tung Wah Committee members were holders of
degrees and official titles. Though wealth determined élite status,
Chinese merchants in Hong Kong and elsewhere still held the
traditional view that these were the ultimate means of bringing
honour and distinction to one's family and ancestors.[16] Honours
were eagerly sought for other reasons too.

All Chinese who had emigrated had violated the Imperial ban
against emigration from the Chinese Empire and were punishable
by death; although by the mid-nineteenth century this ban existed
chiefly on the books, the threat remained.[17] Merchants in Hong
Kong were at a special disadvantage. Hong Kong, associated with
the humiliation and ignomony of the Opium War, was a sore
point for Chinese officials. They regarded Chinese going there
during and after the War as collaborators. In later years, they
resented it as a haven for Chinese criminals, and were ever aware
of the anti-dynastic triad societies.[18] They believed that 'traitor-
ous merchants' in Hong Kong were supplying the Taipings with
arms, food, and clothing, and that after the fall of Nanking,
Taiping leaders retired there to continue their conspiracies.[19]
They detested smuggling from Hong Kong; but they detested
even more the Hong Kong merchants' inclination to hide behind
foreign officers who spoke on their behalf, and used the prowess
of the British Empire against their own government.[20]

Of course, if Hong Kong merchants had no dealings with
China, the problem would not be serious; but with China's proximity, they maintained very close ties through the family, clan,
business, and property, all being susceptible to the vagaries of
Mainland officials. For the merchants, any commerial dealings
with China depended on their good will too. In short, compared
to other Overseas Chinese, those in Hong Kong were most
vulnerable. On the symbolic level, the purchasers of honours
showed their loyalty and good will; the purchase could be seen as

a form of peace offering. On a pragmatic level, the title and honour offered a modicum of protection from prosecution and persecution. In fact, once the first generation of Chinese merchants had consolidated their economic base, it was common for their sons to sit for the Civil Service Examinations, and a number of the Tung Wah Directors had earned their degrees the 'orthodox' way.[21]

One may even allege that the Tung Wah's own existence created further demand for honours in Hong Kong. As Wang Tao, himself an 'orthodox' degree holder, observed, every New Year, Committee members would appear in full official 'regalia', each eager to outrank the rest.[22] This was repeated at the annual inauguration of the Board of Directors.[23] How embarrassing it would be for any Committee member unable to turn up in a Mandarin robe! Apparently the Committee members believed such trappings helped to assert their élite status. At least, they impressed the ignorant and humble masses who, unsure whether official Chinese authority extended to Hong Kong or not, submitted readily to the authority of merchants in Mandarin guise.

This development in Hong Kong coincided with another in China. The sale of honours as a means of raising government revenue expanded during and after the Taiping uprisings; unfortunately, as sales increased, income dropped. In the 1870s prices were further reduced and certain criteria relaxed to encourage purchase.[24] Even the right to wear peacock feathers, originally instituted as a reward for meritorious services on the battlefield, could be bought for between Tl. 500 and Tl. 1,500.[25] Another important development at this point was discovery by Chinese officials of the wealth of Overseas Chinese merchants and their enthusiasm for honours, and salesmen of honours proceeded to Nanyang and Hong Kong to ply their trade and did a brisk business.[26] This made honours more accessible, and further enabled Hong Kong merchants to consolidate their élite status.

Fourth, the Committee's status was elevated by yet another recent development in China. Traditionally, merchants occupied a despised position in society and suffered many disadvantages. By late Ming and early Qing, however, their social position began to improve and from the nineteenth century onwards, this tendency was accelerated.[27] By the 1870s both the court and individual officials recognized the contribution merchants in China and abroad could make both by helping to build a modern economic infrastructure and by donating defence and relief funds.[28] The term *shenshang* ('gentry-merchants') was used more and more frequently, and in Hong Kong it became common.[29] The term depicted a merging of classes, as gentry entered trade to become merchants and as merchants purchased degrees and official titles to become gentry;[30] both these tendencies reflected the rise of the merchant class. But there might be another connotation reflecting another dimension of the development.

It seems that the term *shenshang* was also used to equate merchants with the gentry, acknowledging the former's elevation to local élite status once associated primarily with the degree-holding class. In Hong Kong, the Tung Wah Hospital's Directors were referred to as *shendong* (literally 'gentry Directors') and the Po Leung Kuk's Directors, *jushen* (literally 'gentry of the Kuk').[31] One of the Hospital's own Chairmen used the English term 'gentry' of Hong Kong[32] to describe them. In a way this may be explained by the fact that many Committee members of these two institutions were degree/title holders and so could legitimately be called *shen* in the narrow sense of the word. But they were not *necessarily* all degree/title holders, and it is more logical to conclude that the term *shen* was used because they performed functions comparable to the gentry's in China, and in doing so, made them their peers.

Significantly, even Chinese officials referred to the Tung Wah Committee as *shen*. A plaque presented to it in 1884 by Chinese officials including Li Hongzhang addressed its members as *shendong*.[33] In correspondence, the Treasurer of Guangdong addressed them as *jinshen*, another common term for gentry, and reminded them that as such, they had certain social obligations to fulfil.[34] (See Appendix VI.) In other words, *shen* was no longer exclusively reserved for the official-gentry class, but increasingly applied to others, including merchants, able to serve the community with equal efficacy.

The 'official' status of the Hospital Committee with reference to the Hong Kong government, obtained almost by accident, was equally instrumental in making this local élite. It was constituted by ordinance, and though this recognized only its work as a hospital committee, it was easily misinterpreted by the common people as a mark of authority in other areas as well. In addition, the personal attention three successive Governors paid to it highlighted its 'official' nature and enhanced its prestige.

Governor MacDonnell, we have seen, took a personal interest in the Hospital. Besides laying the foundation and declaring it open, he also started the tradition of visits by Governors to the institution. His retreat in the face of Leung On's protest must have greatly elevated the Hospital Committee's position in the community's eyes. For his own reasons, he continually sang the Committee's praises before the Colonial Office. These unprecedented public statements of endorsement for a Chinese concern in Hong Kong obscured any fears he might have had of the Committee, obviously a formidable combination of wealth and power, becoming over-powerful.

The Hospital's status continued to grow under MacDonnell's successor, Arthur Kennedy, who appreciated the value of co-operating with the Chinese élite in managing the Chinese community. The European community did not take this kindly. Kennedy received deputations from the Hospital Committee so regularly that the *China Mail* jealously described them as 'the order of the day',[35] and his accessibility to the Chinese prompted the *London and China Express* to remind him that familiarity bred contempt.[36]

The Hospital saw its heyday under the next Governor, John Pope Hennessy, who supported the native community in Hong Kong, as he had in other colonies, with near fanaticism. While irritating the Colonial Office and the local European community, he inspired gratitude from the Chinese. Recognizing their economic importance, he took steps to make compatible their social and political positions. In 1878 he appointed Ng Choy, one of Tung Wah's founders, the first Chinese Justice of the Peace, and, in 1880, the first Chinese Legislative Councillor.[37] This historic decision, made without London's approval, was a landmark in the history of the Chinese community, giving it a new sense of importance.

Hennessy gave the Chinese a willing ear, especially to the Tung Wah Hospital Committee whose advice he actively sought. He invited its members to social functions at Government House, and each new Committee was presented to him annually. From 1880, the list of Directors and the annual accounts were published in the Government *Gazette*, now with a Chinese version, further enforcing the impression of its offical status.

Thus, in effect, for the first 14 years of its existence from 1869 to 1882, the Hospital received on the whole friendly and sympathetic support from the Governors. It was a grace period when it established its credibility and position *vis-à-vis* the government and the Chinese community which stood it in good stead during 'lean years' when Governors were less supportive or downright hostile.

It is interesting at this point to contrast the Tung Wah Hospital with its contemporary, the Wa T'o (Huatuo) Hospital Committee. This hospital, or rather, dispensary, was established in Wanchai around 1867, and at one point had attempted to join the Tung Wah as a branch hospital.[38] Though on occasions it too had pretensions to speak on behalf of the Chinese community, its supporters being only 'the lower classes of Chinese shopkeepers'[39] it never enjoyed the same official recognition or social standing. Perhaps it was exactly because of its powerlessness that the *China Mail* suggested in 1879 that it should be used as a counterweight to the over-powerful Tung Wah.[40]

Acting the Role of Local Élite: Civic Centre and Bridge with Government

The Tung Wah Hospital's establishment enabled the emergence of a new local élite, but it was what it could effectively do for the community thereafter which consolidated and sustained its élite status.

As if anticipating the role they would play, the Founding Directors made special provisions which in effect made the Hospital a civic centre. Ordinary members and members of the community were entitled to bring forth 'matters of public interest' and 'philanthropic questions' for discussion and, as we have seen, there were detailed instructions regarding the procedure of meetings. Attendance at the meetings varied, but when there were important items on the agenda, several hundreds might attend. Significantly, the public not only could initiate matters for discussion, but could also vote on the resolution. No distinction was made between Hospital matters and other matters. This tradition was carried on into the twentieth century.[41]

Public meetings had been held at the kung-so, often under the chairmanship of kaifong leaders; with the new Hospital's completion, meetings were held there under the chairmanship of the far more prestigious Hospital Committee.[42] Like the kung-so, the

Hospital provided more than a physical venue. People bringing matters before the Committee were seeking authority, guidance, and leadership. Where necessary, the Committee brought the matter to the government's attention. In this it performed the valuable and essential function of acting as a channel of communication between the Chinese community and the colonial authority.

The I-ts'z episode illustrated the lack of communication between them. The newspapers were correct in charging the government with being oddly ignorant of what went on among the Chinese. Thus, Leung On's petition laying down the conditions for the Chinese Hospital's operation set a new pattern of relationship with the government. Assertive and confident of their representativeness, he and his Committee claimed to reflect the Chinese community's views. They were the spokesmen and guardians of distinctly Chinese ways of doing things and established the Tung Wah's subsequent role.

The Registrar General, a Chinese-speaking officer to be accessible to any Chinese with a complaint, however humble, was supposedly a bridge between the Chinese and the government. In practice, holders of the office often held other posts concurrently and more often than not there was no full-time officer tending to the Chinese. In 1878 the office was even held by John Gerrard (acting) who knew no Chinese at all.[43] Thus the Chinese who went to the Registrar General's office were at the mercy of clerks, whose corruption and officiousness were notorious.[44] Besides, the majority of the Chinese were uneducated and ignorant of the foreign ways of the colonial government; for them, the existing channels were irrelevant. Once the Tung Wah was founded, they went to the Committee instead. In fact, the development of the Registrar General's office, the main instrument for the management of the Chinese, was, from the start, interwoven with the Hospital's own.

The Chinese Hospital Ordinance empowered the Registrar General to inspect its accounts and monitor its administration. Given the Committee members' social standing, he had to deal with them personally instead of leaving them to clerks, and they commanded much of his attention. Soon, even the Committee found it unsatisfactory working with the Registrar General, a fairly junior official in the 1870s, and sought direct access to the Governor, the real source of power. In time, the Registrar

General was bypassed as the humble Chinese went to the Committee, which they found more sympathetic and approachable, and a more direct channel to the Governor.

One Voice

Between the Hospital Committee and the government, a wide spectrum of topics was broached. Some of course concerned the Hospital specifically, such as funds, vaccination, *post mortem* examinations, exemption from amputation, and so forth. But most issues concerned the Chinese community in a more general way. They were wide-ranging — from typhoon shelters, street lighting, and road repair to gambling, adultery, emigration, brothels, land speculation, mercy for criminals, and bankruptcy laws,[45] to name only a few, and nothing concerning the Chinese community seemed to be beyond its province.

Many of the issues reflected fundamental problems and the frustration and anxiety of Chinese living under a foreign regime. They reveal the basic nature of Hong Kong society as well as the value of the Hospital's work.

One problem was the conflict between Chinese customs and British law. The Chinese held dearly to Elliot's proclamation of 1841 which allowed them to keep their own customs, regarding it as the safeguard against the tyranny of incomprehensible laws. Naturally there was much tension between British law and Chinese customs, and marriage laws were a particularly burning issue which the Committee was eager to resolve.

In Hong Kong, Chinese men were free to have as many wives and concubines as they could afford, but the legal rights enjoyed by husbands in China over their wives were not upheld by the English court. This gave them no protection in cases of adultery, it not being a criminal offence in Hong Kong, or in cases of desertion, since women were regarded as free agents.

The Chinese men's dilemma was highlighted by a dramatic case in January 1873. There was great excitement when the second wife of a Chinese of standing left her husband for another man, taking some jewellery with her. The husband admitted he had 'lent' her the jewellery, but nevertheless brought charges against the lover for receiving stolen goods — the only way he could take vengeance. The jury acquitted the defendant. Chinese public opinion was so outraged that the accused had to be smuggled from the Supreme Court to save him from being lynched.[46] It was in the wake of this that the Tung Wah Hospital Committee took the matter to the Governor, asking for a law against adultery. Governor Kennedy refused on the grounds that Hong Kong's laws could not be inconsistent with England's.[47] The Committee was too shrewd to accept this, knowing that in India there were separate marriage laws for Indians, and could see no reason why this could not be so in Hong Kong.[48] The Chinese were persistent because to them marriage was a pillar of society and legal sanction was essential for upholding it. It reflected the basic positions of men and women at home, in society, as well as in the whole moral framework. The government was equally persistent in its refusal. Its officials apparently had no wish to help Chinese men enslave their wives and concubines with public money.

The matter continued to disturb the Chinese and in 1883 the Hospital Committee again brought the matter before the Governor, Sir George Bowen.[49] This time it asked the Governor to send women who had deserted their husbands back to China where they would be restored to their husbands — forceably no doubt — or to make desertion a criminal offence. Bowen turned down the proposal for the same reason as Kennedy.[50]

Another bone of contention was the Night Pass system which was applied only to the Chinese, who, not surprisingly, were outraged by this blatant discrimination. They also queried its effectiveness in combatting crime. Most of all, respectable Chinese resented the indignity of being classified with the commonest coolies and being locked up all night when found without passes.[51] As if to rub salt into the wound, another ordinance was passed in 1870 making it compulsory for Chinese to carry lanterns when out at night, and it is easy to imagine the outrage and bitterness that resulted.

In May 1873 the Hospital Committee took up the matter in the name of the Chinese community.[52] It pointed out the contradiction that while the government refused to adopt Chinese laws to be applied only to Chinese, for example regarding adultery, it had no qualms about creating laws in Hong Kong applicable only to *them*. Its request was modest — to dispense with the lanterns. But as the European community insisted that the Light and Night Pass system was the best safeguard against an onslaught of Chinese criminals, the request was refused. The grievance remained, and the matter was to be discussed even more bitterly at the Hospital's hall in 1895, as will be seen.

The Committee also spoke out on commercial matters. Though the Chinese as a rule found English laws vexing and interfering unduly with their lives, on occasions they actively sought protection by asking for new laws. In 1874, due to a spate of bankruptcies and abscondings, a meeting was held at the Hospital to discuss the problem arising from the absence of any law requiring the registration of partners of companies.[53] It was customary for foreign firms to publish the partners' names voluntarily, but even then, in case of bankruptcy, complications could arise. Among Chinese firms the situation was far more confusing. Each Chinese used a plethora of names, making it difficult to identify him. To add to the confusion, the partner of a business was sometimes given as a trustee or a firm instead of as an individual. Consequently, when a business was in trouble, it was often impossible to locate or identify the responsible parties.[54]

A petition was subsequently sent to the Registrar General in the name of 'the Board of Directors of the Tung Wah Hospital and other merchants' for a notification ordering all shops to register the names of partners, managers, and their respective villages of origin, and any change of partnership. No corporate names were to be used for registration. In this way, they hoped to increase the confidence of potential investors and help trade prosper.[55] The Committee also raised the matter with the Governor on subsequent occasions, and he finally instructed the Attorney General to draft an ordinance.

The law drafted turned out to be more expensive and cumbersome than the Chinese had hoped. One might say that the initial Chinese request for regulation had backfired. Partly due to their objections and partly due to official doubts about its effectiveness, the entire draft ordinance was withdrawn. The problem of registering Chinese partners remained unresolved for many years.[56]

Adultery, Night Passes, and registration of companies were only some of the countless issues the Hospital Committee discussed with the government over the years, selected here to demonstrate the wide range of subjects it raised on behalf of the Chinese community. After all, they were not issues normally associated with hospitals and show how far the Hospital had digressed from medical business to the community's more general needs. The Chinese turned to the Committee in their anxiety and frustration, treating it as a rallying point where incoherent ideas were made articulate, where the feelings of anonymous individuals assumed identity, and where fragments of opinion were forged into forceful, collective action. There, differences of opinion could be remoulded into a modicum of consensus. Despite the Hospital Committee's occasional failure in persuading the government, it nevertheless provided security for those with common grievances.

Chinese went to the Hospital Committee not only to seek a spokesman; very often they went simply to seek advice on subjects affecting the community. Since the Committee consisted of some of the most sophisticated and dynamic business men in Hong Kong, it would be easy to assume that one could benefit from their experience and wisdom as they congregated at the Hospital. One could also assume that, given their influence, any decision with their blessing would be effected more easily. Their presence strengthened the sense of community, both *vis-à-vis* the government and the foreign community.

One meeting at the Hospital which attracted much publicity, perhaps undeservedly, took place in 1878 during the governership of Hennessy. The Governor, affected by the current humanitarian view of criminals in Europe, abolished the public flogging of prisoners in Hong Kong. Subsequently, crimes, including very serious ones, increased. Exasperated, the European community planned a public meeting to discuss the law and order situation and call for stricter punishments.[57]

The day before the public meeting, the Chinese met at the Tung Wah Hospital to discuss whether *they* should attend it, especially when some Chinese merchants had also signed the requisition to convene it. They decided on attending despite some anxiety regarding the procedures of European meetings. Fortunately, Ng Choy, a Founding Committee member, who a year previously had become Hong Kong's first Chinese barrister, was on hand to answer some of the queries, and suggested asking the promoters of the public meeting to allow for an interpreter so that the Chinese might understand the main substance before voting on the resolution.[58]

The *Daily Press* reported the 'secret meeting' at 'the Tung Wa Hospital (the Chinese Government Offices in the colony)'. The writer assumed that the Chinese were under the impression that the public meeting was to be a personal attack on Hennessy so that, being his great friends, they planned to sabotage it by attending *en masse* to out-vote the Europeans. To forestall this, he called upon 'every gentleman' in the colony to attend the public meeting to prevent the European residents from being out-voted.[59] Thus, even before the public meeting started, the newspaper had stirred up bad feelings.

It turned out to be unpleasant enough. As a larger crowd than expected appeared at the City Hall, the meeting had to be adjourned to the open air, where the Europeans formed a tight circle, leaving the Chinese at the periphery. It seemed a deliberate attempt to keep them out of the action, especially when their requests for interpretation were ignored, and most of them, being able neither to hear nor understand what was going on, departed in a body.[60] The following day, the *Daily Press* gloated over the conspirators' failure to ruin the meeting.[61]

The resolution of the public meeting was forwarded to London. A month later, the Hospital's Chairman presented a memorial on behalf of the Chinese community to the Secretary of State giving their own views on the state of public security in Hong Kong.[62] An opportunity for the different communities to act in unison for the common good had unfortunately been missed. Instead, hostility was intensified and the public meeting became a subject of indignant letters to the press from both sides for weeks afterwards.

The episode illustrates how the Europeans saw the Tung Wah as a centre of Chinese intrigue. The communities were normally sufficiently isolated from each other to pre-empt friction. They moved on different planes but there were times such as this when they confronted each other, thanks partly to the provocation of the English-language press. As each side closed its ranks, the Hospital's role as the champion of the Chinese cause was highlighted and confirmed. Crises and conflicts drive people to seek security and one of the Hospital Committee's claims to community leadership was in providing just that.

It would be naïve to assume that there was complete harmony or homogeneity within the Chinese community or even within the Hospital Committee itself, but the Hospital did minimize dissent behind an ostensibly united front. It would be equally naïve to assume that the Committee was never challenged by other

Chinese groups, but it is significant that in the period under study, such rivalry never developed into open strife.

The existence of the Tung Wah Committee, though overshadowing the Man Mo Temple Committee, the kaifong committees, and other such bodies, did not make them redundant. On the contrary they continued to carry out their own functions at their own levels. The Tung Wah Committee only created an additional echelon at the top of the hierarchy of Chinese organizations by having a broader base of support, higher social standing, and greater influence with the government. In fact these other organizations were pillars supporting the Hospital rather than rivals challenging its dominant and senior position in the community.

The Hospital Committee as Judge

When disputes arose in traditional Chinese society, people often avoided formal magistrates' courts and appealed to their community leaders as judges and arbiters instead. Under a foreign regime in Hong Kong this tendency became more pronounced. Local leaders such as the Man Mo Temple Committee and kaifong committees had been the preferred 'tribunals', and with the Tung Wah Hospital's establishment, people took their cases to its Committee. Every day a number of disputes were submitted to it for settlement. An appointment would be made for the parties to meet and consult with one of the Committee members who investigated the matter and judged the dispute. No fee was charged for the service, and the decisions or judgements were generally accepted as fair and impartial.[63] The existence of this system was common knowledge among the Chinese, and they made no attempt to hide their preference for its arbitration to the official courts'.

Some of the cases presented to the Committee involved Chinese social practices which basically conflicted with English laws and could not be adequately handled by an English court. For instance, men whose wives had deserted them or had committed adultery, and masters whose apprentices had run away, would go to the Hospital Committee for justice.[64] Often, when *muitsai (meizai)*,[65] that is, girls sold as maid servants, had deserted, or were decoyed and taken away, the owners would seek help from the Hospital rather than the police.[66] These cases had one thing in common. Whereas English law recognized all adults as free agents, the Chinese did not. There were varying kinds and degrees of bondage operating in Chinese society over wives, concubines, apprentices, *muitsai*, sons, brothers, nephews, and so forth which were incomprehensible and repugnant to English law. But these social principles had to be upheld, even in Hong Kong, and the Tung Wah Hospital Committee, like other local leaders in China, was guardian to them. In other words, the Committee enabled Chinese in Hong Kong to have justice dispensed according to accepted Chinese principles wherever the legal machinery of the British could be bypassed.

Commercial disputes were also taken to the Committee because of its expertise in such matters. One interesting case occurred in 1873, involving a claim for insurance premium.[67] The shroff of the North China Insurance Company, the creditor, took the matter to the Committee, and Ch'an Sui-nam (Chen Ruinan), one of the Founding Directors, was especially called in to preside. The master of the Kin-loong shop, the debtor, however, ignored the judgement which was not legally binding, and the Insurance Company was forced to take him to court. There, it became clear why some Chinese cases were better settled outside.

When the case opened, there was total confusion over the defendent's identity, for though the debt was incurred in the name of the Kin-loong shop, there was no evidence that the man in the dock was the owner, or even one of the owners — the predicament resulting from the lack of an efficient system for business registration. The common Chinese practice of using a variety of personal names is a complete mystery to foreigners; and the mystery deepened when the defendant claimed that he was not the wanted man because the court had spelt his name differently.

The judge, overwhelmed by the confusion, resorted to calling in Ch'an Sui-nam, who identified the man in the dock as the Kin-loong's owner and that was that.[68] The point is that Chinese practices were different, to say the least, and it was often easier for certain cases to be settled within the Chinese community where people were familiar with each other as well as with their own *modus operandi*. The result was that it enhanced the Committee's prestige, and gave the impression that it was part of the official administration. There were other cases when desperate attorneys, with the consent of the magistrate, simply referred their cases to the Committee.[69]

People involved in court cases frequently asked the Committee to intercede with the government on their behalf, a common practice in China.[70] The ordinary Chinese saw the Committee members in a confusion of images; they were regarded as Mandarins, because of their Chinese official titles, deriving their authority from China; they were also seen as semi-officials in Hong Kong, deriving their authority from the Hong Kong government. Their position was indeed ambiguous but the confusion of images could in fact maximize their impact on the average Chinese regarding the extent of their alleged authority.

Hong Kong officials were aware of the 'court' sessions at the Hospital, and that summonses issued for witnesses were similar to those of a regular court's.[71] There was of course no legal obligation for persons so summoned to appear, but the fact that they usually did reveals that, to them, the Committee had great authority. More interestingly, the plaints addressed to the Committee were in the style of official documents addressed to the governing authorities, clearly indicating the native community's impression of its official status.[72]

Despite the community's assumptions, the Committee had no real official status. It had no legal, magisterial power, and no one had to accept its verdict. But this did not deter it from doing what it believed to be necessary, whatever the circumstances. On occasions, when it could not bring the 'guilty' party to justice, the alternative was to sue him, employ a solicitor, and hope that justice would be done in the English court.[73] This meant that it would arbitrate and persuade where its influence and moral authority sufficed, and appeal to the state's coercive power where they did not. This concern with justice was one of its most crucial functions as a community leader, and its willingness to enlist the state's service strengthened its position.

Philanthropy, Funds, and China

Another expected quality of local leaders in Chinese society was the ability to organize and contribute to philanthropic activities. The Tung Wah was undoubtedly the one institution in nineteenth-century Hong Kong providing the most comprehensive and valuable welfare service. Its charitable work, which extended beyond Hong Kong, and its success in fund-raising became legendary, boosting the prestige of the Hospital Committee not only locally but also in the eyes of Chinese officials, with major political and social repercussions.

In 1877 floods in Shanxi brought widespread famine which eventually spread to other northern provinces. Though keen to relieve famine, the Chinese court could do little, as their coffers were depleted by war indemnities, rebellions, and subsequent rehabilitation. As it became obvious that existing sources of relief could no longer cope with disasters of such an unprecedented scale, Li Hongzhang,[74] then Governor of Zhili and Superintendent of Trade for the Northern Ports, as well as the most powerful official in China, searched frantically for new funds, and was eager to test Chaozhou merchants, including those trading in Hong Kong and Nanyang, as potential sources. He instructed Ding Richang,[75] Governor of Fujian, to appoint Gao Tingjie[76] and Ke Chenjie, two Chaozhou merchants with expectant official titles, to help raise funds in these places.[77] The North China famine in fact marked a turning point in the Chinese court's attitude toward Chinese overseas, with its discovery of them as a valuable source of financial, political, and moral support.

Gao Tingjie, better known as Kao Man-hua (Gao Manhua) in Hong Kong, was one of the Tung Wah's Founding Directors and a leading Nam Pak Hong merchant. Ke, known in Hong Kong as O Chun-chit, another Nam Pak Hong merchant, had been Director in 1874 and Assistant Director in 1873 and 1875. The Tung Wah Hospital, so closely associated with both, was enlisted to help in the fund-raising, lending its prestige and experience. The effort was most successful, for together with several charitable societies in other cities, a monumental sum of Tl. 500,000 (approximately $665,000) was raised.[78]

In appreciation, Zeng Guoquan, Governor of Shanxi, presented the Tung Wah with a plaque in 1878, praising it for its charitable spirit.[79] But a grander acknowledgement came from the Emperor himself. As was customary, Li Hongzhang memorialized the throne recommending awards for the various associations for their efforts. Consequently an imperial decree was issued commending their work and proclaiming that tablet-scrolls be awarded them. The Tung Wah Hospital received one inscribed with the words 'shen wei pu you' — 'god's majesty protects all'. The god referred to was the Martial God, Guan di; the court had mistaken that he was the Hospital's patron god, as he was of so many other Chinese merchant associations. The scroll was handed to the Governor-General of Guangdong and Guangxi and then down through the ranks of local officials until it was finally forwarded by the Magistrate of Xin'an to the Hospital Committee in Hong Kong.[80]

A dispatch giving specific instructions accompanied the scroll: the characters on it were to be engraved on a tablet to be hung at the shrine of the Martial God, and the Committee was ordered to report the day it arrived. The acknowledgment was duly made by O Chun-chit, Kao Man-hua, Leung On, and three others. The scroll was received on 19 February 1879, and on 25 February the tablet with the engraved characters was raised in the great hall.[81]

Besides the four main characters, there were six small ones enclosed in a seal, 'Guangxu yubi zhi bao' (literally 'by the Imperial brush of the Emperor Guangxu' [Reigned 1875–1908]).[82] One can imagine the excitement this sign of imperial favour on a distant outpost of the Chinese Empire — as the Chinese themselves saw Hong Kong — must have created, and the pride inspired in the local community.

For the Tung Wah Hospital, an institution barely 10 years old, to raise such a phenomenal sum and be awarded so handsomely by the Emperor must have been a triumph indeed. From 1877, one disaster after another struck China, and drives to raise relief funds were non-stop. The Hospital Committee continued to raise large amounts for many years thereafter, becoming, as it were, a regular feature in China's welfare system.[83] It also organized and administered funds raised overseas, making use of that network of Chinese voluntary associations in which it occupied such a central position.

Consequently, Chinese officials became increasingly aware of Hong Kong's importance. As China's economy modernized, and as it slowly became part of the international system, there were many functions which Hong Kong merchants — wealthy, patriotic, public spirited, and placed at the junction of East-West exchange — could perform for it. In time, Chinese officials would look to the Hospital Committee for various services. These official connections, in the eyes of Hong Kong residents, were signs of Imperial favour which enhanced the Committee's prestige. To the merchants, these were opportunities to further make peace with the Chinese government and lose some of the stigma of being outcasts and traitors. Hong Kong government officials, however, frowned on them as seditious and a threat to the very existence of British rule in Hong Kong; from 1882, they took positive steps to expose and weaken these connections. In time too, the Committee members found that Chinese officials could be too close for comfort, and realized that it was not easy to please both the Hong Kong and Chinese governments at the same time.

But, for the moment, the Hospital Committee was riding high, basking in the benevolent favour of the Emperor of China, and entrenched as the élite of the local community.

Chinese Emigration

Some of the Hospital's most valuable work was connected with emigration. World demand for labour after the prohibition of slavery and the gold rush in Califorina and Australia were the driving forces behind Chinese emigration. As early as 1852, no less than 30,000 Chinese from the districts around Canton embarked for San Francisco from Hong Kong.[84]

As Chinese emigration expanded, so did the abuses and the suffering. Kidnapping, decoying, and the purchase and sale of human beings — 'pigs' as they were called — became outstanding traits. Life on board ship was so harsh that mutinies by the human cargo became commonplace.[85] At Amoy, the most important emigrant port until 1852, the literati were so incensed that they posted notices warning people against the trade and, fearing the mob, European emigration agents moved their offices south to Hong Kong and Macao.[86] The Chinese government, forced to admit implicitly that emigration could not be entirely prohibited, took steps to regulate it, and the Emigration Convention drawn up in 1866 in effect suspended the recruitment of contract labour from the Chinese Mainland for a number of years, further driving the trade to the British and Portuguese colonies.[87]

The British, while eager to mobilize Chinese labour to work in colonial areas like the West Indies, were also committed to devising regulations to mitigate the evils of the 'coolie trade'. In 1855 the Chinese Passengers Act was passed to ensure that emigrants went voluntarily and that conditions on board were adequate.[88] From 1868 Peruvian agents became so active that Hong Kong appeared set to become the contract labour centre.

The Colonial Office, aware of the abuses associated with contract labour, especially in Cuba and Peru, instructed the Hong Kong government to pass further laws. Ordinance 12 of 1868 declared 'the detaining or carrying away by force or fraud any Chinese for the purpose of the coolie trade' to be a felony. Ordinance 4 of 1870 gave the government power to prevent any Chinese passenger ship from departing without a licence from the Governor. Finally, the licence was to be granted only to ships with destinations within the British Empire, where it was assumed the emigrants' contracts would be properly overseen.[89]

By the early 1870s both the Chinese and British governments were actively regulating emigration; local conditions in Hong Kong, however, made the implementation unsatisfactory. To begin with, Governor MacDonnell was sceptical about the abuses. When confronted by Rutherford Alcock,[90] the British Minister at Peking, with reports about emigration abuses at Hong Kong, he criticized him for taking newspaper reports too seriously.[91] Basically, he could not contemplate prohibiting emigration, one of the colony's main businesses, for the sake of eliminating abuses.

Much also depended on the persons actually enforcing the laws: the Harbour Master, who was also Emigration Officer; the Registrar General; and the Colonial Surgeon. Their staffs were small with few senior officers knowing enough Chinese to detect abuses. Even fewer were really concerned about the fate of emigrants, who seemed so transient and incidental to Hong Kong. The problem was so immense and the abuses of such endless variation that no government official, even with the best intention in the world, could hope to improve the situation significantly.

The immense vested interest also made the suppression of emigration abuses unlikely. In 1852 the 30,000 passengers who left for San Francisco paid a total of HK$1.5 million in passage.[92] The profit not only went to steamship companies but also to coolie broker firms and crimps, many having secret society connections. There were contractors who fitted the ships and supplied stores and provisions. For the export traders, every additional Chinese going abroad meant an extra potential customer for Chinese foodstuff, clothing, and opium.

Besides, from the colonial government's point of view, it was really the Chinese government's responsibility to protect its own people and safeguard its own laws.[93] Since 1866 the Chinese government had actively tried to check abuses. Kidnapping was severely dealt with. In 1872 the Guangdong authorities even used land and sea blockades to force the coolie trade out of Macao.[94] In 1873 the Tsungli Yamen appointed a commission to investigate the conditions of Chinese workers in Cuba, one of the main and most horrible destinations.[95] The Commission's report led the Chinese court to send Ministers and Consuls abroad, marking a watershed in China's diplomatic history. The historian Robert Irick's study of Qing policy toward emigration succeeds in refuting the old allegation that the Chinese government was not concerned with the fate of Chinese emigrants.[96] It provides a valuable frame of reference in our study of the Tung Wah's involvement with Chinese emigration.

The Chinese government could do little in Hong Kong. It was beyond the pale of Chinese officials and, in the absence of a Chinese Consul, the matter was left to the Chinese community's conscience. Ultimately it was left to the Tung Wah Hospital Committee with its wealth, expertise in organization, government connections and, above all, the local élite's moral obligation to oversee society's well-being, to deal with the problems of emigration in Hong Kong.

Tung Wah and Emigration

One of the Tung Wah's first 'debut' involved emigration. In October 1870 mutiny broke out on the *Nuovo Penelope*, carrying 300 emigrants destined for Calloa, Peru. One of them, Kwok Asing (Guo Yasheng), was finally arrested in Hong Kong and charged with murder and piracy.[97] Chief Justice John Smale,[98] however, discharged him on the grounds that since he had been kidnapped for emigration, he had a right to regain his liberty, even by killing the officers on board the kidnapping ship.[99] When Kwok was released, the Hospital Committee gave him shelter.[100]

Disaster on board another emigrant ship soon followed. The *Dolores Uqarte*, which left Macao with 650 coolies for Peru, was set on fire. Some 600 on board were killed.[101] The survivors were returned to Hong Kong, again to the care of the Hospital Committee. A subscription was raised to repatriate them, and the Hospital sent their names, places of origin, and other personal particulars to the Hall of Sustaining Love in Canton to trace their relatives. The steamship company was persuaded to charge only half-fare and the remainder of the donation was distributed among the men.[102] The Chinese paper, the *Zhongwai xinwen qiri bao*, moved by this act of compassion, declared on their behalf: 'My father and mother have given me life; the Tung Wah has given me my second life.'[103] This must have accurately expressed the profound gratitude of the rescued men and the appreciation of the Chinese community as a whole. These incidents set a new pattern of activities for the Hospital, for subsequent emigrants in distress, wherever they were, looked to it for shelter, relief, repatriation, and other forms of protection.[104]

The Hospital Committee also exposed abuses in the emigration trade. In August 1871, receiving an anonymous appeal to save some 200 men 'sold' as coolies for the United States, it immediately alerted the Registrar General and, finally, those found unwilling to emigrate were allowed to leave the ship. As a result, the government preferred charges against the American agent to his Consul for having broken Hong Kong's emigration laws and the Registrar General was told not to allow anyone in whom this agent had any interest to emigrate.[105]

This telling evidence that emigration abuses did exist in Hong Kong put pressure on Governor MacDonnell; he took action but his gestures did little to check the abuses. The Chinese leaders waited until Governor Kennedy arrived to present a document entitled 'A Correct Statement of the Wicked Practice of Decoying and Kidnapping' containing a detailed account of the vices of the Macao emigration trade,[106] and during several meetings they convinced him that abuses occurred in Hong Kong's emigration trade too.

As a result, three ordinances were passed in 1873 to check abuses, the most relevant being Ordinance 6 which expressly forbade the decoying of persons from China to Hong Kong for the purpose of shipment to some outside port, such as Macao. It also provided for better protection for Chinese women and girls, whose sale to the California market was becoming notorious.[107]

The Hospital Committee capitalized on the new Governor's co-operativeness. For some time it had taken matters into its own hands by employing detectives to stop kidnappers. In early 1873 it sought his sanction and asked the government to pay the detectives' salaries, while it undertook to employ proper and trustworthy men. It suggested increasing the number of detectives from two to six, paying $20 to the two head detectives, and $10 to the others. Kennedy agreed, even suggesting giving them papers to prove their authority, and offering the help of the Registrar General and the district watchmen.[108]

The scheme proved amazingly effective. Every day two or three kidnap cases were brought before the magistrate and a number of persons were saved.[109] The detectives extended their activities to Kowloon and out-lying villages to look out for kidnappers operating in small boats between Hong Kong and Macao.[110] Though Acting Registrar General Tonnochy had thought six detectives too many, Kennedy, apparently satisfied with their work, was willing to pay for them.[111]

The unusual success reveals several salient points. Up to January 1873, not one case had been brought to court under Ordinance 12 of 1868 which made kidnapping for emigration a felony. Since it is inconceivable that such crimes had not occurred before that date and then suddenly proliferated, we can only conclude that in the earlier period they had simply gone undetected. This was due to MacDonnell's complacency and to the notorious inability and unwillingness of the Hong Kong police to detect Chinese crimes.[112] In these circumstances the Chinese had to fall back on their own resources, and now, armed with Kennedy's sanction, the Hospital Committee could throw its power and influence behind the project while its detectives could deploy their ability to the full. It was the new attitude and strategy that made the difference.

The Tung Wah Hospital continued to keep vigilant over kidnapping for the rest of the nineteenth century.[113] As a result of this as well as the abolition of contract emigration from Macao in 1875, the establishment of the Protector of Chinese in Singapore in 1877, and increasing emigration restrictions in many countries from the mid-1870s, kidnapping gradually decreased.[114] The Hospital's detection work became so well known that individuals and associations in different parts of the world sent kidnap cases for it to solve. Requests also came for it to find persons who had been decoyed or had run away from home, or had simply lost their way.[115]

The Hospital Committee undertook to combat other forms of deception in the emigration trade too. One was the credit-ticket system by which passage was advanced to an emigrant who then continued to work for the creditor until the sum had been paid off, which could be a long time. Thus, when the Committee exposed the fact that it took as long as two years for an emigrant to work off his passage in the sugar plantations of the Sandwich Islands (Hawaii),[116] Hennessy took its advice and prohibited emigration from Hong Kong to those islands.[117]

There was also fraud through misrepresentation. In 1875 the Committee exposed a broker recruiting labourers for Acheen in North Sumatra who claimed that the Harbour Master would guarantee the terms of the contracts. This was of course untrue since contract emigration to places outside the British Empire had been banned from Hong Kong since 1870. Indeed, the Harbour Master should have been prosecuting the agent rather than endorsing his contracts.[118]

Sometimes the real destination was misrepresented. In November 1875 an anonymous placard denounced a broker for telling people that they were going to Tonkin (Northern Vietnam) while the real destination was Deli in Sumatra,[119] where working conditions were miserable. The placard appealed to the Hospital Committee to save the 500-odd victims.[120] The Registrar General, informed by the Committee, went on board and re-examined the emigrants, most of whom subsequently left the ship and were taken to the Hospital for repatriation.[121]

The Committee members were personally active. They interviewed both the victims and offenders of illegal emigration. They employed lawyers for plaintiffs in some cases and attended court to give their moral support.[122] They not only saved the victims but also ensured that justice was done, for it was the local élite's duty to relieve suffering as well as uphold social justice and maintain its moralizing influence in society. No wonder appeals for help went to the Hospital Committee rather than directly to the government.

It also showed great concern for the emigration of Chinese women as prostitutes. As few Chinese men took their wives abroad with them, the demand for Chinese women was desperate. A girl bought in Canton for $50 could be worth $1,000 in San Francisco.[123] It was a complicated business. When women were kidnapped, the case could be prosecuted as such. When they were sold, it was more difficult to prosecute because the sale of persons, especially young girls, was an accepted practice among Chinese,[124] illegal only when the girl had been sold for prostitution. It was also complicated when the women emigrated voluntarily to become prostitutes. From the Hong Kong government's point of view, they were perfectly free to travel and follow the profession of their own choice. After all, prostitution was legal in Hong Kong. Some officials even felt that they were better off in San Francisco or elsewhere where they might have a chance to get married.[125] But the United States and Canadian governments began to frown on Chinese prostitution as a form of slavery and organized crime so that respectable Chinese and, later, Chinese Consuls checked the traffic with the Hospital Committee's help.[126]

The problem was brought to Kennedy's attention in 1872 when he was told of several hundred women being sent from Hong Kong to San Francisco to be sold as prostitutes.[127] Despite existing laws against the detention and decoying of women, it was difficult to determine when these had been committed. If it was difficult to find out from men whether they were emigrating voluntarily, it was nearly impossible to extract the truth from Chinese women trained to give certain answers. As Harbour Master Thomsett admitted, though he knew that most women emigrants were purchased on the Mainland and exported for prostitution, so long as they claimed that they were going voluntarily, as they had been instructed, there was little he could do to help them.[128]

With Kennedy's support, a new system evolved. Whenever a steamship was about to leave with large numbers of Chinese, the Hospital's Committee members would go on board or to the Harbour Master's office to conduct a general enquiry and ascertain that no women were shipped off for immoral purposes.[129] When uncovered, such cases were referred to the Registrar General for prosecution. Thus the Committee became even more directly involved with the administration and, not surprisingly, in many minds it had acquired quasi-official status.

The Committee's value was further confirmed by the United States Consul's reliance on it to regulate the emigration of women from Hong Kong. In 1875 a Supplementary Act of Congress prohibited the emigration of Chinese women into the United States for immoral purposes,[130] which greatly added to Consul D. H. Bailey's headache. For years he had tried to distinguish voluntary emigrants from involuntary ones, a most exasperating task, and now he had to distinguish respectable women from prostitutes, an impossible one. He could expect little help from Hong Kong officials since prostitution was legal there. Besides, the acting Governor, J. Gardiner Austin, believed that with such an abnormally high ratio of single Chinese males, the US government should not discourage the emigration of Chinese females.[131] Bailey looked elsewhere for help.

Assured of its good faith and efficiency,[132] Bailey turned to the Hospital Committee and found it eager to co-operate. After several meetings, they worked out a system of joint action.[133] Every female applying to emigrate to the United States was required to fill out a declaration, giving personal details and stating that she had not been decoyed, kidnapped, or forced to emigrate, and that she was not going for 'lewd and immoral purposes'. (See Appendix V.) She was to obtain security from a shop and proceed with the documents to the Hospital Committee, which would examine the evidence and report on the case to the Consul.[134] This placed the onus of preventing Chinese prostitutes entering the US on its shoulders. Not surprisingly it created the impression that unless a woman passenger had received the Committee's permission she was not free to sail for the United States.[135]

There was much criticism of the system, not least of which was that an irresponsible body was given so much power. But the American government must have appreciated the system for it continued for a number of years. The Chinese themselves also appreciated this service. In 1887 the China Consolidated Benevolent Association of Victoria, British Columbia, asked the Committee to prevent prostitutes from going to Canada by the same means,[136] apparently assuming that it had legal as well as moral authority to regulate emigration.

However close the vigilance, many Chinese prostitutes did manage to reach the United States. When discovered, they were sent back, at first by Chinese voluntary associations and later by Chinese Consuls, to the Tung Wah Hospital in Hong Kong, which undertook either to repatriate them or marry them off. As early as 1873, even before the United States officially prohibited their immigration, Chinese prostitutes had been sent to the Tung Wah Hospital for repatriation.[137] It is clear that at every stage of the emigration business, the Committee was involved.

The Hospital Committee also placed coffins on passenger ships. Deaths on board ship were common, and often the bodies were simply thrown overboard. This was anathema to the

Chinese, but there was little else they could do. In 1877 two deaths occurred on ships along the China coast and in both cases the bodies were cast into the sea. Public opinion was outraged and it was decided that something had to be done. Consultation took place between Wong Kwan Tong (Huang Juntang) of the Tung Wah Committee, the Siemssen Company, and the China Merchant Steam Navigation Company. The outcome was that the Hospital undertook to place coffins on ships travelling between Guangdong and Shanghai, and a special fund was raised to support the operation.[138] The money came mostly from Canton merchants but Chinese officials were also keen subscribers, with the prefects of Guangzhou and Huizhou among the first. In 1885, when Zhang Zhidong[139] became Governor-General of Guangdong and Guangxi, he donated the princely sum of Tl. 1,000 (approximately $1,370).[140]

This was probably the beginning of the *taiping guan* (literally 'coffins to be used in case of emergency') system which the Tung Wah extended to ships bound for other ports as well. Catering to one of the greatest and most basic needs of the Chinese, the practice was deeply appreciated. In 1887 the China Consolidated Benevolent Association of Victoria, after praising the Tung Wah profusely for this service, declared that it too would follow its example.[141]

The Hospital soon established a reputation among Overseas Chinese for the many services it performed, and one of the most popular of these was acting as a centre of information. Besides being a shipping and trading centre, after the telegraph came in 1869 Hong Kong remained for many years the only telegraph terminal in the region.[142] Not till 1882 did Canton, connected to Hong Kong, get telegraphic service.[143] With the English-language newspapers an important source of information about the outside world,[144] relevant materials were reprinted in the Chinese newspapers to be widely circulated in the whole area.

The dependence of Overseas Chinese on the Tung Wah as an information centre is best illustrated in the case of the California community, the community with the closest and earliest ties since most of its members had come from the districts around Hong Kong. For years, people on the Mainland learnt about conditions in the United States and changes in regulations from the Hospital's notices in the Chinese newspapers. In the early 1870s the papers told of the hardship among the Chinese in America, in the late 1870s of Chinese being refused landing, and in the 1880s of anti-Chinese riots.[145] The Six Companies[146] of San Francisco were the main sources of information, and in view of the difficulties, they depended on the Hospital Committee to discourage people from travelling there. In fact this pattern of development was repeated in many other places — Peru, Panama, Costa Rica, Hawaii — where Chinese first struggled with abominable working and living conditions, then discrimination, and finally exclusionism.[147] At each stage, the Tung Wah played a key role in keeping prospective emigrants informed.[148] Chinese Consuls who found the Hospital Committee an effective channel of communication also supplied information, hoping that it would convince people with its influence and credibility.

For this reason, the Hospital Committee was often better informed about Chinese abroad than Mainland officials. The case of Chinese emigration to Hawaii illustrates this well. As demand for labour in Hawaii rose sharply in 1876 with the United States allowing Hawaiian sugar to enter duty free, several Chinese and foreign firms became busy importing labourers to Hawaii.[149] The Hospital Committee, as we have seen, succeeded in persuading Governor Hennessy to prevent anyone from Hong Kong emigrating there, so that between 1878 and 1881 no one did. In the meantime, however, large numbers of Chinese proceeded from Whampoa near Canton, and the China Merchant Steam Navigation Company did good business out of it, especially as the Hawaiian government was subsidizing the traffic.[150]

In Hong Kong, the English-language newspapers queried the Hospital Committee's motives. If, they asked, abuses existed in emigration to Hawaii, why did it not persuade Chinese officials to prevent emigrants from China too.[151] The *Daily Press* even suggested that it was helping the Chinese steamship company gain a monopoly of the trade at the expense of business in Hong Kong.[152]

As usual, the press was over-reacting, and far off the mark. For one thing, many emigrants went to Hawaii on German ships.[153] Secondly, Canton officials were much less well-informed and seemed quite oblivious of the abuses pointed out by the Committee. Even Li Hongzhang, who raised questions about Chinese emigration to Hawaii in 1879, was more concerned that it might be a cover-up for the coolie trade to Peru or Cuba.[154] When asked by Li, Liu Kunyi,[155] Governor-General of Guangdong and Guangxi (1875–79), assured him that everything was above board.

Liu did not discover the truth, long known to the Tung Wah Committee a few hours downriver, until 1881, when Chen Lanbin, the Chinese Minister to Washington, reported on it. But by that time Liu had already left Canton, and all he could do was to advise the Tsungli Yamen to instruct Canton authorities to impose stricter control over emigration. By then much harm had already been done. The Chinese continued to rush into Hawaii and it was only when that country began to impose immigration restrictions from 1884 onwards that the numbers started to fall off.[156]

Increasingly Chinese officials, especially those in Canton, learnt to appreciate the Tung Wah Hospital's usefulness, and not merely as a fund-raiser and operator of the *Taiping guan*. In 1878 the acting British Consul at Canton, H. F. Hance, reported that the Hospital Committee was 'hand in glove' with the 'Prefect of Canton', and claimed that it was chiefly due to its influence that the Chinese took such vigorous action in the Peru emigration case.[157] Unfortunately Hance did not elaborate. But it is likely that he had exaggerated the Committee's influence; at least, as we have seen, high officials such as Liu Kunyi did not seem to be in direct communication with it. It was only when Zhang Zhidong became Governor-General of Guangdong and Guangxi that contact was established on such a high level.

Its relations with the Chinese diplomatic staff, however, started as soon as China began sending envoys abroad. When Chen Lanbin left for the United State in 1878, he took with him Chan Ayin, an early Committee member of the Hospital who later became Consul-General to Havana. A very active member of the Hong Kong Chinese community, he had on many occasions acted as interpreter for deputations to the Governor, and Hennessy was especially impressed by him.[158] Perhaps it was through him that the Chinese diplomatic staff discovered the Hospital's usefulness. In 1882, as we have seen, Chen Lanbin appointed the Hospital the agent for transmitting correspondence for Chinese emigrants.

Another interesting example of Tung Wah's involvement with Chinese diplomats occurred in 1882. The *Mary Tatham* with 600 passengers from Hong Kong was wrecked near Hakodate in April. Li Shuchang, Chinese Minister to Japan, having reported the matter to Li Hongzhang, telegraphed the Tung Wah Committee requesting it to ask Leung Tai (Liang Tai), the charterer, to send another steamer for the passengers.[159] It did so immediately but Chinese officials in Japan grew impatient as Leung took his time and a number of telegrams on the subject went back and forth between the Consul at Yokohama, the Minister at Tokyo, and the Tung Wah Hospital. The Committee continued pressing Leung, and even summoned him to a meeting at the Hospital for him to explain the delay. In exasperation, it approached James Russell,[160] the new Registrar General, asking him to put pressure on Leung to send a ship at once.

Though Russell had some reservations about the quasi-official status of the Hospital Committee and was unsure about the government's policy towards this, he nevertheless complied.[161] In other words, not only was the Hospital enlisted into assisting the Chinese government, Hong Kong officials too were brought in to serve its purposes, with the Hospital Committee as middle man. It had become an integral part of the administration of Chinese officials overseas.

It carried out these and a whole range of emigration related functions partly because it was the local élite, and partly because there was no Chinese Consul in Hong Kong. Very few Chinese diplomats were sent abroad and in Honolulu, for instance, a local Chinese resident was appointed unofficial Consul.[162] In Hong Kong, attempts to establish a Chinese Consul, begun as early as 1869, had been resisted by every Governor on the grounds that a Chinese Consul in Hong Kong would have undue influence on the overwhelming majority of the population.[163] China's proximity was such a real cause for fear that not even an honourary or unofficial Consul was contemplated. As a result, many of the Consular functions devolved on the Tung Wah. The diary of Zhang Yinhuan,[164] Chinese Minister to Washington between 1885 and 1889, reveals how heavily he and his staff depended on the Hospital Committee for providing and disseminating information, and caring for persons repatriated from the United States. In a way, the Hospital Committee was acting as an honourary Consul, but the sheer volume and range of emigration-related business makes its achievement phenomenal.

Chinese emigration gave rise to countless abuses and problems seriously affecting Hong Kong. In dealing with them, the Tung Wah fully acted out its role as the local élite. It displayed not only an amazing ability to organize but also the social, political, and moral influence it could bring to bear. Its work affected Chinese in many parts of the world and in time it grew to be more than a 'local' élite as such, assuming global significance. A pivotal contact point between the Overseas Chinese world and China, the Hospital demonstrated the importance of Hong Kong's position as China's gateway to the world.

The Po Leung Kuk

One of emigration's most permanent effects on Hong Kong was the establishment of the Po Leung Kuk. In 1878 four prominent merchants, natives of Dongguan district, presented a petition to the Governor for permission to found a society to prevent kidnapping and to protect the victims. They asked for authority to employ detectives, offer rewards for arrests, and return the victims to their homes.[165] This later became known as the Po Leung Kuk (*Bao liang ju*, literally 'protect the innocent society'), or the Society for the Protection of Women and Children.

As these functions were already being performed by the Tung Wah Hospital Committee, it would appear at first sight an attempt to set up a rival organization. In fact this new society was proposed, planned, and organized by the Tung Wah Hospital people[166] and after the Po Leung Kuk was established, the two organizations worked together so closely that they were sometimes indistinguishable from each other, giving rise to the expression '*Dong Bao ijia*' — 'the Tung Wah and the Po Leung Kuk are one family'.

Why was it necessary to create a new society? For some time, the Hospital had been criticized in the English-language press for engaging in non-medical functions, and its 'true nature' had been questioned. The press attacked the Hospital's work with emigration, especially of women, attributing to it all kinds of sinister motives. In challenging the Hospital's legal authority for those functions, the press touched a particularly raw nerve because, so far, it had only done so at the Governors' 'pleasure'. To institute a society with the legal authority specifically to protect women and children from kidnapping would legitimize the work of the Chinese community leaders.

The timing itself was significant. The petition was presented in 1878 with unusual urgency. The ostensible reason was that the number of kidnapping cases had increased with the recent alternating flood and drought in China, which had led to poverty and crime.[167] This might be true, but there seems to have been another more pressing reason for action at this particular time. Urgency was due to the introduction of Ordinance 2 of 1875 which made any sale of human beings criminal. Of course, according to English law slavery was illegal, and there had always been laws on the books in Hong Kong against the sale of persons.[168] But they had never been vigorously applied and until 1875 the selling of girls as *muitsai* or concubines, and of boys for adoption was transacted without fuss.

The practice, however, attracted attention when emigration abuses were exposed. In 1871 Chief Justice Smale condemned the coolie trade as slave trade, and created great controversy by declaring Kwok Asing innocent. In the process, other forms of human trafficking were revealed and the Hospital Committee itself fought the sale of women for immoral purposes overseas, and it was partly as a result of its representation that Ordinance 2 of 1875 was passed.[169]

Its efforts, however, seem to have backfired. Much to its dismay, the Hospital Committee found that the Ordinance was directed not only at kidnapping and the sale of 'pigs' and women for prostitution, but at the buying and selling of human beings in every form.[170] One can imagine what an outcry such an indiscriminate formulation of the law would produce among the Chinese. As they put it themselves, it 'put all native residents of Hong Kong in a state of extreme terror'.[171] When the police began enquiring into suspected cases of 'illegal detention', resentment mounted. Although no charges were made so long as it could be proved that the child involved had been properly treated and that the sale had been transacted with the parents' consent,[172] this new Ordinance nevertheless made Chinese householders with adopted sons, bought concubines, and *muitsai* susceptible to blackmail, harassment, and conviction. To make things worse, magistrates had different ideas of which party was guilty. If a child was sold, who was guilty, the buyer or the seller? Who should have custody of the child? Some magistrates found the buyer guilty, others the seller, and these inconsistencies in the interpretation of the law only aggravated the situation.[173]

To the promoters of the Po Leung Kuk, the fundamental issue

was the need to distinguish between *legal* and *illegal* sale of persons. This was clearly spelt out in a second petition presented by Leung On and the Tung Wah Hospital Board the following year.[174] It claimed that past Governors, though aware of the buying of girls for domestic servants and of boys for adoption, had treated the matter with indulgence and had forbidden prosecution. The customs, necessary and respected in Chinese society, had safeguards against the ill treatment of such children and were legal. Evil practices such as kidnapping and the seduction and sale of women for prostitution, however, should be criminal. Invoking Captain Elliot's proclamation, they reminded the government of the right to practise Chinese customs, implying that the Society aimed exactly at maintaining them within legal bounds.

The contradiction was pointed out by Chief Justice John Smale: while the Chinese community tried to suppress kidnapping, their proposed action fell short of attempting to punish those who created the supply and demand — those who sold to, and those who purchased from, these kidnappers.[175] This was a pertinent and pregnant observation highlighting an inherent contradiction of this particular Chinese practice. Yet it was not for the Hospital Committee to resolve it. Rather it was its duty as the local élite to preserve and defend social customs, not to challenge them; to contain contradictions, not to expose them. One of the prerequisites of traditional Chinese community leadership was the ability to uphold common social values, a primarily conservative function. The establishment of the Po Leung Kuk is a noteworthy expression of this function.

Hennessy was largely responsible for making the Po Leung Kuk possible. He gave the promoters the go-ahead to organize themselves and carry out their proposed plans provisionally even before he wrote to London for approval. The draft Rules and Regulations went back and forth between the Chinese meeting at the Tung Wah Hospital and the law officers in order to work out something acceptable to both. The Chinese seem to have aimed at two principles which were not always reconcilable. One was to acquire as much autonomous power for performing the proposed functions as possible, the other to seek government approval and be constituted by ordinance like the Tung Wah Hospital. Government officials, however, were worried that the Society, working with detectives and informers, might become too powerful[176] — certainly they had no intention to create another powerful Chinese society like the Tung Wah Hospital.

Despite Hennessy's lavish recommendations, the Secretary of State for the Colonies, the Earl of Kimberley, remained cautious. When he finally approved of the Society, he took the Attorney General's view that there was no need for it to be constituted by special ordinance. Thus, unlike the Tung Wah Hospital, the Po Leung Kuk was not incorporated by ordinance and did not gain the legal status that its promoters had hoped for.[177] It remained a junior associate of the Hospital.

Despite that, the Hospital's creation of the Po Leung Kuk was no less a feat. It had been founded in the face of strong opposition from John Smale and other sceptical officials and Hennessy's own initial idealistic animosity against slavery and the human trade. The Chinese then converted him to their view that only the *abuses* should be interfered with. When he approved of the proposal for the Po Leung Kuk, Hennessy rationalized that 'As long as they were treated as an alien race it is not surprising that they were allowed to keep up practices alien to our constitution'.[178] But he was begging the question, because the Chinese *wanted* to remain separate, and in allowing the human trade, however 'legal' it might be, he himself was perpetuating this segregation and enabling two social codes to co-exist.

A practice so repugnant to English law and the spirit of liberalism was thus protected in the British colony as a 'Chinese social custom'. In upholding it, the Hospital Committee demonstrated the essentially conservative character of the Chinese local élite. In time, not only foreigners but certain sectors of the Chinese community as well came to regard the practice as barbaric. In the 1920s the Hong Kong government came under strong pressure to abolish the *muitsai* system, the pressure coming from the Colonial Office and the League of Nations, but originating from Christians, missionaries, labour unionists, and women activists, both Chinese and European, in Hong Kong.[179] In changed circumstances, the Tung Wah Hospital and the Po Leung Kuk, the guardians of Chinese customs, appeared as citadels of conservative and benighted forces and were besieged as such. This revealed the rifts that occurred in the Chinese community as it grew increasingly heterogeneous in its political attitude and social values in a period of rapid, radical changes. But in the 1870s the

Hospital Committee, by being instrumental in this entrenchment of Chinese social practice in face of foreign laws, confirmed both its role as champions of Chinese social principles and its leadership status.

Management of the Chinese

As the local élite, the Tung Wah Hospital played a crucial role in the management of the Chinese. This ought to have been the duty of the Registrar General and one may say that their relative importance was in inverse proportion to each other.

In the 1870s the Registrar General's office was a fairly junior one, often held concurrently with other offices. In 1872, besides holding that office, C. C. Smith was also acting Colonial Secretary, acting Auditor General, and acting Treasurer.[180] For long periods the Registrar General's duties were performed by acting officers who, in turn, would be holding other positions. Tonnochy, acting Registrar General in 1876, was concurrently Sheriff of the Supreme Court, Marshal of the Admiralty Court, and Superintendent of Victoria Gaol.[181] This could be a major reason for the weakness of the office, offering an opportunity for the rise of the Hospital Committee. It was a rise, as it were, by default.

The office of the Registrar General disintegrated further under Hennessy, who actively sought to reduce its power. The ostensible reason was economic — costs could be cut by transferring parts of the Registrar General's duties to the Police Department, the Harbour Office, and the Treasury.[182] In effect, the Registrar General would be reduced to dealing only with registration, and his role as Protector of Chinese would disappear. Smith objected to this[183] but he left at the end of 1878 to become Colonial Secretary of the Straits Settlements. John Gerrard, the First Clerk in that office, was appointed acting Registrar General until May 1881, while the substantive appointment remained unfilled.[184] This can be seen as the first stage of the disestablishment of the office. Not knowing any Chinese, Gerrard was unqualified as Protector of Chinese. As Frederick Stewart, the acting Colonial Secretary, discovered, the resulting vacuum was filled by the Tung Wah Hospital Committee, which was 'assuming and exercising the function of the Protector of Chinese'.[185]

Hennessy obviously had other motives for reducing the Registrar General's power. He was persuaded that the existence of a government department dealing with the Chinese as a separate community was a sign of class or racial discrimination which he was determined to abolish. The responsibility of governing the Chinese, together with that of governing the foreign community, he felt, should equally be the Colonial Secretary's.[186] To help the Colonial Secretary deal with the Chinese, he announced his intention to appoint Dr E. J. Eitel, a distinguished Chinese scholar and his great supporter, to be head of the Interpretation Department for £1,000 (approximately $5,400) a year, the highest government salary after the Colonial Secretary's.[187]

The proposed restructuring was extremely unpopular with the Colonial Office, which felt that the Registrar General's post was too important to be reduced and had worked too well to be disrupted.[188] What they did not realize was that by this time the office had *already* been diminished. As for the Chinese secretary, they objected partly as a matter of principle and partly because they would prefer the position going to an Englishman and not Eitel, a German.[189]

The Tung Wah Hospital was another consideration. John Bramston, the assistant Under-secretary of State, having been Attorney General of Hong Kong for three years (1874–76), was familiar with its special position. He pointed out that with the Governor openly favouring it, the ordinary Chinese believed that their business would be put more favourably through the Hospital Committee, resulting in its becoming the main channel of communication with government. He suspected that it had proposed the change as a means of increasing its own influence, and warned against an *imperium in imperio* that would take years to counteract.[190]

Despite the Colonial Office's opposition, Hennessy got his way. Eitel became interpreter. The Registrar General's office remained in name; in practice it was all but abolished.[191] Consequently, the Chinese increasingly brought their business to the Hospital Committee, whose influence did grow, as Bramston had feared.

Interestingly, in Singapore the Protector of Chinese was established in 1877, just about the time when that office in Hong Kong was allowed to disintegrate. This shows how the different opinion and attitude of individual Governors could decide matters on the spot in the absence of a rigid and comprehensive imperial policy toward 'natives'.

The emergence of a widely accepted élite had great value for the government. It went a long way to remedy the endemic problem of the government's lack of communications with the Chinese community. It was used to mobilize the Chinese community's resources. MacDonnell had encouraged the Hospital's Founding Committee because he knew that it was able to tap its resources much better than the government ever could. Kennedy sought the Committee's help to raise funds for a new building for the Central School.[192] An Irishman, Hennessy, was pleasantly surprised to find how much more the Chinese could contribute to the Irish Relief Fund than the Europeans.[193]

The Hospital Committee could also be used to promote the Governor's personal interest. Hennessy for one might have mobilized Chinese support as a counterweight to European hostility. There might be some truth in the allegation that the Hospital Committee was trying to drum up support for the Governor against his critics at the public meeting of October 1878.

Both Kennedy and Hennessy regularly looked to the Committee for advice, to the extent that the China Mail spitefully called it the 'Advisor-General' of the government.[194] Without it as a source of information and advice, problems such as emigration abuses would simply not be solved. Hennessy admitted, 'In this spacious hall [of the Tung Wah Hospital]...I have often taken counsel with my Chinese friends as to what would be the best course to adopt for this colony'[195] and clearly he took its advice. He braved criticism in prohibiting emigration to Hawaii from Hong Kong, helped found the Po Leung Kuk, and granted it a site.[196] Many long-standing Chinese grievances expressed by the Committee were acted upon. It was during his time that the law regarding Night Passes, with which the Hospital had been so concerned, was relaxed. Finally he made one of its Founding Committee members, Ng Choy, the first Chinese Legislative Councillor in Hong Kong.

Just before Hennessy left for England in early 1882, he was invited to a banquet at the Tung Wah Hospital. It was an event of great symbolic significance. Ng Choy, who presided, made the important point that 10 years before, no Chinese would have dared to invite the Governor to a banquet.[197] The gulf between the Chinese community and the government was narrowed, and the Hospital, posing as the local élite, had been instrumental in bringing it about.

Conclusion

The Tung Wah Hospital Committee's emergence as a local élite had enormous impact on Hong Kong's history. For the Chinese community it marked a new era. It carried out the duties of a local élite with unprecendented authority and effectiveness. It relieved suffering in many ways and oversaw the community's general well-being. It upheld Chinese moral principles, maintained Chinese social practices, dispensed Chinese justice, and protected Chinese interests under a foreign regime. Through it, the Chinese community's opinion could be voiced with greater force and coherence, and a sense of purpose, communal pride, and unity was inspired. As its own status rose, it brought a new dignity to the Chinese community as a whole. As Wang Tao observed, the civilizing influence of the Tung Wah Hospital had transformed the whole atmosphere of Hong Kong.[198]

It also brought about new and closer relations between the Chinese community and the government, which became more aware of the value of co-operating with the Chinese community. As the Registrar General's ineffectiveness gave the Hospital Committee a chance to emerge as the 'protector of Chinese', the effectiveness of the Committee further made that office dispensable.

The Committee transformed relations between the communities. Its high profile provoked foreign residents, led by the newspapers, to watch the Chinese suspiciously. By championing the cause of the Chinese community it unwittingly sharpened the contradictions of a multi-racial society.

The impact of the Hospital Committee's work as a local élite was more than local. As the Committee proved its worth to Chinese officials as a source of financial, administrative and, later, political support, its work assumed a China dimension. Finally, its involvement with emigration and with Overseas Chinese claimed for it a central place in the Chinese world both inside China and abroad. These activities not only confirmed the Hospital's historical importance but also demonstrated Hong Kong's significance in the modern history of China.

5

Criticism, Confrontation, and Control

THE Tung Wah Hospital as a local leadership group saw its heyday in the 1870s and the opening years of the 1880s. This chapter will describe how its ascendency was challenged and examine how new circumstances arose to erode its dominant position.

The English-Language Press and Early Criticisms

From the start, hostility towards the Hospital Committee was expressed in the English-language press. In so far as the newspapers affected the European community's opinion, as well as being a means for expressing it, they reflect the relations between the Tung Wah Hospital and that community. Moreover, as the English-speaking sector in the Chinese community grew, the influence of the newspapers became even more pervasive and significant. The basic hostility tended to produce exaggerated and distorted reports, often telling one more about the writers' own bias, and yet, it is also true that in their eagerness to expose the 'misdeeds' of the Hospital Committee they provided detailed and interesting accounts of its activities.

Sometimes the papers were simply petty. When the Tung Wah Directors brought the issues of the Night Pass and adultery to Governor Kennedy, the *Daily Press* called them 'arrogant and presumptuous', finding it 'outrageous that Chinese were impertinent enough to belittle Western culture and to compare merits of Christian and Confucian principles of government with the Governor'.[1] This comment reveals the paper's own arrogance and the Europeans' general sense of racial and cultural superiority.

But there were also fundamental issues involved. Ostensibly, the English-language press disapproved of a 'hospital' taking upon itself non-medical functions. In an editorial, the *Daily Press*, after listing all these functions, concluded that to continue calling such an institution a hospital would be an insult to the common sense of the community.[2] But this actually stemmed from an underlying fear of its immense power. Realizing that the Committee operated as 'a sort of Small Cause Court, Chamber of Commerce, Tribunal of Arbitration, Hong Kong Association, and Advisor-General of the Government'[3] and 'the absolute directors of all native emigration from this port',[4] European opinion was anxious that it had set up an *imperium in imperio* independent of the government — an independent body, responsible to none[5] — and, with its sway over the Chinese population, its was a potentially subversive force.

Basically insecure, the English-language press looked at all the Hospital's activities suspiciously. When it sent survivors from the *Dolores Uqarte* home, was it in order to get them out of the way before they could be properly interrogated?[6] When it checked contract labour, was it because local people would not be getting 'head money' out of this form of emigration?[7] Even its efforts at preventing women emigrating as prostitutes were assigned an evil motive. Was it not done to discourage male emigrants from marrying and settling down so that, obliged to return to China by the shortage of women abroad, the men would be 'squeezed' by the Hospital on their way home?[8]

In contrast, the Chinese community defended the Hospital fervently, both in the Chinese and the English-language press. Far from usurping government powers, the Chinese insisted that the Hospital Committee was serving both the government and the community with its extensive participation in public affairs.[9] Being so numerically preponderant, they needed representation and, in the absence of an official body, they went to the Hospital Committee instead. The Hospital Committee was facilitating the government's access to Chinese opinion and feelings.[10] Never doubting the Directors' competence, honour, and philanthropy, they argued that the Committee conducted community affairs with the same compassion and righteousness with which they ran the Hospital.[11] In short, the Hospital was a subject of constant controversy, an issue through which the tension between the communities manifested itself.

Though well defended by the Chinese community, the Hospital Committee was nevertheless disturbed by the criticisms. In 1875, amid exceptionally vicious attacks on its emigration-related activities, the Committee felt it might be advisable to introduce a separate institution for the non-medical functions it had been performing. It asked the Governor for approval to build a City Hall; he agreed, and promised a site for the building.[12] A meeting at the Hospital was called in November 1875 to discuss the issue; circulars went out before the meeting to influential individuals for their advice and, when it assembled, some three hundred attended, showing how important it was considered.[13]

At the meeting several items were raised and voted on. Despite the Committee's consternation, the meeting voted in favour of its continued participation in community affairs. Leung On especially pointed out that the Hospital's Regulations had provided for it to hold meetings on questions affecting the interest of the Chinese community.

The meeting also voted in favour of the Committee's continued co-operation with the government in such activities as the suppression of gambling and kidnapping, and the regulation of women's emigration. The participants disagreed that there was any usurpation of governmental powers.[14] In other words, the representatives of the Chinese community reaffirmed, justified, and sanctioned all the Hospital Committee's non-medical activities, so severely criticized in the English-language press.

Some of the members, satisfied with present arrangements, saw no need for the proposed City Hall at all.[15] But the Committee pursued the matter. In July 1876 it formally asked the Governor for a part of the Chinese Recreation Ground near the Tung Wah Hospital for the building. Kennedy was agreeable, but the Surveyor General, J. M. Price, advised against it because the ground, granted for the recreation of the public, should not be used for construction purposes. He continued to object despite several modifications in the original building plan, and the Chinese concluded that he was simply being obstructive.[16]

After Hennessy replaced Kennedy as Governor, another petition, signed by 778 persons styling themselves the 'whole Chinese community', was submitted by the old guard of the Hospital — Leung On, Li Sing, Wei Yuk (Wei Yu),[17] Ts'o U-t'ing (Cao Yuting), and Ng Choy — repeating their request for the site at the Chinese Recreation Ground, but this time the land was to be used for a Chinese Chamber of Commerce, 'for the furtherance of intercommunication in commercial affairs', and for the Po Leung Kuk.[18] In February 1882 Hennessy instructed Price to prepare a deed for half of the Ground.[19] This was done, apparently with great reluctance, and delivered to the trustees. But in the meantime, Hennessy left the colony.

William Marsh,[20] the Colonial Secretary who administered the colony from March 1882 to March 1883 and intermittently between then and 1887, felt very differently about the Hospital Committee. He openly challenged its position and brought about the beginning of its decline. As for the proposed site, he found the terms of the lease — a grant for 999 years for a consideration of $15 down, and an annual rent of $1 — objectionable.[21] He was also under the influence of Osbert Chadwick,[22] who had been sent to Hong Kong in late 1881 to examine the sanitary conditions, agreeing with him that the Recreation Ground must be kept intact for health and sanitary reasons. With the Executive Council's approval, and anticipating that of the Colonial Office, Marsh took the rather grave step of suspending Hennessy's instructions to grant the lease.[23]

By depriving the Hospital people of the land, Marsh was in fact frustrating their effort to find alternative 'authoritative bodies' on which to divest the Tung Wah's non-hospital functions. Neither the City Hall nor the Chamber of Commerce was organized, perhaps because the Chinese took the refusal of the site as a sign of government disapproval. At the same time, it provided an excuse for those Chinese leaders happy with the *status quo* to drag their feet.

Consequently, the Tung Wah Hospital continued to play the part of City Hall cum Chamber of Commerce by providing both the meeting place and leadership for community matters. Moreover, despite the establishment of the Po Leung Kuk, in the absence of its own premises, the women and children it rescued were put up at the Tung Wah Hospital, and even its meetings and administration took place there. The two institutions continued to work closely in matters relating to women and children.[24] Thus, despite the will to shake off non-medical commitments, the Hospital Committee was not wholly able to do so. And its critics continued to have a field day.

Early Official Reservations

Though the Hospital Committee proved so valuable to the government, many officials had reservations about it. Even Kennedy, perhaps pressured by public opinion, at times tried to confine it to hospital work.[25] Unable to defend its multifaceted role, he welcomed suggestions for ways to eliminate its social and political functions.

In July 1873 Tonnochy, the Acting Registrar General, proposed having two men elected from each district to help him in municipal matters and take care of the affairs of their own districts. The Governor supported the scheme, and, significantly, he asked for the Hospital Committee's advice. Showing no great enthusiasm, the members said that they would be glad not to have to deal with community matters any more. They warned that there might be some difficulty as those elected might not have the time and disposition to answer the call, and made the interesting point that even the present Chairman of the Board was only induced to accept the post by earnest solicitation![26] Perhaps due to their non-enthusiasm, the scheme was abandoned, not to be revived until 1891.

Kennedy was also concerned that the Registrar General was being totally bypassed. In 1876 he found it necessary to issue a notice reminding the Chinese that they should communicate directly with him through the Registrar General.[27] This was obviously a move to curtail the Hospital Committee's influence.

The Committee's rise became meteoric under Hennessy, and his patronage coincided with the increasing patronage of the Chinese government. While official Chinese cognizance enhanced the Committee's position in the community, it also antagonized local officials and caused alarm in London.

In November 1878, the acting British Consul at Canton, H. F. Hance, raised an alarm over 'the mischievous influence exercised in Hong Kong by the Tung Wa [sic] Hospital'. He cited the opinion of McLeavy-Brown, formerly the Commissioner of Customs at Canton, who had just returned from a visit to Hong Kong, that the Hospital Committee was 'hand in glove with the Prefect of Canton' and 'really managed Chinese affairs in Hong Kong', adding that it was chiefly through the influence of the Hospital and the Prefect that the Viceroy took such vigorous action in the Peru emigration case.[28]

In response, the Secretary of State, Sir Michael Hicks-Beach, wrote a strongly worded confidential dispatch to Hennessy. Referring to Hance's letter, he wrote:

I trust that you are fully sensible of the necessity of restricting the Committee of the Management to their proper functions, and of the inglorious effects which might follow if this institution were permitted to exercise any political influence over the Chinese population of the colony, extensive as that suggested or to become the recognized medium of communication between the Chinese resident and the government.[29]

Obviously, Hicks-Beach took the matter seriously. With China so close, if the Chinese government could exert influence over a body of Chinese controlling the local population, the situation could be menacing. Although up to 1878 Tung Wah–China connections were confined to raising funds and assistance for emigration, after that the connections did become more extensive and political in nature. Hicks-Beach's observation was therefore farsighted and perceptive.

Hennessy, however, took the Secretary of State's letter rather lightly, and even managed to lose it.[30] He did, in a rather halfhearted way, speak of consulting Chinese bodies other than the Hospital Committee,[31] but the effect was offset by his own actions. After watching the decline of the Registrar General's office in dismay, Lord Kimberley, the new Secretary of State for the Colonies, finally instructed the Governor in 1881 to offer the Registrar Generalship, vacant since 1878, to either W. M. Deane, a cadet and Superintendent of Police, Tonnochy, or Frederick Stewart, all of whom had had long service in the administration, spoke and read Chinese well, and were familiar with things Chinese.[32] Hennessy's counter-offer — to let Eitel have the position — the Colonial Office categorically turned down.[33] Hennessy took his time negotiating the appointments. Finally, James Russell, the Colonial Treasurer and a cadet, was appointed in May 1881 as Registrar General, drawing half the usual salary.

Lord Kimberley also instructed Hennessy to restore the Registrar General's former duties and issue a notification announcing that all communications between the Chinese and the government should first go to that officer.[34] Seeing this as a retrograde policy restoring racial discrimination, Hennessy put off issuing the notice, insisting that it would check the prosperity and progress of the colony. When on leave in England he continued pleading his case with Kimberley. He argued that the Chinese were happy with the present arrangement of going to the Chinese secretary, and doubted if Russell's ability to speak Chinese was adequate to deal with them.[35]

Distrustful of Hennessy, Kimberley preferred to hear 'the wishes of those besides the compradores and the directors of the Tung Wa [sic] Hospital'; but even this came to nothing.[36] It was clear that as long as Hennessy remained Governor, no matter what the local press, the Colonial Office, and his own officers might say, the Tung Wah would continue to be a vital channel of communications between the government and the Chinese. The powers given the man on the spot were great. London might call the tune, but the Governor could dance as he pleased.

Official Pressure

Hennessy left Hong Kong in March 1882. For those anxious to put the Tung Wah Hospital in its place and those simply with an axe to grind with the former Governor, the time for action had come. With Governor Marsh hostile towards both, the change in policy became immediately apparent. It started with his withdrawal of the site Hennessy had granted for the Po Leung Kuk and Chinese Chamber of Commerce. In June he launched a more frontal attack. Writing to Lord Kimberley, he said,

There seems to be little doubt that for some time past the Hospital Committee have not limited themselves to these [that is, charitable] purposes. They appear to have been recognized by the Chinese as a kind of tribunal to which petitions for redress of grievances should be addressed and in fact to have exercised the duties, of which the Registrar General was relieved, of Protector of Chinese. Public sittings were held occasionally and summonses to witnesses to appear were obeyed as if issued by a regular court of justice.[37]

He enclosed three reports from James Russell, the new Registrar General, to support the allegations.

The first two referred to the Hospital Committee sitting 'as if they were a bench of magistrates', and to how 'a citation from the Directors is as readily obeyed as one from the Supreme Court'.[38] Russell pointed out that the Hospital had been assuming functions never contemplated by the Chinese Hospital Ordinance and queried whether 'an eleemosynary body with any propriety [could] convert itself into a political institution or assume the functions of a Court of the Colony'.[39]

The Attorney General's minutes on the reports expressed similar suspicions. Agreeing with Russell that unless the Hospital was carefully watched it could become a 'very mischievous association', he contended that its ambitions were clearly shown in the Po Leung Kuk rules it originally submitted.[40]

No doubt many officials had found the Hospital's work irregular, but with Hennessy abetting it, there was little they could do. Once Marsh's attitude became obvious, they were only too ready to speak their minds. There may even have been an element of vendetta against Hennessy.

The third report referred to the Hospital's correspondence with Chinese officials relating to the *Mary Tatham*, which Marsh thought was most decisive. Remembering Hicks-Beach's letter, he was now able to prove the allegation that the Hospital Committee was working closely with Chinese officials. While feeling strongly that these practices should be stopped, he did not think any abrupt steps should be taken. One consideration was that the government had never warned the Hospital Committee against such proceedings, and the open manner in which it conducted itself showed that the Chinese did not regard these practices as wrong or illegitimate.[41] This is significant, showing clearly how the former Governors' tolerance had induced the development of the Hospital Committee's role as community leaders.

Marsh suggested taking a more tactful line by issuing a notice announcing that the Registrar General's former functions had been restored.[42] Seeing this as a way to redirect Chinese business from the Hospital Committee, Kimberley agreed. He instructed Marsh to be cautious, tactful, and discreet in case the Chinese were alarmed that the government was making a radical change of general policy. He was also to take Hicks-Beach's dispatch of 1879 as the basic guideline regarding the Hospital, and gradually to confine it to its proper operations which were so valuable.[43]

Even before Kimberley's reply went out, an incident occurred prompting Marsh to immediate action. The Registrar General informed him of a petition presented to the Hospital Committee. A shoemaker involved in a case of fraud was taken to court, and he petitioned the Hospital to intercede with the judge who, the shoemaker feared, might fail to see the truth; and the Hospital told him that his statement had been considered.[44] Not only did Russell object to the Hospital interfering with legal proceedings but also to the style used in the petition — it was that used in official documents addressed to the governing authorities. This clearly shows that most Chinese residents regarded the Hospital Committee as such.[45]

This was the status the Hospital Committees had been openly enjoying for over a decade. But now Marsh, in a position to decide matters, considered the matter too urgent to await the Colonial Office's advice. With a new Committee coming into office, he believed it was time to lay down the line once and for all.[46]

The Colonial Secretary duly wrote to the Hospital Committee pointing out that the Governor was prepared to receive any Chinese representation either directly or through the Registrar General, and he hoped the Directors would refuse to accept any appeals made to them. He reminded it that according to the Ordinance the Hospital had no powers to interfere with the functions of a properly constituted court.[47] In fact, the government would no longer tolerate the Hospital interfering in any matters beyond the charitable. Thus, for the first time since its establishment, the government formally defined the Hospital's activities and restricted its influence. It was the beginning of a more direct confrontation between them as officials reviewed the problem of the management of the Chinese.

Restoration of the Registrar General; Constitutional Reforms

As soon as Marsh took office he started restoring the Registrar General's former duties[48] which, as has been seen, had been increasigly performed by the Hospital Committee.[49] Soon, he reported that the restored system was working well. He cited the opinion of two leading Chinese, Fung Ming Shan (Feng Mingshan)[50] and Wei Yuk, who reported that the Chinese themselves were very pleased with the present arrangement since Russell could read Chinese petitions himself and dispose of the more trifling ones on the spot.[51] Frederick Stewart also reported that the Chinese considered it 'a high privilege' to have an officer of Russell's standing, experience, and judgement to consult. A petition by members of 'every section of the Chinese community' also applauded the restoration.[52] The one person who refrained from joining the general applause was Ng Choy, confirming suspicions that he had been the original instigator of Hennessy's scheme to reduce the Registrar General's office.[53]

More significantly, the Tung Wah Hospital itself expressed satisfaction with the restoration to the acting Governor when members of the out-going Committee and the new Committee called upon him in August 1882, adding that they hoped the function of Protector of Chinese would not be taken away again.[54] For Marsh this was the ultimate proof that he had made the right move. Even Robert Meade at the Colonial Office observed, 'This is important, coming from the Tung Wa [*sic*] Hospital.'[55] The timing is interesting. Delivered only two weeks after the Colonial Secretary's warning letter, this commendation from the Hospital Committee was perhaps to reassure Marsh that it had no political ambitions. It was, one may say, a peace offering.

Just as the Registrar General's office was settling down, James Russell resigned. Marsh insisted that the vacancy must be filled by a senior officer or the post would become a sinecure one.[56] He might have added that, otherwise, the Chinese would be going to the Hospital Committee again. His choice was Frederick Stewart, whom he described as patient and considerate with the Chinese. Marsh was sure he would be very popular. The Colonial Office accepted the nomination.

This was the beginning of a gradual upgrading of the Registrar General's office. Not only was it strengthened by the appointment of an experienced officer, it was further elevated constitutionally under Governor Sir George Bowen, who made the Registrar General an *ex officio* member of the Legislative and Executive Councils. Approving this change, the Colonial Office staff agreed that the Registrar General must sit on the Legislative Council as 'the mouthpiece of the Chinese community'[57] and the Secretary of State, Lord Derby, concurred that this would properly mark the importance of the office.[58]

In April 1884 the office was further re-organized when Gerrard, the first clerk, retired. Bowen took the opportunity to suggest abolishing the position of first clerk and installing an assistant Registrar General instead. N. G. Mitchell-Innes, a passed cadet who knew both written and spoken Chinese, was recommended for it. He was given preference over the Portuguese registration clerk partly because the latter did not read Chinese and partly because his English training was thought to enable him to take a proper view of many questions relating to personal freedom which frequently occurred.[59] The new situation was a far cry from the days when the office either barely had a full-time head, or had one who knew no Chinese. Now it was headed by two highly qualified officers who could cover each other even when one was on leave.

In July 1884 Bowen further enhanced the position by raising the Registar General's salary, arguing that a post requiring a knowledge of the Chinese language, laws, and customs should be better paid than officers of minor departments.[60]

Bowen, arriving in 1883 with a wealth of experience in constitutional reforms, was keen to introduce them to Hong Kong too, and many of them were to affect the Chinese community's development as well as the Hospital's.

In May 1883 there were four unofficial members in the Legislative Council, two of whom were paid officials. All four were appointed by the Governor. Bowen abolished the unpopular practice of giving unofficial seats to government officials. The number of unofficial members was raised to five. To satisfy demand for representation, one of the unofficial members would now be nominated by the Chamber of Commerce and by the Justices of the Peace. At least one of the five was to be Chinese. Frederick Stewart, who had been sitting on the Council as an unofficial member, was made an official member in his capacity as Registrar General.

After informally sounding out the Chinese, Bowen nominated Wong Shing (Huang Sheng),[61] who had the widest support for the Chinese seat. He approved of him as a 'Chinese gentleman of high character, good education and of large property', and Wong was willing to be naturalized as a British subject to sit on the Legislative Council. Educated in Hong Kong and Massachusetts, Wong had served Li Hongzhang in China and at the Chinese legation in Washington. With such experience Bowen felt he would be able to 'look at Chinese affairs with English eyes and English affairs with Chinese eyes'. A Founding Director of the Tung Wah Hospital, his long residence in Hong Kong and activity in the community won him support among the Chinese, which Bowen saw as an additional asset.[62]

The two newly created 'functional constituencies' — the Commission of Peace and the Chamber of Commerce — were fairly cosmopolitan in make-up. Ng Choy became the first Chinese Justice of the Peace in 1878,[63] and by the end of 1883 seven out of 79 were Chinese.[64] Of the 34 members of the Chamber of Commerce, two were Chinese.[65] As the number of naturalizations and the number of Chinese able to understand and appreciate the British way of government grew[66] these avenues for political participation — the Legislative Council, the Commission of Peace, and the Chamber of Commerce — became viable and attractive alternatives to bodies such as the Tung Wah Hospital. They were also attractive to Chinese professionals basically excluded by the Hospital Board's merchant-based structure. As these government-created avenues to power and social status evolved, the relative position of the Hospital Committee declined.

In the meantime, the Colonial Office staff monitored with interest every sign of the growth or diminution of the Hospital Committee's influence. Indeed, for the first few months after the Colonial Secretary's warning letter, the Committee seems to have decided to lie low. A deputation calling upon the Governor in January 1883, though comprising many of its members, including the Chairman, Ho Amei, seems to have taken care not to call itself a Tung Wah Hospital deputation.[67] They presented a memorial signed by 1,176 of the principal Chinese residents complaining about the government's inability to suppress gambling and sly brothels, that is, unregistered brothels. This pleased Bramston who thought it showed that the Chinese were learning to bring their grievances directly to the government, and not to the Hospital Committee.[68] The Secretary of State, Lord Derby, instructed Bowen and his officials to continue encouraging the Chinese in this direction.[69]

Still, it was not in the government's interest to deprive the Committee of all its influence. Its usefulness had not disappeared overnight. The Governor continued to receive deputations from the Hospital Committee as spokesmen for Chinese opinion, and the Registrar General continued to defer to it on many issues. One was the perennial problem of 'unfortunate women' — for example, the difficulty of identification for registration under the Contagious Diseases Ordinance and in order to prevent brothel slavery.[70] One solution was to introduce photographs, still a novelty in the early 1880s. Russell, realizing that any innovation would be resented, anticipated strong resistance from brothel keepers. To pre-empt this, he consulted the Hospital and the Po Leung Kuk Committees and, with their approval, he was 'fortified in my opinion that it will work by the unanimous opinion of the Chinese Committee'.[71] In other words, with their approval, he was more confident that the brothel keepers would comply. The government was clearly prepared to harness the Hospital's influence for its own ends.

Indeed, keeping the Hospital Committee's influence within bounds was one of the government's primary tasks. Its dilemma was exactly this: how to exploit the Hospital's ability to maintain social order without abdicating its own administrative powers. This dilemma was clearly manifested in 1884 when strikes and disturbances led to a show-down between the government and the Hospital Committee.

The 1884 Strikes and Riot

Since 1882 Sino-French hostilities over Annam had been building up tension in South China. Anti-French sentiments were widespread in Hong Kong,[72] and Bowen reported these feelings among the leading Chinese after a meeting with the Tung Wah Committee.[73]

These feelings climaxed with the French bombardment of Tamsui and Foochow in August 1884. In response anti-French strikes broke out in Hong Kong in September.[74] Zhang Zhidong, a prominent member of the pro-war party, was sent south to become Governor-General of Guangdong and Guangxi. Convinced that people in Hong Kong and other outlying areas could be mobilized to support China's war effort, he issued proclamations calling on them to be patriotic and sabotage the French,[75] fuelling the already intense hostilities felt by Chinese in Hong Kong.

On 11 September dockers at the Hung-hom docks refused to work on French ships,[76] thus starting a series of strike actions against the French, including refusal to provision French ships, to transport French cargo, and even to serve the prospective French Resident at Hue at the Hong Kong Hotel.[77] Zhang's proclamations notwithstanding, there is evidence that these actions in Hong Kong were spontaneous demonstrations of patriotism.[78]

Marsh, again acting as Governor, opposed the strikes. Several of the boat people who had refused to carry goods for French ships were fined heavily at court, creating great *furor* among the

Chinese community. The fines were blatantly illegal and immoral. According to Section XVII of Ordinance 8 of 1858, persons could be punished for asking for more than the regulated rate, but in these cases, the boat people were not asking for higher wages but simply refusing to work. Even the Colonial Office pointed out the fines would give the Chinese the impression that the government was being pro-French.[79] As a result the strike spread to a wide range of trades and crafts.[80] The injustice of the fines had transformed the strike from an anti-French one to an anti-government one.

On 3 October skirmishes broke out.[81] The actual fighting lasted only a few hours but the strike persisted. To prevent further 'rioting', Marsh called in the East Kent Regiment, the 'Buffs', to patrol the streets. More significantly they were quartered at the Tung Wah Hospital,[82] ostensibly because it was located in the populous Tai-ping-shan area. But there may have been more complex reasons for this.

The Chinese leaders had made no secret of their anti-French sentiments. There were also rumours — and they seem to have been nothing more — that the strikes were controlled and assisted by Chinese of position, wire-pullers in the background who prolonged, if not excited, the disturbances.[83] It was even believed in some circles that the Tung Wah Hospital itself, with the guilds, had provoked the disturbances to create a chance to usurp government powers.[84] While it is impossible to tell whether the Governor believed these rumours, it is very likely that the troops were stationed at the Hospital as a show of force, even to hold it as hostage until the disturbances were controlled. One can imagine the Committee's reluctance to accommodate them.

Different parties tried to end the *impasse*, and on the second day after the riot present and former Committee members of the Tung Wah Hospital and others requested to see Frederick Stewart to find a solution. Marsh thought the leading Chinese were beginning to change their position because, as merchants, they were sustaining losses.[85] Moreover, unbeknown to him, some of the leading merchants, including members of the Tung Wah Committee, had received instructions from Zhang Zhidong to end the disturbances.

The meeting fully manifested the complex relationship between the Hospital Committee and government with its mixture of jealousy, suspicion, and jockeying for position. The customary courtesy was absent. The Chinese made it obvious that they thought the government was handling the whole thing badly.[86] Leung On had been asked to draft a Chinese proclamation calling people to resume work, but Stewart found it objectable because it contained words to the effect that the government had pardoned the rioters on the intercession of the Chinese leaders and had accepted terms suggested by them. Clearly they wanted to create the impression of being instrumental in settling the dispute.

Leung also made other suggestions: that the troops be removed from the Hospital and that the Directors of the Tung Wah should call a public meeting to persuade the people to return to work. Alternatively, the Tung Wah Directors could issue a proclamation to that end.

Stewart opposed them all, declaring that this was not a matter that concerned the Tung Wah Hospital Directors as such. In fact, he told them point blank that to accept Leung's proposals would amount to the government abdicating its powers to the Hospital.[87] In short, the charges fired for so many years in the English-language press, or aired in confidential dispatches to London, even hinted politely to the Tung Wah Committee in 1882, were now thrown straight in its face. Though on this occasion the purposes of the government and the Hospital Committee were ostensibly the same, there were other interests so conflicting that they lost sight of any common ground. The meeting ended without resolution and the tension remained.

By this time all parties realized that the main obstacle to an amiable settlement was the fines. Marsh took the rather unusual step of offering to remit the fines to anyone who wished to apply for them. No one did. In fact he heard that someone else had gone about refunding the cargo boat people.[88] It must also have surprised him to find work resumed on 5 October.

Meanwhile, the Chinese newspapers reported that the strike had been settled through the Tung Wah's intercession with the government.[89] Zhang Zhidong himself reported likewise to the Tsungli Yamen, adding that the Hong Kong government had remitted the fines, and were paying damages to those killed during the riot.[90]

The interesting question is, who had repaid the fines?

It is tempting to allege that the Hospital Committee had. Eager to resolve the situation, and eager especially to be seen to have resolved it, it must have seen the remitting of the fines as the easiest and most expedient way out. If this was so, we can logically conclude that the Tung Wah had proven itself extremely effective in fulfilling the government's object to end the strike. Unorthodox though the measure was, it was nevertheless effective and imaginative.

But to the government and the European community at large, the Tung Wah's efforts were dishonourable. The issue was even brought up in the Legislative Council when T. Jackson[91] of the Hong Kong and Shanghai Bank and an unofficial member, denounced the Tung Wah Hospital's ambitions at a Council meeting. 'I think it ought to be publicly stated beyond all doubt that there is but one government in this colony, and that is the Executive — that there is no body of Chinese gentlemen between the government and the people.'[92] Referring to the Chinese newspaper report that the settlement was due to the Tung Wah Hospital, he went on to declare:

It should be publicly stated this day in council that these gentlemen of the Tung Wa [sic] Hospital are merely members of a charitable organization and their powers begin and end there. They appear to wish to arrogate to themselves something more and to assume a position which is not permissible and which they are certainly not entitled to. I hope we will hear no more of the gentlemen of the Tung Wa [sic] Hospital in connection with matters of this kind.[93]

It was also declared that the situation was more dangerous because the trouble-makers were not the ignorant lower classes, but the influential and wealthy members of society — the so-called 'better class Chinese'.[94]

The 1884 episode developed into nothing less than a showdown. Despite common goals, the clash of interest was only too real. The significance of stationing the troops at the Hospital was both real and symbolic. It showed the government's determination to put the Hospital in its place. It was no accident that in the two following years it energetically confined the Hospital's influence and suppressed its connections with China. The 1884 crisis must have been an object lesson prompting it to build alternative bridges to the Chinese community and bypass an intermediary which might turn out to be too powerful and ultimately working for opposing interests.

One dimension of the Tung Wah's activities causing particular anxiety and highlighted by the 1884 strike and riot was its connections with Chinese officials. It was a major factor hardening the government's determination to suppress it in the 1880s.

Zhang Zhidong

The Tung Wah Hospital's connections with China grew closer during Zhang Zhidong's Governor-Generalship in Guangdong and Guangxi (1884–89). Being in the south, he began to appreciate Hong Kong's importance both in itself and in relations to Overseas Chinese, especially those in Nanyang, whose emigration and trade were basically centred on Hong Kong.[95] As he discovered the Hospital Committee's many uses, he grew increasingly dependent on it.

In 1884, Zhang mobilized the people in Hong Kong to support China's war effort by sabotaging the French, and by supplying arms and information about the enemy. He was so sure that Chinese merchants there would act as informers that he rejected the proposal to send agents (tanyuan) to Hong Kong as unnecessary.[96]

One of the most energetic 'agents' was Ho Amei, better known in China as He Xianchi. Educated at the Anglo-Chinese College in Hong Kong, he had spent some years in Australia and New Zealand, involved in mining and the importation of Chinese labour. Back in Hong Kong, he worked as a clerk in the Registrar General's office between 1869 and 1872 before going into a number of enterprises. His relations with Chinese officialdom began in 1868 when he served for six months in the Chinese Imperial Customs; later he joined the Guangdong Provincial tax bureau. In 1882 he became a principal in forming the Wa Hop (Huahe) Telegraph Company, established to build a line between Canton and Kowloon, while he was promoting a modern waterworks in Canton. By 1884, when he was busy sending telegrams to Zhang Zhidong regarding French movements and the general situation in Hong Kong, he had also become one of the most prominent Chinese community leaders — Chairman of the Tung Wah Hospital (1882) and the Po Leung Kuk (1883, 1884). As secretary to the On Tai (Antai) Insurance Company, he also sat on the Chamber of Commerce, the first Chinese to do so.[97] Thus the suspicion that 'better class Chinese' might be keeping close, even subversive, connections with Canton was completely justified in Ho Amei's case. He best demonstrates the ambiguous position of the Chinese resident in Hong Kong and the complex and awkward nature of extraterritorial loyalty.

Eventually, Zhang relied on Chinese merchants in Hong Kong to check the strike. He had been censured severely by the Tsungli Yamen when the British protested against his provocative proclamations.[98] When the strike and disturbances broke out in Hong Kong he was naturally blamed for them, and he needed to absolve himself. Once the riot was over, he reported to the Tsungli Yamen that he 'had secretly telegraphed Chinese merchants in Hong Kong, persuading them to "*shi ke ji zhi*" ('put a stop to [the disturbances] when the time was appropriate').[99] He went on to report that with the Hospital Committee's mediation, the Hong Kong government repaid the fines, released those arrested, paid damages for the killed, and agreed to tolerate Chinese refusal to unload French ships.[100] Evidently he was pleased with the outcome and satisfied with the Hospital Committee's work, while keen to impress upon the Tsungli Yamen that he too had played a part in bringing the incident to an agreeable conclusion.

The use of the phrase '*shi ke ji zhi*' is significant. It implies that the disturbances could be tolerated until they became excessive. Indeed, it could even imply that these merchants had initiated the disturbances and could terminate them whenever they chose. Did the Tung Wah Hospital Committee initiate the disturbances? Interestingly, the *China Mail* correspondent at Canton insinuated that it might have started the troubles with an eye to rewards from the Chinese government,[101] but this seems to be purely vicious speculation. Though it was sympathetic to the strikes the evidence indicates that the strikes were spontaneous, and the local Chinese leaders' role was more in providing moral support than in actively inciting them.

Did the Committee try to settle the dispute to comply with Zhang's instructions? It would seem from the negotiations with Stewart that it was primarily aiming to maintain social order in its capacity as community leader; in addition, as merchants the members of the Committee's financial interests were damaged, while the approval it might win from the Canton authorities could be an important added incentive.

The Tung Wah Hospital's part in ending the strike remains a mystery, and ultimately the solution rests on who had repaid the fines in the government's name. Perhaps this will never be known. But in the present context it is sufficient to know that Zhang Zhidong *believed* that the Committee had mediated successfully. He was impressed by its effectiveness and, perhaps, its political clout. He must have been pleased to think that it had acted upon his instructions and, with this assumption, he proceeded to demand from it various services. From 1885 his attitude towards it became increasingly imperious.

In 1885 the Hospital again brought credit upon itself by raising over $100,000 for flood relief in Guangdong,[102] once more proving its worth to the Chinese court and its officials. Zhang memorialized the throne and a second imperial tablet bearing the inscriptions '*wan wu xian li*' (all creations benefit [from its benevolence]) was presented to the Hospital.[103] However, this very fund would lead to another show-down, this time between the Hospital and the Chinese government, as we shall see.

Zhang made use of the Hospital's well-established connections with the many Overseas Chinese associations, and the Hospital became the intermediary between Chinese officials and Overseas Chinese. In 1886 it even took part in negotiating a Chinese Consul for the Philippines.[104] The Directors' experience with the outside world made their advice invaluable to Zhang. It also served him well as a transmitter of information. One of the most interesting messages came to the Hospital Committee in February 1886 in an urgent telegram from the 'Chinese Guild' and the Chinese Consul-General in San Francisco, reporting on the recent ferocious anti-Chinese riots there by Irish immigrants. It was requested to issue proclamations warning Chinese against going to the United States and to forward a telegram to the Hall of Sustaining Love and Zhang Zhidong in Canton.[105] Zhang became worried that anti-foreign feelings might erupt in Canton or Hong Kong. Keeping aside his own antipathy to foreigners, he told merchants to discourage anti-foreign agitation and asked the British to keep H.M.S. *Midge* in Canton.[106]

In addition, he telegraphed instructions to the Tung Wah Hospital to help prevent trouble. Since the Chinese and American governments would be negotiating directly, he felt it would be harmful to excite the local population with information about the riots in America, which would certainly lead to agitation and diplomatic complications; anti-American activities in China would only bring on reprisals on Chinese in the United States. Seeing posters describing the riots appearing in Canton, he asked the Committee to find out whether they had been brought from Hong Kong, and urged it to prevent people from sending them. It was told to reply immediately.[107] Zhang was obviously treating the Tung Wah Committee in the same way he treated local élite groups in China. In his eyes, it not only could gather and disseminate information, but also restrain people's movements — that is, it had wide semi-official authority over the local population. Local leaders in China often assisted officials in maintaining public order — exactly what Zhang was asking of the Committee. Of course, as has been seen, the Hospital Committee *was* almost similar to local élites on the Mainland but for one very important difference. It was in Hong Kong, on British soil, and under British sovereignty; Zhang did not seem overly conscious of this reality, and the possibility that he could be infringing upon British territorial sovereignty did not seem to have crossed his mind either. Or, if it did, he was not unduly bothered by it. It was such indiscriminate imposition of authority by Chinese officials on the Tung Wah which caused diplomatic dispute.

In an overseas context, the Committee had been asked to do what a Consul would have done. The network of Chinese officials at home and abroad was very incomplete, and officials regularly commandeered the services of civilians — most frequently community leaders — to serve as missing links. Being in Hong Kong, the Tung Wah Hospital's position was often pivotal, and so long as it remained the focal point regarding information, funds, emigrants, repatriation, and so on, it was of special value to the Chinese government.

The absence of a Chinese Consul in Hong Kong not only meant extra responsibilities for the Committee, it also enhanced its position as the local élite. In Singapore, where a Chinese Consul was established in 1877, his influence overshadowed that of the local leaders, taking over many of their earlier duties in the protection of Chinese.[108] In Hong Kong, however, without a Consul, the task and role of protecting the Chinese, and the concomitant élite status, remained unchallenged with the Tung Wah Hospital. At the same time, its role was a dual role — indeed an ambiguous one. There were matters which concerned its members as community leaders which also involved Chinese officials, emigration being a prominent example and, consequently, it found itself carrying out instructions from the Chinese government. It complied as long as their interests coincided, especially when these official connections boosted its standing in the local community. When differences of opinion and clashes of interests occurred, its ambiguous position became problematic.

The Relief Fund Controversy

Much that went on between Chinese officials and the Hospital happened beyond the knowledge of the Hong Kong government. Since these activities were generally well reported in the Chinese newspapers, government ignorance was actually due to a lack of interest. Minutes of meetings and all correspondence were carefully kept and could be produced on request. Most importantly, tablets from the Emperor and Chinese officials were prominently displayed at the Hospital's hall, testifying to their connections. The government was responsible for not knowing more and sooner of its activities. Or, as in Hennessy's case, the Governor approved of them and saw no cause for alarm. However, after 1882, with Marsh explicitly opposing its extra-Hospital activities, the Committee adopted a lower profile, and did not volunteer information.

It was British policy to guard the sovereignty over Hong Kong jealously against any external political influence on the Chinese population there, but it is clear that their policing effort was weak. We have seen how the alleged collaboration between the Tung Wah Hospital and Canton officials in 1878 alarmed the Colonial Office. A scenario with Canton officials ruling the Chinese in Hong Kong through the Tung Wah haunted them.[109] And yet when Marsh reported on the *Mary Tatham* case in 1882, the news was received with near nonchalance. Lord Kimberley regarded the matter calmly, maintaining that the *Mary Tatham* case, though perhaps irregular in detail, was 'productive of good'.[110] Clearly, to him, not all Tung Wah's connections with Chinese authorities should be condemned. But they did make the Colonial Office more determined to define the Hospital Committee's functions.

In the spring of 1885 severe floods devastated Guangdong province. The Tung Wah responded immediately by sending boatloads of food to the victims. It also started a fund which soon grew to $100,000, donated by Chinese in Hong Kong, Singapore,

Peru, and other places overseas. The money was spent on rice, which was distributed among the distress areas by relief parties under the Tung Wah Hospital's supervision. The total sum expended was about $70,000, leaving a balance of about $30,000.[111] The flood had seriously damaged the embankments, but as the Canton government was too poor to pay for repairs, Ho Amei informed the Provincial Treasurer of the balance of the relief fund held by the Tung Wah, and suggested using it for this purpose.[112] Finding it a good idea, Zhang Zhidong was keen to force it through quickly, fearing that unless the money should be transferred soon, it would be lost for ever.[113] A dispatch requesting the sum was therefore sent to the Hospital in September 1885.

When James Stewart Lockhart, acting Registrar General, heard about this, he at once sent for the Chairman and Vice-Chairman about the matter, and read the dispatch for himself. Dismayed by the demand, he told them that Chinese officials had no control over them, an institution founded by British law in a British colony. They in turn declared their intention to ignore the instructions.[114]

A meeting was held at the Hospital. A resolution was passed not to send the money to Canton but to apply it only to its original purpose, namely, the relief of future distress. Until then the balance would be banked under the supervision of the Chairman, Kwan Hoi-chun (Guan Kaichuan).[115] The Tung Wah Hospital had been successful in raising large sums for charitable purposes precisely because of its integrity — it had so far ensured that money was not misused, or commandeered by corrupt officials[116] — and, naturally, this integrity must be maintained. The Hospital was liable to prosecution by donors if the funds were disposed of arbitrarily.[117] Besides, once the Hong Kong government had actively intervened, the Committee could do little else.

On 12 December, Kwan and the Vice-Chairman, Lo Ch'i-t'in (Lu Zhitian), showed Lockhart another dispatch from the Provincial Treasurer, which announced that Zhang Zhidong had memorialized the Imperial throne to request that an honorary tablet be awarded the Hospital for the recent fund-raising.[118] They asked for Lockhart's instructions and were told not to do anything until they heard the acting Governor's decision, and not to receive any communication from the Chinese authorities unless sent through the proper channel, the British Consul at Canton.[119]

However, on 31 December, Lockhart discovered in the Chinese newspapers that the tablet scroll had been received in the Tung Wah two days before. He immediately sent for Lo, who denied the newspaper report. After further investigation, Lockhart discovered that Lo 'was mistaken'; the tablet scroll was sent by a messenger from the On Tai Insurance Company, where Ho Amei was secretary, and was later received by the Chairman at the Hospital in the presence of the other Directors. Lo insisted that he knew nothing about the matter and that, if he had known, he would not have received it.[120] Lo, of course, was not 'mistaken'; he was simply lying, and the fact that he was forced to lie reflects the predicament the Hospital Committee had been forced into between the Hong Kong government and Chinese authorities.

Lockhart and Marsh objected to the whole business for several reasons. One was the direct communication between the Hospital and Chinese officials. Another was the style the Chinese officials adopted in all the communications, one normally used by a superior to command those within his direct jurisdiction. Marsh also objected to the 'unwarrantable tone' which he was convinced was calculated to encourage the beliefs that Hong Kong was held by the British government only on sufferance, and only as a purely temporary arrangement, and that the Hong Kong government was subordinate to Canton authorities — beliefs already prevalent among residents in Hong Kong. The reference to Hong Kong as part of the province of Guangdong further convinced Marsh and Lockhart of their dishonourable design. With the Chinese officials treating the Hospital as an institution subject to Chinese government's orders, they feared that an *imperium in imperio* would be created, amounting to an invasion of British territorial sovereignty.[121]

The person playing a leading part in this episode was again Ho Amei. The tablet scroll and the accompanying dispatch were sent to him, opened by him, and acknowledged by him on behalf of the Hospital. When confronted by Lockhart, Kwan denied that Ho had been authorized to do so,[122] which is not impossible, but it should also be noted that when the tablet scroll did arrive at the Hospital, the Directors had not turned it down. Understandably they did not wish to refuse such a high honour; perhaps no one dared to do so. Thus Lockhart lamented,

I regret to say that the Committee of the Hospital which is composed of respectable merchants with whom this Department has always maintained the most cordial relations do not appear to realize the gravity of their action in receiving official despatches [sic] from Chinese Mandarins and, though I have again and again pointed out to them that by so doing, they are encouraging an invasion of the territoriality of a British colony, they seem to think that because they do not pay any attention to the despatches [sic] sent, they are not in any way acting improperly.[123]

Nor did they ignore the dispatches. The characters were duly inscribed, and the tablet was then hung in the hall, as instructed.

Lockhart believed that such invasion of territoriality should be taken seriously, otherwise it would become more difficult to control the large Chinese population in Hong Kong.[124] Marsh, on the other hand, was inclined to let the matter rest as far as the Directors of the Tung Wah were concerned, realizing that they were under pressure from Chinese officials.[125] Both were determined that from then on all future correspondence should only go through the proper channels.[126]

But events were to overtake their decisions.

On 2 January 1886 Ho Amei published an article in the *Huazi ribao* giving an account of the recently received Imperial tablet scroll, and rebuked those who thought the Tung Wah Hospital had no right to receive it.[127] He asked why it should be regarded wrong for 'their superiors [to] proclaim their beneficial acts to encourage them' when the Hospital had excelled in charitable works. Citing a previous occasion when another tablet had been presented, he asked why there was no remonstration then.[128]

It was as if Ho had thrown down the gauntlet at the government. As he had always shown himself aggressive and outspoken, it is difficult to ascertain whether he had done so on instructions from the Canton authorities or out of his own sense of righteousness. One result of his article was to alert the government to the existence of the earlier Imperial scroll of 1879 and an investigation was immediately instigated;[129] all the objections Hong Kong officials saw in the latter presentation were found applicable to the earlier situation. More urgently, Ho had openly challenged the very political and diplomatic principles the Hong

Kong government was so eager to uphold. Marsh could no longer leave the matter alone.

He took action by writing to N. R. O'Conor, the British Chargé d'affaires in Peking, asking him to obtain from the Imperial government a disavowal of the Canton officials' actions. He enclosed their original dispatches, taken from the Hospital, to show him the 'unwarrantable tone'. This removal of its records must have been a severe loss of face for the Hospital Committee.[130]

When the matter reached London, it caused considerable concern. Aware that 'the connection of this body with the Canton authorities had been a constant source of complaint', the Colonial Office staff felt that a new strategy was needed.[131] Hitherto, they had depended on the Governors to restrain the Directors, now the Directors themselves were not in control of the situation. In fact, neither was the Colonial Office, which admitted it could do nothing to save the family members of Hong Kong residents in Canton from being squeezed[132] — an admission of the British government's inability to provide adequate protection. Ironically this demonstrated the need for continued appeasement by Chinese residents in Hong Kong.

The Colonial Office realized they should be directing their remonstrances at the Chinese government instead. It was now a matter for the Foreign Office. But before O'Conor could make representation, events took a rather strange turn.

The Hospital Committee never replied to the Treasurer to inform him of the resolution not to send the money, and the Canton authorities repeatedly sent letters pressing payment. Kwan, disturbed by the whole business, called another meeting, but because of the gravity of the issue it was decided that no answer could be given without mature consideration.[133]

On 23 February, while in Canton on business, Kwan was suddenly summoned by the Treasurer. He panicked. Too terrified to appear, he entrusted a friend to present for him the resolutions passed at the first meeting. After this, two more summonses came, both of which he dodged. Finally, the Board of Reorganization[134] headed by the Treasurer sent another dispatch repeating the demand for the fund in a most threatening tone.[135] Kwan, whose wife, children, and property were in Canton, attempted to resign his chairmanship. But members refused to accept it; instead they further confirmed the earlier resolution.[136] Desperate, Kwan turned to the acting Governor to accept his resignation, but Marsh was of course not in a position to do so.[137] The last dispatch from the Canton authorities deserves close analysis. It began by telling the Hospital Committee members that as *jinshen* (gentry), they were naturally benevolent, and an official dispatch had already been sent to praise them for their good works. It was of course flattering for them to be recognized by Chinese officials as 'gentry', but in this instance they were reminded more of their duties than of the honour. They were told that as gentry, they ought to yield the balance of the fund to defray the embankment costs, as instructed. For not bothering even to reply to the repeated requests, they were rebuked for being callous and lax, perhaps a reminder that the gentry had certain standards to maintain.[138]

To show that the Board of Reorganization meant business, the letter ended with the warning, 'Do not try to make excuses or cause delays, lest such behaviour causes you inconvenience.'[139] The peremptory and threatening tone was obvious. But it also demonstrates the subtle complexity of the Chinese officials' relations with the Tung Wah Hospital. They could dangle before the Committee's eye things they craved — official recognition and gentry status. They could also hold out what they feared — reprisals on the Mainland. It becomes clear that by a combination of flattery and threats — the carrot and the stick — Chinese officials tried to get the Committee to toe the line.

For Marsh, this was the last straw. The episode confirmed all fears of Chinese official interference with local residents and the pressures they could bring to bear. It became a test case,[140] and a test of strength between the governments of Hong Kong and Canton. Marsh believed that the prosperity of the colony was largely due to the feeling of security of Chinese residents, and warned that unless some guarantee was obtained against such assumption of jurisdiction in the future such feeling would be undermined.[141] It is interesting how 'the prosperity of the colony' has been used throughout Hong Kong's history to justify anyone's policies.

The Chinese authorities naturally saw things differently. They regarded Chinese in Hong Kong, and anywhere else, as Chinese subjects with obligations to the Imperial court; surely they did not seem aware of, or subscribe to, the clear distinction made by

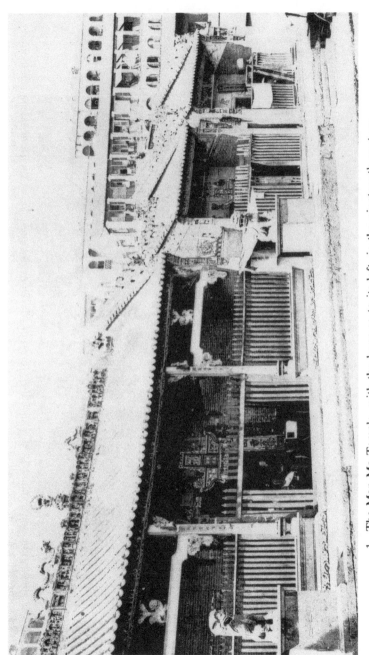

1 The Man Mo Temple, with the kung-so to its left, in the nineteenth century.

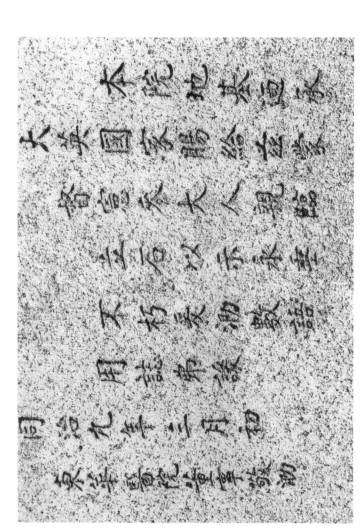

2 The foundation stone, dated 1870, indicating Governor MacDonnell's presence at the stone-laying ceremony. Photograph taken by the author.

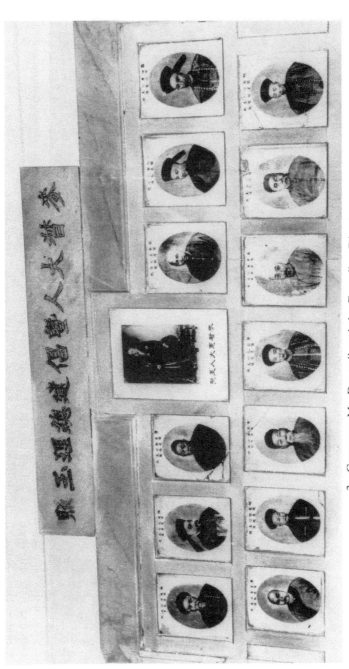

3 Governor MacDonnell and the Founding Directors.
Source: Tung Wah Group of Hospitals

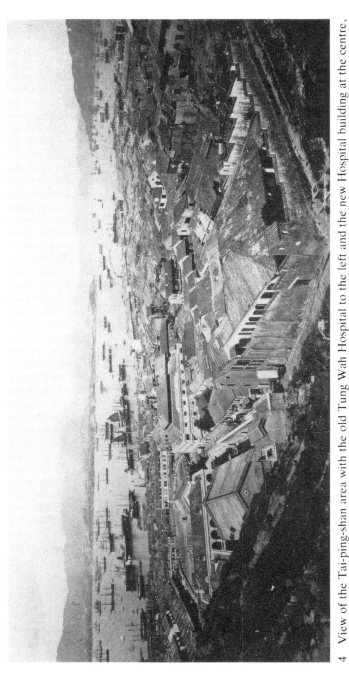

4 View of the Tai-ping-shan area with the old Tung Wah Hospital to the left and the new Hospital building at the centre, around 1900. The open area behind the old Hospital is the Chinese Recreation Ground.
Source: Hong Kong Museum of History

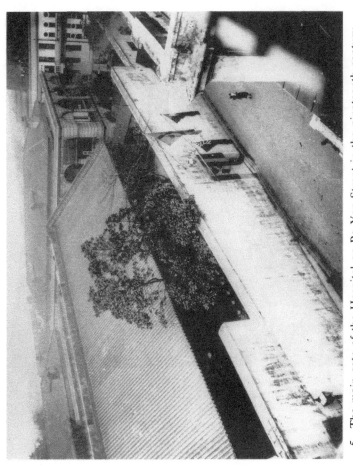

5   The main gate of the Hospital on Po Yan Street in the nineteenth century.
Source: Tung Wah Group of Hospitals

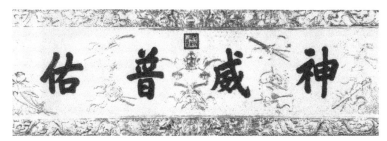

6　The plaque bestowed by the Guangxu Emperor in 1879.
Source: Tung Wah Group of Hospitals

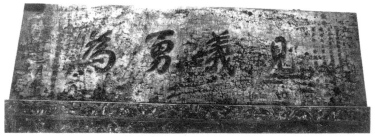

7　The plaque presented by Li Hongzhang and others in 1884.
Photograph taken by the author.

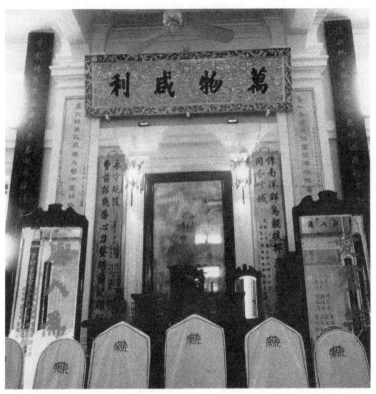

8 The plaque bestowed by the Guangxu Emperor in 1885 in the Hospital's hall today. The picture below is that of Shennong.
Source: Tung Wah Group of Hospitals

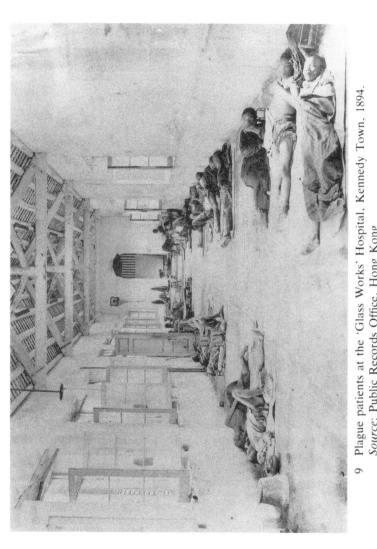

9 Plague patients at the 'Glass Works' Hospital, Kennedy Town, 1894.
   Source: Public Records Office, Hong Kong

the Hong Kong government regarding territorial sovereignty. Besides, wasn't it splitting hairs to distinguish between using the money to relieve distress and using it to prevent further distress by repairing embankments? In any case the money was raised not only by the Tung Wah but also by other institutions, and some of them seem to have been annoyed that the Tung Wah Committee had unilaterally decided how it should be spent.[142]

The Hospital Committee was in an unenviable position. It is tempting to ask, had it not been for the government's interference, would it have gladly yielded to Chinese official demands? This we shall never know. But we do know that this episode did not resolve the ambiguity of its position as the Hong Kong government had hoped.

Yet, even during all this trouble, and despite the Registrar General's warning, the Hospital Committee remained in close contact with Zhang Zhidong and the Chinese diplomatic staff. It is difficult to discern whether this stemmed from fear of Chinese officials or commitment as the local élite, or a sense of duty as Chinese subjects. In this instance, at least, they found themselves caught between the British and Chinese authorities — the perennial dilemma of Chinese, especially the élite, in Hong Kong. If they could at times bask in the Chinese Emperor's benevolence as well as enjoy the Hong Kong government's recognition, at others, the ambiguity became a double-edged sword. Things could backfire, and they could fall between two stools. No wonder the Directors were furious with Ho Amei for his suggestion.[143]

O'Conor took up the matter with the Tsungli Yamen. In a note to it, he reiterated the Tung Wah's efforts to raise funds for Chinese charities, pointing out that the Hospital Committee, responsible to the donors, was not free to expend funds except for the specified purposes. Being a corporate body in Hong Kong, it was entitled to British protection, and under no circumstances would the Treasurer be justified in commanding or threatening its Chairman, especially in demanding the monies for other purposes. O'Conor complained about the language used, especially by such a senior official, who could hardly plead ignorance. He suggested that the Tsungli Yamen should instruct Canton against further interference in this matter and against further annoying Mr Kwan and his family. In conclusion, he warned that while the Tung Wah Hospital had been extremely active in charitable matters, such actions by the Treasurer could check these 'charitable instincts',[144] a subtle reminder that this valuable fund-raiser might cease to be as co-operative in the future.

Nothing was said about territorial sovereignty or jurisdiction and O'Conor's tone was much more moderate than either the Foreign or Colonial Offices had hoped.[145] But O'Conor had good reason for this. At the time, the British government was complaining about a more serious case concerning the landing of Chinese officials in Hong Kong to make an arrest.[146] The problem of extradition and of Chinese officials' rights to make arrests in Hong Kong territory had been a long-standing one, and apparently he wanted to concentrate on this case where the breach of sovereignty was more obvious, without letting the Tung Wah case cloud the issue.[147]

In reply, the Ministers of the Tsungli Yamen curtly stated that a telegram had been sent to Zhang Zhidong calling upon him to instruct the provincial Treasurer not to 'act in this manner'.[148] This O'Conor forwarded to Marsh; copies of the document were then forwarded to the Tung Wah Hospital.[149] It is not known how much satisfaction this produced there. The Colonial Office, however, was clearly disappointed that the 'laconic reply' contained no apology,[150] and asked the Foreign Office to take it up further. But Sir John Walsham, who had become British Minister at Peking in the meantime, proposed not to, being satisfied that the Chinese government had already sent the telegram to Zhang Zhidong,[151] with the result that the Tung Wah issue did not develop into a major diplomatic confrontation. The episode did, however, attract a lot of attention, with everyone keen to see the outcome. Local residents had much at stake, as any sign could affect their security and status in the colony as well as in China. It must have ended as an anti-climax for all concerned.

Despite the tension and unpleasantness between the Hospital Committee and Chinese officials, their connections were not severed. Quite the contrary. The Imperial tablets still hung proudly in the Hospital's hall. In the preface to the *Zhengxinlu* of 1886, the Directors humbly and profusely thanked the Emperor for his benevolence.[152] On a practical level, the Tung Wah Committee continued communicating directly with Chinese officials at home and abroad on philanthropic matters. But things were different, and circumstances did change after 1886. After this, Zhang Zhidong began pushing vigorously for a Consul in Hong Kong;[153] he must have realized that the Tung Wah was no substitute for one. However willing to co-operate, the Committee came increasingly under the watchful eye of the colonial government, and its usefulness to the Chinese government was narrowly circumscribed. The attempt to raise it to an instrument of Chinese administration on a higher level was aborted.

Bypassing the Tung Wah, I

However, after all that, the anomaly remained — the only institution able to speak on behalf of the general Chinese community was a hospital committee — and something had to be done. No one was more disturbed about it than the Hospital itself. As has been seen, it had created the Po Leung Kuk in 1878 on which to devolve its work on women and children. As early as 1875 it had tried to divest some of its functions on a City Hall and again, in 1880, on a Chinese Chamber of Commerce, but neither of these scheme had been successful.

In 1888 the Hospital Committee and its associates revived the idea of a Chamber of Commerce.[154] Its promoters, including Ho Amei, Li Sing, and Wei Yuk, all past Directors/Chairmen of the Tung Wah Hospital, and Ho Kai, raised funds for a building and a petition was sent to the government, again for a grant of land.[155] In a memorandum to the government enclosing its draft rules and regulations the secretary, Ho Kai, admitted that the Tung Wah Hospital hall, used frequently by merchants as a meeting place, was 'unsuitable and improper'.[156] The implication was not only that it was improper to use the Hospital as a venue but also for it to deal with extra-hospital affairs; that its role should be curtailed, and that the Chinese leaders were prepared to accept the curtailment. He went on to list all the advantages this could mean to the government.

The government could easily find out Chinese views and feelings on any particular subject through the Chamber composed of 'the most reliable representatives of the Chinese community' and reach the lower classes through it.[157] In short, it would be the ideal substitute for the Hospital Committee. And, there was an added advantage; its wholesome and public influence would 'to a great extent prevail over the secret and often improper influence of trade guilds',[158] a real bogey to Europeans.

Its openness was provided for by Rule no. 4, empowering the

Chamber's Committee to invite certain government officials to become honorary members.[159] This was an extraordinary provision, since government officials had never been so associated with Chinese organizations nor with chambers of commerce, and was obviously designed to allay fears of conspiracy and sedition.

Lockhart liked the idea and for him, too, the Tung Wah Hospital Committee was a major consideration. He shared Ho's objections to the Chinese holding meetings there, 'which is by no means suitable for that purpose, and which in that account often prevented the meetings from enjoying as much publicity as was desirable'. He might be implying that there was too much of an in-house atmosphere about the meetings there; with the Committee's influence predominating they could hardly be 'open'. He also liked the idea of admitting officials to the Chamber, for though they were unlikely as honorary members to take an active part they could nevertheless counsel and advise and, more usefully, check any members from assuming authority and usurping functions not belonging to them. Referring again to the Hospital, he wrote, 'Difficulties of this kind were once experienced in connection with the Tung Wa [sic] Hospital, to which petitions in some cases repaired, as if to a regularly constituted tribunal, and it appears to me a wise thing in the interests of all concerned, to prevent any chance of such a recurrence in the future.'[160]

He supported the proposal and urged the government to grant the land. Recalling Chinese discontent in 1882 when the land grant was withdrawn, he hoped that by granting land this time round they could be reconciled.[161] Frederick Stewart, acting as Governor, agreed, and his experience as Registrar General must have made him see the advantages of such a chamber. He recommended granting the land, a piece of waste ground near the Tung Wah Hospital,[162] and the Colonial Office agreed.

The Chamber of Commerce took a long time to materialize; there are no records to explain the delay, though internal disagreement among the Chinese was a possibility. Nothing more was heard about it until January 1896 when the newspapers announced its opening.

Bypassing the Tung Wah, II

Chinese officials, realizing the Tung Wah Hospital's limitations, continued to press for a Chinese Consul, and in 1890 the Foreign

Office finally agreed. In Hong Kong all the old arguments against a Chinese Consul were reiterated. Lockhart protested strongly that it was the money of the local Chinese the Chinese government was after, not their welfare, and claimed that he would be spending his time keeping a watch on the Consul, and protecting the Chinese *against* him. But Imperial interests overrode colonial ones, and the Foreign Office gave the Chinese the go-ahead. The Chinese appointed Tso Ping-lun (Zuo Binglong), who had proved himself so successful as Consul in Singapore. But in the end the scheme fell through and no Chinese Consul ever came to Hong Kong.[163]

As far as the Tung Wah Hospital was concerned, a discreet distance was kept with Chinese officials, and its contacts were restricted to the 'philanthropic'. Its role as community leader was also transformed by a number of other developments. Some were intentional and institutional. These included the expansion and consolidation of the Registrar General's office. The creation of a permanent Chinese seat in the Legislative Council, and of the Chamber of Commerce and the Commission of Peace as functional constituencies, provided alternative avenues for ambitious Chinese. In 1886 the appointment of a Chinese Sanitary Board member added one more such avenue.

Ho Kai was the first Chinese to sit on the Sanitary Board. He had returned to Hong Kong after qualifying both as a doctor and a lawyer in Britain. In 1883 Bowen had mentioned him as the only other possible nominee for the Chinese seat in the Legislative Council other than Wong Shing, but he was passed over for being too young and too Westernized to be acceptable to the Chinese community.[164] His medical background made him the ideal appointment for the Sanitary Board, and in that capacity he was able to display his personal dynamism much more than Wong did in the Legislative Council. He might be Westernized, but this did not deter him from fighting for what he believed to be Chinese causes. He proved that the Sanitary Board could be made a forum for a wide range of issues as he spoke on racial discrimination and social inequality, a forum where the voice of the Chinese community could also be heard.[165]

Ho's appointment was significant. As a public figure, he represented a new type of Chinese community leader. English-educated, he appreciated the advantages of the British legal and administrative machinery. He was aware that the government's 'great mistake' was in 'treating Chinese as if they were Europeans',[166] and yet he was also painfully aware of the problems of Chinese social values and political practices, and was eager to eliminate abuses and offer ideas of reform. His reformist ideas made him one of the most influential Chinese reform thinkers of the late Qing period. Significantly, too, he was not associated with the Tung Wah, though both his father and brother-in-law, Ng Choy, were on its Founding Committee. He never became a member, and being a professional rather than a merchant he would have found it difficult to squeeze himself on to the Board of Directors. The distance might also have ideological roots. An admirer of English ideas of personal freedom, he must have found its patriarchal approach rather disconcerting, and it is not surprising to find him in conflict with some of the more conservative Chinese leaders, such as Ho Amei.[167]

The government continued its efforts to reach out to the Chinese. In 1891 Lockhart recommended to Major-General Barker, the Officer-Administering-the-Government, the appointment of 12 prominent Chinese gentlemen as the District Watch Committee to co-operate with him in administering the District Watch Fund. Since 1866 only informal and unimportant committees had advised on the District Watch Force, but the new District Watch Committee was of a very different character and status.[168] Its real functions were much wider than the declared one, and in 1892 Lockhart wrote that the Committee's advice 'on several important questions connected with affairs of the Chinese community has been a great help to the Department'.[169]

Of the 12 members of the first Committee, seven had been members of the Tung Wah Hospital Committee and three had been members of the Po Leung Kuk Committee; only two, Ho Fuk (He Fu)[170] and Ho Kai, had none of these affiliations. It must have been difficult finding influential and respectable persons who had not already served either of these institutions. Their appointment makes it all the more obvious that the government's intention was to reorganize them into a new body whose legitimacy was derived from the government and responsible to it, and to direct their social position and influence to the government's own end.

Another institutional development that portended ill for the Tung Wah Hospital was the reconstitution of the Po Leung Kuk. Europeans had always been suspicious of it, and in 1892 they renewed their attack, charging it with corruption and fraud, and an unofficial Legislative Councillor, T. H. Whitehead[171] even called it a 'secret society'. As a result, the government set up a committee to enquire into its workings.[172]

The committee reporting in February 1893 cleared it of all the charges. It recommended that it should be given a legal status by ordinance. More importantly, it created a Permanent Board of Directors consisting of not less than five and not more than 10 persons nominated by the Governor, including the Registrar General as ex-officio President and the Chinese Legislative Councillor as ex-officio Vice-President. In addition, there was to be an annually elected Committee.[173]

From one point of view it might be said that the Po Leung Kuk had emerged stronger from the struggle. It was now incorporated by ordinance, like the Tung Wah Hospital, a status it had sought in vain 11 years before. But by the same token its autonomy was severely curtailed. Though Lockhart, both as Registrar General and personally, had been deeply involved with its workings long before 1893, the new constitution placed it in a very different relationship with the government. It was the price it had to pay for its survival, and a sign of the times — a sign that the government was reluctant to let such as influential 'voluntary association' remain completely autonomous. The independent body had been almost reduced to a minor, self-funding department of government.

These institutional changes show a tendency toward integration, and was complemented by a simultaneous transformation, one more subtle and amorphous, among Chinese residents in Hong Kong.

Ho Kai was the archetype of a new generation of Chinese in Hong Kong and some other Chinese cities, who through prolonged contact with the outside world had acquired new values and attitudes. This can be partly accounted for by the formal education in Hong Kong schools. We may cautiously generalize that an English education provided a key with which Chinese persons with the right disposition might look at the world in new lights. It might enable them, at least, to read about the outside world and read the constant criticism of China and Chinese ways in the local English-language press, which could be tools for reassessing their own social and political values and beliefs.

The English educated élite became the target group to whom

the government turned in its efforts to integrate Chinese elements into its governing structure. This policy might have raised the value of an English education, resulting in the rapid rise of student numbers towards the late 1880s. In the Central School alone, which produced some of the most progressive thinkers, the number jumped from 634 in 1888 to 919 in 1889 to 1,062 in 1892.[174]

Besides formal education, the general situation in Hong Kong itself could have been another factor in transforming the attitudes and values of Chinese. Aspects of Hong Kong society which had impressed men such as Wang Tao, Guo Songdao, Kang Youwei, and Sun Yat-sen[175] — the orderliness, the dynamism, the efficiency, the opportunities for cultural exchange, the personal freedom, and relative freedom from corruption and injustice — were all parts of the atmosphere which local thinking Chinese breathed. When they wrote on the subject, the British system of constitutional monarchy was held up as a paradigm of reform, and they generally appreciated Hong Kong's own system of government for offering a fair share in political participation. The steady flow of applications for naturalization from 1881 testifies to the desire among Chinese to take advantage of the channels of political and social advancement the Hong Kong government offered.[176] Of course the social tensions were still there and foreigners were still confronted with a mixture of hatred and grudging admiration; but it did not prevent these Chinese individuals from being receptive to some of the more positive qualities of 'Western' life.

If lesser men were unable to articulate their feelings and ideas as well as Ho Kai and Hu Liyuan,[177] they nevertheless shared them. The 1870s and 1880s were periods of ferment in China's intellectual history. Hong Kong itself played an active role in advocating reforms through its newspapers, particularly the *Xunhuan ribao*, where Wang Tao's ideas were mainly published. Both Wang and Ho Kai highlighted the superiority of the Western, mainly British, political and administrative systems, while ridiculing those who stubbornly followed the old ways. By the late 1880s these ideas had become a part of Hong Kong's intellectual atmosphere. The Sino-Japanese War of 1894, which forced the reassessment of Chinese political values on the Mainland, must have made the Chinese in Hong Kong look at the British system even more positively. In short, the intellectual and cultural changes in Hong Kong freed Chinese from being culturally bound in the sense that they no longer believed that being Chinese entailed the blind following of old attitudes, values, and practices — or that by acquiring new ideas they became less Chinese. Historians have identified this transformation in Chinese history as the transition from culturalism to nationalism,[178] and Hong Kong was one of the places where this process occurred early. The formation of the Furen Wenshe (literally 'support virtue literary society') in Hong Kong in 1892, dedicated to the revitalization of China through reform and revolution, and having as its motto *Ducit Amor Patriae* ('Be wholeheartedly patriotic') is perhaps the most significant testimony to this development.[179]

The new institutions provided new opportunities for this new breed of men. But we must not assume that either the men or the institutions made the Tung Wah Hospital obsolete or redundant overnight. On the contrary. As long as it remained a symbol of élitism and charity, its attraction remained, and many of these 'new men' served on it. What did happen, however, was, as we shall see, that they brought tension to the Committee as they confronted the 'old guards', representing a microcosmic version of the cultural conflicts between the old and new gradually taking place all over China itself. The new men often showed themselves more amenable to government suggestions, partly because the state could reward them with social and political advancement, and partly because, intellectually and emotionally, they were genuinely sympathetic and receptive to them. It started a long-drawn-out process of change as the concept of community leadership based on the conservation of traditional values gave way to the concept of leadership based on dynamism and progress.

That changes in personnel were as vital as institutional changes is manifest in the Registrar General's office. Frederick Stewart's appointment in 1883 transformed the post. Competent and sympathetic, he personally enhanced an office already elevated constitutionally. But it was his successor, James Stewart Lockhart, acting from 1884 to 1885, and holding the office substantively from 1887 to 1901, who stole the show. Widely recognized as a Chinese scholar, he was, like many sinologues, more Chinese than the Chinese. Finding him approachable, the Chinese began to take before him matters concerning missing wives, children, and young girls, even domestic and business disputes[180] — showing their confidence in him to deal with matters connected with Chinese family morals and business ethics. If the barrier between the government and the Chinese had been a cultural and linguistic one, Lockhart proved that it was not insurmountable. One of the Tung Wah Hospital's claims to community leadership had been their moral authority to arbitrate in family and business affairs; the Registrar General's ability to fulfil the same function must have gone some way to undermine its Committee's monopoly on moral authority, and therefore its leadership status.

More significantly, Lockhart could see that Hong Kong's prosperity depended increasingly on the Chinese commercial and business élite, making it difficult to preclude them from political power,[181] and knew that their support could be enlisted to the government's advantage. Unlike Governor Hennessy, his approach was cool, rational, and constructive. It was he who reorganized the District Watch Committee and saved the Po Leung Kuk. The next chapters describe how he helped to reorganize the Tung Wah Hospital to save it from abolition.

Conclusion

Much of the friction between the Hospital Committee and its critics stemmed from conflicting interests and conflicting views of community leadership. While the Chinese wished to maintain their own ideals and practices, foreigners, both through fear and ignorance, refused to accept them.

Traditionally, the Chinese government had depended on local power groups, giving them a wide berth to control those within their 'jurisdiction'. Without actually administering the law, they purported to uphold moral and commercial norms. In a society where authority permeated every stratum, men, each belonging to some hierarchy of political and social relationship, subjected themselves to the authority of informal power groups.

Of course, there were always grey areas where their powers were less well defined. Even in China, the relationship between the state's formal power mechanism and the local élites' informal one was full of tension and, occasionally, the former, feeling itself threatened, had to restrain the latter.[182]

In a colony the latitude the government was prepared to give to informal native power groups was much narrower. The Hong Kong government, jealously guarding its sovereignty and monopoly in judicial matters, had no intention of letting a native organization usurp its power. There were also other important considerations. With China looming large across the borders, and the Chinese constituting an overwhelming majority of the population, government was ever wary of any Chinese group becoming the Chinese government's agent in any way. China's proximity and refusal to accept Hong Kong as foreign territory were two fundamental facts governing the fate of Hong Kong that the British and Hong Kong governments had to live with. Moreover, as few Chinese regarded Hong Kong as foreign territory, they insisted on keeping their own customs and value systems, and on having their own community leaders provide a framework within which these could be maintained.

The Tung Wah Hospital Committee had grown powerful in the political vacuum of the 1870s and 1880s; after that, the government sought to fill that vacuum with bodies less autonomous and more manipulable and, unlike the Hospital, constituted specifically to perform social and political functions. It began to appoint Chinese to the various Councils, Boards, Commissions, and Committees, and reinforced the Registrar General's office. All these moves reflect a more mature and coherent policy in the management of Chinese, the benefit of accumulated experience. In a broad sense one can see a general tendency towards more extensive, and more organized, government, which in the Hong Kong context meant more direct government of the Chinese. Another tendency was towards integration, as members of the Chinese community were consciously recruited as instruments of management.

At the same time, centrifugal forces within the Chinese community grew as men with new ideas and approaches to things emerged. Though not necessarily critics of the Tung Wah Hospital, they were instrumental in slowly modifying its function and role in both negative and positive ways. By joining the new government institutions they showed them to be avenues to political power and social status, viable alternatives to the Tung Wah Hospital Committee. By joining the Hospital Committee, they brought subtle changes to it, both through realizing new concepts of community leadership and through adjusting its relations to government.

Thus, by the early 1890s, it seemed that the Hospital Committee's decline had begun and its predominance would inevitably end.

Then the plague broke out in 1894.

6

Crisis: The Plague, 1894

CRISES — be they floods, wars, economic collapse, epidemics — bring out the best and the worst in people. They tear down the façade of rationality shored up by the routines of daily life, which are themselves disrupted. Formalities that cushion the shocks of contact between individuals and between institutions disintegrate, the contacts turning into naked confrontation. In the panic and mass hysteria, the contradictions of society — racial discrimination, social and legal injustice, cultural conflicts — normally subdued and tolerated, are accentuated and become unbearable. However well maintained in normal times, the social fabric could become irredeemably torn apart. The willingness to consult and compromise is displaced by the instinct to dictate and crush opposition. As the subtle jockeying for position and exertion of influence are reduced to open struggle for control, power relations are rearranged.

The bubonic plague of 1894 had exactly these effects on Hong Kong society and, for the Tung Wah Hospital above all, it marked a turning point. As a hospital, it naturally became involved right from the start, but the plague also led it to a bitter confrontation with the government which ended not only its autonomy in medical matters, but also its final autonomy as an informal power group.

The Plague

When the bubonic plague struck Hong Kong in May 1894, it should have surprised no one. For one thing, from February at least, a 'mysterious disease' had been causing great numbers of deaths in Canton — between 200 to 500 each day in the following three months.[1] There was heavy traffic between Hong Kong and Canton, 90 miles upriver and several hours of boat ride away, disregarding political boundaries. In an average week, over 11,000 passengers came to Hong Kong from Canton.[2] On special occasions the numbers multiplied and it was reported that on 2

March that year, 40,000 Chinese had gone to Hong Kong to watch a Chinese New Year procession[3] — and this was while the plague was raging in Canton. With the commercial and demographic ties between the two cities so close it seems strange that the Canton epidemic had not alerted the Hong Kong authorities to take precautionary measures earlier.

The plague should have come as no surprise for another reason. There were people who had for years, indeed decades, been appalled by the dreadful sanitary conditions of the colony, and by the government's inactivity, prophesying disaster. Successive Colonial Surgeons had complained of the drainage system, the overcrowding and filth of Chinese residential areas, even the atrocious habit of keeping pigs in homes.[4] The government had reacted mostly with inertia, despite the occasional effort by individual Governors such as Richard MacDonnell to deal with public health. The Chadwick Report produced in 1882 highlighted some of the worst sanitary problems in Hong Kong, and recommended fundamental changes.[5]

Early public health laws, though passed, had remained largely unimplemented. One pat rationale for inertia was that the Chinese should not be unnecessarily aggravated;[6] the other was economic. The Chinese, it was alleged — strangely enough by the Chinese themselves — did not mind living in poorly ventilated, dark, damp, and cramped conditions. Landlords who aimed at maximizing their returns naturally supported this line of argument. They warned that if open spaces and other architectural stipulations designed for better sanitation were enforced, it would drive up rents, implying that the low wages upon which the colony's economy depended would also be forced up.[7] Consequently, the Public Health Bill, which could have fundamentally improved the colony's sanitary conditions, was passed in 1887 in a very diluted form.[8] In short, the sanitary conditions remained dreadful, and Hong Kong was extremely vulnerable to epidemics.

It was only on 26 April 1894, two months after it had first appeared, that Police Inspector Quincey reported to the Sanitary Board on the Canton epidemic.[9] Lau Wai Chuen (Liu Wei-chuan),[10] a Chinese Sanitary Board member and Chairman of the Tung Wah Hospital, minuted that 'precautions must be taken',[11] and Ho Kai felt that a meeting must be called. None was called until 10 May, by which time several cases of plague had already broken out in Hong Kong. In the meantime, Dr Ayres, the

Colonial Surgeon, took concrete steps by sending for more information about the disease from the British Consul in Canton, and sent the acting superintendent of the Civil Hospital, Dr J. A. Lowson[12] to Canton for a closer look.[13] On Lowson's return, the first case of plague was officially certified on 8 May. Two days later, Lowson was ordered to visit the Tung Wah Hospital to inspect some cases there.[14]

This was rather unusual because, for all practical purposes, the Tung Wah Hospital was out of bounds to Western doctors except the Colonial Surgeon. Lowson's first visit proved to be the beginning of a bitter struggle between the Chinese Hospital and the medical authorities. He found about 20 persons affected by the plague, all in an advanced stage, and all from the neighbourhood around the Hospital.[15] At a Sanitary Board meeting that afternoon, Ayres suggested immediately introducing infectious disease precautions, although, at this point, he had not confirmed that the disease was an infectious one. These precautions included house-to-house visits to search for infected persons and the removal of such persons for isolation, checking of cleanliness and disinfection, provision for special grounds for burial, and so forth. There was no objection to this, but his suggestion to take patients on board the hospital ship, the *Hygeia*, which was originally designed to isolate smallpox cases, was queried.[16]

Ho Kai pointed out that the Chinese would surely object to the *Hygeia* and suggested a place ashore instead; the two European doctors, however, were convinced the ship was far more suitable. They felt that if Ho Kai and other Chinese leaders would see the *Hygeia* for themselves and be satisfied, and if patients were allowed to take their own attendants, they might be persuaded to go.[17] Events were to prove that opposition to the *Hygeia* was much more vigorous than either Ho or Lowson had anticipated, and would become the main bone of contention in the days to come.

Questions about the Tung Wah Hospital were also raised. J. J. Francis,[18] another unofficial member of the Sanitary Board, noted for his pugnacity, asked the President, Lockhart, how it was that no one had suspected several cases coming from the same house on Bonham Strand to be plague. The answer was that very sick persons were often taken to die at the Tung Wah without giving valid addresses, and it was not immediately obvious that the deaths had occurred in the same neighbourhood.

Secondly, it became clear that the cases Lowson diagnosed as plague were not identified as such by the Tung Wah doctors.[19] These facts were not pursued then, but they were to become major points of debate.

The next day it was declared that the Sanitary Board would administer the necessary sanitary measures and a Permanent Committee was formed for that purpose. The plague thus brought the Sanitary Board, after several years of obscure inactivity, into action and into the limelight, much as the cholera epidemic of 1848 had brought the General Board of Health to life in England.[20]

The sanitary measures were not well received. It was easy enough to bring the *Hygeia* off Praya West, and the China Merchant Steam Navigation Company even offered their wharf for its use.[21] But it was another matter trying to move patients there from the Tung Wah Hospital. All day on 11 May their resistance was virulent, and no one was taken against his will.[22] The deep-seated Chinese fear of Western medicine, and of Western doctors in particular, which had necessitated a Chinese Hospital in the first place has been described; now those fears were rekindled by new developments. Isolation as a precautionary measure against infectious diseases was strange enough to the Chinese, the idea of being taken on to a ship was even more incomprehensible. No wonder rumours that patients would be shipped off to Europe to be ground into powder for medicine for the royal family spread with amazing speed.[23]

Though Lowson blamed the Tung Wah Hospital authorities for obstructing the removal,[24] it seems that the main resistance came from the patients themselves. In the meantime, the Man Mo Temple Committee had distributed over 10,000 copies of a circular containing the observation and prescription of a Chinese doctor, one Yu Yau-chuen, who allegedly had cured a number of plague victims in Yunnan.[25] This might have strengthened the patients' eagerness to be left in the hands of Chinese doctors.

After a long meeting with the Tung Wah Hospital Committee, Ayres conceded that the Tung Wah's own doctors could go to the *Hygeia* and treat Chinese patients there under Western medical supervision. Perhaps it was this which made the majority of the Committee, after some wrangling among themselves, accept the proposal.[26] In the afternoon, the 'leading Chinese in the community' attempted to persuade the patients to go to the *Hygeia*[27] but with little success. By five in the afternoon, 36 had been taken on board, two of whom died.[28]

Resistance

The idea of the *Hygeia* split the Hospital Committee. In fact, it might have simply magnified and made public a dormant conflict between those more sympathetic to government policies and Western approaches to things, and those against any form of government interference or change. The former were led by Lau Wai Chuen, the current Chairman, compradore of the Hong Kong and Shanghai Bank, and owner of an Australia and California trading company. Naturalized as British in 1891, he was appointed a Justice of the Peace, a member of the Sanitary Board, as well as a member of the District Watch Committee the following year. Not surprisingly, he was amenable to the Sanitary Board's suggestions and more ready to accept the idea that, in a crisis, pragmatic action took precedence over Chinese prejudices. As soon as he learnt of the Canton epidemic, he advocated taking precautions. Others of the Committee challenged his views, leading the *Daily Press* to lament that, imbued with 'anti-foreign feelings', others on the Committee could not be as co-operative as Lau; indeed it suggested that they were stirring up resentment among the common people.[29]

In fact their objections to government interference are understandable even without invoking the idea of 'anti-foreign feelings'. From the beginning, the Hospital had insisted upon autonomy and operating the Hospital according to Chinese principles, that is, by Chinese doctors, using Chinese medical treatment and modes of organization. No wonder this forcible removal of patients — such a blatant affront to the Hospital's autonomy — should be so resented. They also feared that this was only the thin end of the wedge for more intervention, and when Surgeon-Major James of the Army Medical Staff went on duty at the Tung Wah Hospital on 15 May to detect plague cases, their worst fear was confirmed.[30]

As the patients resisted being moved, widows, orphans, relatives, and friends besieged the Hospital for redress, and at times the mobs became violent.[31] Besides being a great discomfort to the Hospital, this was above all humiliating. For two decades the Hospital had assumed the role of the Chinese community's protector, and though in the last few years this role had diminished, the government's interference now flagrantly exposed its impotence. The resistance of the plague victims and their relatives and of some of the Hospital Committee members fed on each other. The more the victims fought, the more the Committee felt obliged to uphold their wishes. The more firmly the Committee stood against the government, the more the sufferers felt their protests justified.

A Tung Wah Hospital doctor did go aboard the *Hygeia* as agreed but finding that he had to report to the Civil Hospital's superintendent, he went away and never returned.[32] Perhaps he disliked the idea of being supervised by Western doctors; more likely, he believed that with their interference, he would not be able to treat patients properly. For whatever reason, no Chinese doctor came again, even though Lowson made an effort to let them know they were welcome. Consequently, the *Hygeia* was left entirely to Western doctors.

If Western doctors were dreaded by the common Chinese people, never were they more so than at this time. Rumours abounded regarding the atrocities they committed — that they cut up pregnant women, that they took out the livers of children[33] — the usual anti-foreign, anti-missionary tales that had floated about the China coast for decades, now regenerated by the horror of the plague. The frustration of the Chinese masses might have been aggravated by the Tung Wah Hospital's inability to continue shielding them from Western doctors. The tension grew so great that Western doctors engaged in plague work felt it necessary to carry revolvers when they reached the excited neighbourhood of the Tung Wah Hospital.[34]

There was immediate resistance against the house-to-house visits; sporadic at first, it soon became widespread.[35] Many cases of plague were not reported as required by law partly to avoid these visits; in fact, it appears that every means was adopted to hide and disguise plague cases. Victims were removed from house to house to evade the search parties. According to one report a dead person was propped up at a mahjong (*majiang*) table to hoodwink the intruders.[36]

To reinforce the visiting teams, men from the Royal Engineers and the Shropshire Light Infantry were enrolled as special sanitary officers.[37] On the next day, 19 May, resistance 'broke

bounds'. At first, houses to be visisted were blockaded, and
sanitary officers stoned; by the afternoon, it had become so
unsafe that all visits were called off, only to be resumed the
following day under strong police guard.[38]

These house-to-house visits, so disruptive to people's lives,
would have caused resentment in any society at any time. When
public health measures were first introduced on a large scale by
the government in England in the mid-nineteenth century, they
were resisted on the grounds of the loss of liberty. They represented another dimension of the changing relation between the
state and the individual in English history.[39] But in Hong Kong
the resistance was not in the name of the individual but of the
community. One might even say that the opponents of the visits
saw them as a wholesale assault on the privacy of the home and
the sanctity of Chinese cultural values.

Chinese objections to Western treatment were naturally exaggerated by the general hysteria. Nor did the disruptive sanitary
measures calm the community's fears. Grave doubts of their
effectiveness precluded the majority of Chinese from lending
support to a difficult but *perhaps* worthwhile cause. The transi-
tory nature of the population and its basically emigrant mentality
perhaps also discouraged people from sacrificing their immediate
security and comfort. The situation certainly strengthened
Chinese unwillingness to give up old beliefs and to try to understand new ideas and methods.

Intrusion into the home was particularly inexcusable in Chinese
eyes. With their strange notions about the foreigners' sexual
appetites and habits, respectable girls and women, who generally
saw very little of foreign men in any case, and certainly never
expected to be physically examined by them, became very
anxious. In addition, there must be some truth in the complaints
against the search parties. Some were alleged to have asked for
'squeeze'; soldiers and sailors turned sanitary officers did not
always behave at their best; theft was suggested, as was unnecessary damage of property during disinfection.[40] One may even
assume that in a colonial situation, the search parties, burdened
with a filthy and depressing task, would tend to be more arbitrary
and callous than otherwise.[41] Most damning of all, not being
experienced medical men, they were not always able to recognize
plague symptoms, especially in the badly lit quarters of a Chinese

tenement building; and visits were specifically scheduled for late at night to ensure that people would be indoors. As a result, people not suffering from plague had been removed. Thus the protests were not only against the visits *per se* but also against the callous and high-handed manner in which they were carried out. Inevitably, the Tung Wah Hospital became involved. The violence against the visitation squads spilled over as the mob gathered at the Po Leung Kuk, just across the street from the Hospital, and broke its windows.[42] This was clearly a demonstration against the leading Chinese, who had proved unable to protect their community, and was perhaps also meant to force them to push the Chinese case more vigorously.

On 20 May a large meeting was held at the Hospital, with Lau Wai Chuen in the chair. About 70 members of leading firms and some 400 others attended; also present were the Superintendent of Police, F. H. May,[43] and the Colonial Surgeon. The main issue was the sending of patients to Canton. Irritated and fearful of the medical treatment imposed on them, many patients wanted to go to Canton instead of remaining in Hong Kong. Lau pointed out that requests had been made for taking these people to Canton by special launches, but May claimed that Canton officials prohibited this. This was 'received with strong marks of dissatisfaction', presumably because the Chinese at the meeting doubted him and took it as the government's excuse to prevent Chinese from leaving Hong Kong. Lau suggested that he would personally apply for permission from the Governor and Canton officials. His proposal to send a petition signed by all the leading firms of Hong Kong was unanimously agreed.[44] May then went on to explain the government's actions and to dispel rumours.

In the midst of this, reports came that Lau's shop had been sacked and he hurriedly excused himself. A howling crowd met him outside, stoned him, and overturned his sedan chair. In this state of indignity, he ran back to the Hospital for shelter. A mounted contingent of armed Sikhs had to be sent for before the agitation calmed down.[45] But the point had been made. It is a telling indication of the crowd's intense indignation that all the Tung Wah Hospital's aura could not protect its Chairman from such humiliation. Perhaps one could say that this aura, which had been fading gradually since its heyday, was rapidly dimmed in the crisis.

Government versus Tung Wah

The ugly mood of the populace prompted the government to forestall further violence. Later that day the Hospital, with the government's permission, issued a notice stating that from then on patients would no longer be taken to the *Hygeia*, but to the 'Glass Works' factory at Kennedy Town, where a temporary hospital had been set up with Tung Wah doctors. It asked people not to fear the house visits, and to bring forward their dead.[46]

The concession, coming so late, satisfied neither the community at large nor the entire Hospital Committee. On 20 May an exodus for Canton began, at the rate of about 1,000 people every day.[47] They were leaving not to escape the plague, which was still rampant in Canton, but to escape Hong Kong's plague measures. According to a Western doctor in Canton, nothing more than street cleaning had been introduced there by way of sanitary measures.[48] There were also stories that Canton doctors were successfully curing the disease.[49] Most fundamental of all, many people were in fact making their way back to die and be buried with due ceremony in their native land. To be dumped into a 'dead box' with quicklime and buried in a grave without ceremony, which was the fate of plague cases in Hong Kong, was perhaps the worst fate imaginable.

Deciding to battle on without their Chairman, Committee members of the Tung Wah petitioned the government to modify the sanitary measures, and finally obtained an audience with the Governor. It is a remarkable stroke of fate that at this crucial juncture, the helm of government should be in the hands of one as insensitive as Governor William Robinson (Governed 1891–98),[50] a fact which accounted for much of the bitterness in the government's encounter with the Chinese leaders.

They reiterated their demands: one, that the house-to-house visits should cease; two, that sick people should be allowed to return to China; three, that all patients on the *Hygeia* should be sent to the 'Glass Works' hospital; and four, that all sick persons should henceforth be sent there.[51]

Robinson answered their demands point by point. Sick people could choose to go to any hospital they liked, he explained, because the government was not forcing them into any particular one.[52] In fact this was only partially true, and he contradicted himself when he went on to say that he could not approve of transferring patients from the *Hygeia* as it was dangerous moving them about, and he could not take the responsibility for any loss of life. In other words, as far as patients already on the ship were concerned, there was no alternative.[53] Strangely enough, like May, Robinson also claimed that it was the Canton authorities who were keeping patients away while he had nothing to do with it. He was again contradicting himself. Despite the large number of Chinese leaving for Canton — and many sick people had also managed to sneak away — officially all plague cases had to be reported to the Hong Kong medical authorities and, once reported, the victims were kept under surveillance and isolation, with guards posted to prevent them from slipping away. In this way, plague victims were not free to go *anywhere*, let alone Canton.

The house-to-house visit was the most sensitive issue of all.[54] Such visits, Robinson argued, were absolutely necessary, for without them the dead bodies would never have been discovered. Consideration would be given to women and children and damage would be recompensed, but the visits would continue. Indeed, they would be reinforced by additional sanitary inspectors.[55]

This confrontation has been described in some detail to emphasize the irreconcilable situation. The Governor was clearly getting down to basics by telling the Chinese deputation that Hong Kong was a British colony and as they had chosen to reside in it, they must admit to British laws and methods of sanitation. He positively declined to listen to their requests. He reminded them of their duties as Hong Kong residents to help the government in this terrible crisis, not to obstruct, or allow their countrymen to obstruct, its efforts.[56]

The Tung Wah leaders left disgruntled but relentless. Despite the Governor's negative attitude, the Hospital, with its tradition of relieving suffering and of protecting the Chinese community's interests, would not accept defeat easily. It was necessary to regain their self-esteem and re-establish their credibility in the eyes of the Chinese masses. If the Governor was intransigent, so were they. They persisted, working at those points where the Governor's resistance appeared weakest. Focusing on getting permission to remove patients from the *Hygeia* and transfer them to Canton, they went about achieving these aims in various ways.

Yet, ironically, it was also at this juncture that the division within the Chinese community became manifest.

The Tung Wah Hospital's own Chairman was among the first to admit that sanitary precautions were necessary and supported them in face of opposition from the Committee and the mob. But he was not alone. Other Chinese also recognized that, though unpleasant, these sanitary measures were indispensable, and some actually helped the sanitary inspectors in their task.[57] Moreover, they were prepared to criticize those who objected to them. In other words, the crisis had led to a rift within the Chinese community as different sectors adopted different attitudes. While the lower classes resisted by strike and riot, some of the educated classes stayed aloof.

One critic was Tse Tsan Tai (Xie Zuantai).[58] A government clerk born in Australia and educated at the Queen's College in Hong Kong, he was a staunch reformer and revolutionary. In 1892 he founded the Furen Wenshe with his friends to plan and organize revolution against the Manchu and, from 1895, he was involved with Sun Yat-sen's revolutionary movement. As a social reformer, he attacked such practices as fengshui, foot-binding, opium smoking, and slavery,[59] and was obviously intolerant of any sign of ignorance and social backwardness.

Outspoken and articulate, he often used the English-language newspapers as a forum for his reformist thought. With the English-language press blaming the Chinese community for the disturbances he came forward to speak on behalf of his 'more able countrymen'.[60] He asserted that the disturbances had been created by the 'ignorant coolie classes' and showed his eagerness to draw the line. He regretted the Tung Wah Hospital's support for them, lamenting that 'it must be known and regretted that it [the petition to the Governor] was unfortunately inserted in order to please and appease the angry, ignorant and riotous mobs composed of the coolie classes'.[61] In short, speaking as a self-styled intelligent and morally superior Chinese, he not only condemned the ignorant mob but also its ill-advised supporters, the Tung Wah Hospital Committee. Characteristically, he considered that leaders of the community should be leading it in a more progressive and enlightened manner instead of feeding its ignorance.

Similar views were expressed in a letter signed by 'A Chinaman', who wrote to correct the *Hong Kong Telegraph*'s report by

pointing out that the Tung Wah deputation did not represent all
the Chinese in the colony. He claimed that he and others regarded the sanitary measures as 'wise and justified', and hoped
for the 'triumph of the available forces of the government over
ignorance, fanaticism and ridiculous jealousy', and that 'the
adoption of stringent measures in the future' would prevent
another epidemic.[62]

These were important signs that the 'constituency' of the Tung
Wah was shrinking as the Chinese community's social and cultural attitudes began to change. While never completely homogeneous, it certainly was becoming even less so. It was no longer
valid to assume that there were common values shared by all
Chinese and that the Tung Wah Committee by defending them
was speaking on behalf of the whole community. Where once the
Tung Wah's Directors had been generally regarded as energetic,
competent, and honourable, now they were associated with
'ignorance, fanaticism and ridiculous jealousy' by other
Chinese.[63] It was not that the Hospital Committee itself had
essentially changed, only that they were now under the scrutiny
of new eyes. It was the first occasion since its inception that
Chinese residents in Hong Kong publicly disassociated themselves from the Committee and disputed its representativeness as
Chinese community leaders.

The atmosphere grew tense as the relationship between the
government and the Hospital deteriorated. On 23 May, cargo
boats refused to work.[64] Ostensibly the boatmen did not want to
be recruited into transporting plague corpses. But they could also
be protesting against the government's refusal to concede to
Chinese demands and the escalation of the house-to-house visits.
The *Hong Kong Telegraph* suggested that the Chinese were playing 'the same old game,'[65] that is, every time they found themselves in conflict with the government, they would begin by going
on strike, then close their shops, and finally throw stones. The
Telegraph also suggested that the Tung Wah Hospital and Po
Leung Kuk were encouraging and permittting the lower classes to
break out into open rebellion.[66] There is no evidence for this but
it seems that even the government suspected it. On 24 May the
Governor ordered the gunboat *Tweed* to be anchored 'opposite
to the Tung Wah and the Tai-ping-shan'.[67]

This is reminiscent of 1884, when troops were quartered at the
Tung Wah Hospital during the disturbances. Government was

flexing its muscles again and, again, the pressure was on community leaders, rather than on the populace in general, to restore order. This only made reconciliation more impossible. As in 1884, the government and Chinese leaders shared the aim of maintaining order, but there were too many clashing interests and divergent views, too much suspicion and ill will to make the maintenance of order a matter of first priority.

Diplomatic Confrontation

Developments in Canton added a new dimension to the episode, involving the Tung Wah Hospital, yet again, in a Sino-British confrontation. Soon after the plague broke out in Hong Kong, placards began appearing in Canton. Some, merely warning people against going to Hong Kong because of the plague, were innocuous enough.[68] Others were more malicious. Gruesome stories were told of how Western doctors cut up pregnant women and scooped out children's eyes to make medicine.[69] More unfortunate still, local English papers connected the Tung Wah Hospital people with these placards. The *Hong Kong Telegraph* labelled them and others as 'traitors' for spreading these rumours, remonstrating that as long as the 'would be satraps of the Tung Wa [*sic*] Hospital and Po Leung Kuk had their own way and lived in the belief that Hong Kong was a Chinese city and they were its dictators, no cloud could possibly rise on our political horizon....'[70] Again, these were sheer allegations, but it is interesting that the plague had highlighted the Tung Wah Committee as leaders of the ignorant masses against government, so that any sign of resistance was alleged to have emanated from that master-mind.

Robinson flew into a rage. He could not understand how after more than 50 years of British occupation and 'benign, not to say paternal, government, Chinamen resident in this British Dependency could be found who were ignorant enough to believe such statements, and treacherous enough to give them currency'.[71] He immediately telegraphed the British Consul at Canton asking that such placards be suppressed at once; in addition he wanted the Governor-General of Guangdong and Guangxi to issue proclamations to denounce them as false.[72]

The correspondence between the Hong Kong Governor and the Consul at Canton that went back and forth in the next few days reveals the basically different viewpoints of the colonial and diplomatic services. It left the Governor exasperated with the lack of support. In fact neither the Consul, Byron Brenan, nor the Governor-General, Li Hanzhang,[73] could understand Robinson's position. Brenan and his Vice-Consul believed that he had not considered Chinese feelings enough, and found some of the drastic measures unwarranted.[74] Moreover, Brenan did not want to see his ill-advised actions create anti-foreign feelings in Canton, that is, trouble for himself, and warned that 'recent events have shown that the sentiments of the Chinese residents of Hong Kong is a factor which has to be reckoned with, and that the danger of riding rough-shod over this sentiment can extend beyond the limits of the British colony'.[75] Above all, he had no wish to let this jeopardize his carefully cultivated relations with Li Hanzhang.[76] In short, this was the classic attitude of British Consuls in Canton over matters regarding Hong Kong.

Li Hanzhang, brother of Li Hongzhang and himself an official of outstanding achievements, had even less reason to comply. The Tung Wah Hospital had kept him informed of goings-on in Hong Kong and of the general mood of the Chinese there, and he seems to have genuinely sympathized with their plight.[77] It would be natural for him to share some of their prejudices against Western medical and sanitary practices. Furthermore, he could not be expected to take instructions from the Governor of Hong Kong. Thus, though he agreed to issue a proclamation, he took care that it would serve *his* purposes.

The proclamation announced that conditions in Hong Kong regarding plague patients were improving, that patients including those on the *Hygeia* had been either transmitted to the Tung Wah Hospital or, interestingly enough, were 'provided with a passage back to China, as each individual preferred'. People were told not to listen to idle stories, as 'all are free to come and go as they wish'.[78]

These statements were actually more wishful thinking than accurate. These were conditions which the Tung Wah Committee had been demanding all along and which the Governor had so insensitively rejected. By distorting the truth, Li was actually forcing the issue. He was making at least one point clear — if plague patients were disallowed from leaving for Canton, it was not due to objections from Canton. The pressure was shifted back on to Robinson.

Li's intentions become even clearer when he proposed to Brenan on 29 May that all Chinese patients should be given the option of returning to China, where they could, at worst, die amongst their friends and be buried on Chinese soil, and that patients on the *Hygeia* should be allowed to go ashore to the Chinese-run hospital.[79] It also becomes clearer that he was simply transmitting the message of the Hospital Committee which, in desperation, had appealed to the Canton authorities for help.

Li Hanzhang's action must have made the Committee members glad to have turned to him, for not only did he offer to open the gates of Canton to plague patients, he even magnanimously offered to send proper ships for them.[80] At a time when Robinson was at his most uncompromising and apparently most despotic, Li's thoughtfulness and solicitude stood in sharp contrast. Li seems to have been unusually careful to avoid repeating Zhang Zhidong's diplomatic *faux pas*, and to avoid giving the impression that he was interfering in the government of the Chinese in Hong Kong, or that he was extending protection to them because they were 'Chinese subjects'. But many must have been grateful for his concern.

Brenan forwarded the request informally, but Robinson wavered and sulked at Li's omission of 'any public expression of his indebtedness' to the Hong Kong government for the concession of transferring patients from the *Hygeia*, which was being implemented in the meantime.[81] On 19 May all the Chinese patients on the ship had been removed to Kennedy Town, and when Lockhart wrote to Brenan, apparently on Robinson's intructions, he carefully pointed out that this was done to meet the Chinese community's wishes and not to concede to Li's request.[82] The point might seem petty but it was a political point Robinson was determined to make, a crucial point in the struggle for the allegiance of the Chinese residents in Hong Kong. As Lockhart pointed out on his behalf, to give the impression that the Governor had given in to Li's request would be tantamount to 'a concession of British sovereign rights'.[83]

But the point was not even accurate; to the cynical, it was downright dishonest. Chinese patients were in fact taken away from the *Hygeia*, not in deference to the Chinese but on instruction from Lowson, in his capacity as acting Superintendent of the Civil Hospital, who, expecting that Europeans might soon be attacked by plague, wished to reserve the ship, which was more comfortable, for them.[84] It certainly gives the lie to Robinson's earlier argument that the Chinese should not be removed from the ship because it might kill them! It is difficult not to conclude that the Governor was inconsistent and arbitrary while keen to claim as much credit as possible, and one wonders which, the well-being of the colony, the misery of plague victims, or his own vanity and desire to establish authority, concerned him most.

Another issue was the removal of plague patients to Canton, one of the Hospital's earliest demands, but the authorities continued to insist that all reported cases be confined to hospitals in Hong Kong. In fact several attempts were made to help them leave. As early as 26 May there were rumours that a charitable institution in Canton had offered to send a boat for them, but nothing came of it.[85] A few days later, Ho Amei formed a committee which included Lau Wai Chuen to help send patients to Canton. He wrote to the Sanitary Board on 2 June, informing it of their plans, and asked to be assured that the police and sanitary officers would not interfere.[86] The Board, most of whose members opposed the proposal, referred the matter to the government, which made no response. Equating silence with rejection, Ho dismissed the committee on 7 June.[87]

On that day, Ho Amei wrote an angry and frustrated letter to the *Hong Kong Telegraph*. He could see why the government should try to keep plague out of Hong Kong by examining passengers from Canton, he wrote, but he could not see why it should object to patients *leaving*, when neither the Canton authorities nor the friends of the sick objected to it. To keep the plague victims in Hong Kong would only allow the disease to spread and infect Chinese and foreigners alike and, he wrote sarcastically, as his family was there, he had to look after their safety as well as his interests in the colony.[88] Ho had logic on his side; the Governor's stubborn objection to letting plague patients leave was indeed incomprehensible and inexcusable.

Another appeal came from several compradores of large firms who promised the Governor that if they were allowed to move the sick to Canton they themselves would remain in the colony instead of joining the general exodus.[89] This is another manifestation of the concerted effort by Chinese leaders to meet the community's wishes. Robinson finally yielded. If nothing else, the compradores had made him look at economic realities. The quarantine measures against Hong Kong by many ports had hit shipping and emigration drastically.[90] With between a third to a half of the population gone, there were disastrous economic repercussions.[91] Coolie labour was becoming scarce; many shops were closed and goods were unclaimed from the godowns — one firm alone had £70,000 worth of unclaimed kerosene on hand.[92] The colony was in fact grinding to an economic standstill and obviously something had to be done.

When the Governor finally gave his permission on 9 June he caught many people by surprise. They could not believe that Canton authorities, with their own hands full with plague patients, would want a fresh supply from Hong Kong; neither could they believe that the medical staff would allow it.[93] But the boats for the victims arrived the following day;[94] the gunboats *Kwong-kang* and *On-lan* were reportedly chartered by the Tung Wah Hospital.[95] On 13 June the first batch of patients were sent to China.[96]

Why did the Hospital Committee fight so hard to send plague patients to China? The *Hong Kong Telegraph* gave the infantile explanation that because its doctors could not cure them in Hong Kong, it was better that they should be shipped off to a place where no records of their deaths could be kept.[97] Perhaps a more realistic explanation can be found in the Hospital's genuine desire to alleviate the anguish of the common people, who had opposed every sanitary measure introduced by the government. This was not the first time the Committee had come forth to ask the government for more understanding of Chinese problems. For 25 years it had tried to present Chinese cultural biases to the government, and when these were brought to a frantic pitch in this crisis, its earnestness was also transformed to fanaticism. Realizing that the house-to-house visits would certainly not be abandoned, the Committee members concentrated their efforts on obtaining concessions more likely to be granted, to bring some relief at least. Winning Li Hanzhang's support must have greatly boosted their morale.

But the government's permission to ship patients to China was not met with rejoicing, as one might have expected. After all the wrangling and manoeuvring, when it did come, it brought little relief. If it came as a victory to the Hospital Committee, it was at best a pyrrhic victory. This was partly because each transfer had to be registered so that infected houses would be identified for cleansing and disinfection.[98] At the same time, new sanitary measures had been introduced aggravating the general frustration. With the new by-laws, many houses were declared unfit for habitation and closed, and the inhabitants simply expelled.[99] Many of these residences were in the Tai-ping-shan district, and the Governor mentioned that the whole district would be destroyed to make room for better-planned houses, to end threats from the plague for good.[100]

The dislocation of people and the whisper of wholesale destruction of Chinese homes kept excitement in Hong Kong at a high pitch, and tension spilled over into Canton. On 12 and 14 June 'anti-foreign' riots were reported in Honam.[101] Placards appeared claiming that if Tai-ping-shan were burnt down, Shameen, the foreign enclave in Canton, would be set on fire.[102] Once again, events in Hong Kong had direct repercussions in Canton.

This time, instead of approaching the Hong Kong Governor, Li Hanzhang wrote to the Tsungli Yamen, blaming the Hong Kong government's policy for the disturbances. He warned that if Hong Kong officials were not made to change their policy, anti-foreign feelings in Canton might get out of hand.[103] The matter had finally reached Peking.

Tung Wah — More Humiliation

In response, the Yamen's Ministers approached O'Conor, the British Minister at Peking, and made a rather unusual request. Disclaiming any intention to interfere improperly with the colonial authorities, they asked him to telegraph the Hong Kong Governor to suggest that the Chinese Hospital Committee issue a notification to the people explaining the object and aim of the sanitary measures.[104] It is significant that the Tsungli Yamen recognized the importance of letting the people understand the purpose of the sanitary measures, something the Hong Kong government had not seriously attempted. In this respect, both Chinese officials and British diplomats showed more sympathy than the Hong Kong government. Secondly, the Yamen showed that it recognized the Tung Wah Committee's leadership role and the effect a proclamation it issued might produce.

O'Conor duly telegraphed Robinson, suggesting that he should consult 'popular prejudices as far as possible'.[105] Robinson instantly sent for the Tung Wah Hospital Directors. He informed

them of the Yamen's anxiety concerning the unrest in Hong
Kong and Canton, and of its suggestion that they should issue a
notification which would 'calm people's minds'.[106]
   He then proceeded to tell them what he thought should be put
in the notice and, to make sure that the Directors would not
adulterate the message, he instructed them to submit the draft for
his approval before posting the proclamation.[107] In effect, he was
dictating to them. If anyone should wonder at his readiness to
comply with the Yamen's request, the explanation lies in his
adeptness in manipulating the situation to his complete advantage.
   Thus, the following proclamation was composed, approved,
and issued throughout the colony and Canton:

The Tung Wa [sic] Hospital of Hong Kong, having learnt that placards
and wild rumours have been profusely spread and published through
Canton, which have excited the minds of the people and almost created
serious disturbances, puts up this notice in order to allay suspicion, for
the Hospital is well acquainted with Western doctors, who have always
treated patients of all classes with the greatest care, kindness, and
compassion; moreover great harmony now prevails between the Western
and Chinese doctors in the treatment of the patients. The rumours
current in the streets and the placards published there are all false and
forged. Let every one be careful to be in no degree misled by these
rumours.[108]

   The irony is only too obvious. For the Tung Wah Directors
who had so vigorously resisted the sanitary measures and Western doctors to have to issue such a proclamation must have been
painful and humiliating. Clearly everything in it contradicted all
they believed and felt. It negated all their attempts to press the
government for concessions, especially to return patients to the
care of Chinese doctors, and made a mockery of their efforts at
recruiting the sympathy and support of Canton authorities. There
had been *no* harmony among the Tung Wah and Western doctors; rather, conflicts had arisen over the administration of the
'Glass Works' and other hospitals nominally operated by the
Tung Wah doctors but in reality supervised by Western medical
staff. This was why Li Hanzhang retorted that though the Hong
Kong government had agreed to adopt Chinese methods, it was
an empty promise. Dr Lowson's own reports show that the hostilities among Chinese and Western doctors were mutual and
intense.[109]

As the *Hong Kong Telegraph* observed, the Tung Wah Hospital had no alternative but to submit to the Governor's request. To refuse would be tantamount to admitting that either they had approved of the infamous anti-foreign propaganda, or had themselves circulated it.[110] Robinson, having made the Directors look ridiculous, was exceedingly pleased with himself. He reported to the Colonial Office that 'the Tung Wa [*sic*] Hospital Committee have in my presence, and publicly admitted, *though no such admission was absolutely necessary*, [my italics] except perhaps to calm the fears of ignorant and illiterate Chinese, that the treatment of the sick by English doctors was as it always is, and ever will be, characterized by the greatest kindness and humanity'. He thought it good tactics because such an admission 'forthcoming from such a source was valuable at the moment and doubtless had a good effect'.[111] But he deceived no one. Even the Colonial Office staff could not help commenting that 'he had practically dictated the proclamation which ostensibly was issued by the Tung Wa [*sic*] Hospital'.[112]

It is doubtful if the proclamation changed Chinese attitudes toward Western doctors, reduced anti-foreign feelings, or won sympathy for the government's sanitary measures. If anything, it would only have highlighted the Governor's insensitivity and unscrupulousness and made his confrontation with the Tung Wah Hospital more irreconcilable.

On 23 June a Chinese hospital, converted from an unoccupied official building, was opened at Lai-chi-kok (Lizhijiao) on Kowloon Peninsula, just across the border. It was said to be the branch of a Canton hospital and funded by Ch'an Sui-nam, one of the Tung Wah's Founding Directors.[113] Once opened, plague patients from Hong Kong started going there. It was popular probably because it was free of Western doctors, and it was much easier for patients' families to visit them there than in Canton. Besides, going to Canton, they still needed to register their infected premises. So, during the first few days, a large number of patients turned up.

As its own hospital was increasingly coming under the supervision of the medical authorities, the Tung Wah Committee also saw this as a viable alternative, and actively hired boats to take patients across.[114] This went on until the Hong Kong police discovered the Lai-chi-kok hospital, and a police cordon was introduced. Boatmen caught carrying patients across the harbour were prosecuted for failing to report plague, or for not having the necessary clearance papers.[115] From the government's point of view, this was aimed at keeping a record of plague cases, but the Chinese saw it as prosecution for going to the Lai-chi-kok hospital at all. Tension mounted again.

At this point, the Hong Kong General Chamber of Commerce took the matter up with the government. Concerned with the loss of business, it was anxious to prevent matters from deteriorating.[116] After meeting with it, the Governor issued a circular withdrawing the cordon, notifying all who wished to go to Lai-chi-kok to report themselves at the Kennedy Town Wharf where two junks would be ordered to transport them. The Permanent Committee of the Sanitary Board was asked, in a letter from Robinson, to make the necessary arrangements.[117]

The Tung Wah Hospital Committee, apparently pleased with the new policy, lost no time in taking advantage of this apparent softening of the Governor's attitude. It promptly suggested amending the arrangements for the greater comfort, safety, and convenience of the sick.[118] Its response, as it turned out, was premature.

The Permanent Committee's reply to Robinson's letter took him by surprise. Its chairman, J. J. Francis, flatly refused to have anything to do with transporting patients to Lai-chi-kok. He argued that while Canton was far enough away, Lai-chi-kok could be a source of re-infection, and he objected strongly to the lax manner of burials there.[119] Thus another opportunity for the Hospital Committee to help plague patients was inadvertently lost. With this reply too, a new situation obtained. The confrontation between the Governor and Chinese community leaders was overshadowed by the one between the Governor and the Sanitary Board's Permanent Committee. Where only a few days previously Francis had written to the newspapers praising the Governor's support for the Board, they were now at each other's throats.[120] For the next few days the recrimination they hurled at each other filled the newspapers, as if to provide comic relief to the misery of the plague.

The official conveyance of patients to Lai-chi-kok was suspended.[121] To break the *impasse*, Robinson finally proposed requesting the Governor-General at Canton to improve sanitary conditions at Lai-chi-kok, and gave the Permanent Committee to understand that once conditions there were satisfactory, he would allow patients to proceed regardless of its opinion.[122] In the meantime, a special patrol was sent to prevent people from crossing the harbour.[123] Action was taken at the Lai-chi-kok hospital. On 12 July, after Francis had visited the hospital, the Permanent Committee finally agreed to provide junks to take patients across.[124]

By this time the plague was abating. The number of cases fell, and Chinese began returning to Hong Kong.[125] The conflict between the Tung Wah Hospital and the government gradually subsided. Many of the demands urged upon the government were slowly being met. On 12 July an official announcement was made reassuring landowners of the Tai-ping-shan district that should the government resume their properties, they would be properly assessed and paid for.[126] This announcement had a calming effect on the property-owning class. Then, on 4 September, a clean bill of health for the port was returned.[127]

Repercussions — A Thankless Job

The plague had devastated the colony. Over 2,500 plague victims had died.[128] At one point over 100,000 people had left the colony.[129] The epidemic had also left the Tung Wah Hospital exhausted by attacks from many fronts.

Never popular with the foreign community, the Hospital invariably became the focus of hostitily in any racial confrontation. The plague was from the beginning identified as 'Chinese', not only because it had originated in China, but also, more tellingly, because it was carried by Chinese and recognized as a consequence of filthy, poor, Chinese habits. Neither the government nor the local English-language press disguised the fact that the main object of the sanitary measures was to prevent plague from spreading from the Chinese to the European community. Criticizing the government for making too many concessions to the Chinese community, the *Hong Kong Telegraph* commented that 'though the Chinese may perhaps be allowed to kill themselves with their epidemic, they must not and shall not be allowed to kill us also'.[130]

This abusiveness was well matched by the Governor's insensitivity when he spoke to the Legislative Council. While he welcomed orderly, industrious, and useful Chinese to the British colony, he declared that it was the government's duty not to let the health of 'the community' suffer in any way 'by their residence amongst us'.[131] The Chinese were clearly identified as a threat to the health of 'the community', that is, the European residents. As Consul Brenan at Canton observed, the Governor and the English-language press seemed to object to being more considerate of Chinese feelings because to do so would be 'selling their birthright in Hong Kong to the Chinese'.[132]

The we/they dichotomy became pronounced from the Chinese point of view, too. Sanitary measures were only applied to Chinese quarters, although non-Chinese had also fallen victim to plague.[133] It has been noted how the Chinese resented those measures — the house-to-house visits; the cleansing, disinfection, and expulsion from homes; the Western medical treatment; the emergency burials. The atmosphere provided fertile ground for rumours, which were spread not only in Hong Kong and Canton, but also in Amoy and Shanghai as well. A crisis like the plague, not surprisingly, brought up latent anti-foreign feelings along the South China Coast. The generosity and compassion of the Governor-General of Guangdong and Guangxi highlighted the intransigence of the Hong Kong Governor.

The Europeans' attacks were malicious. As on other occasions, the 'better class Chinese' were perceived as master-minds and instigators of trouble. The *Daily Press* condemned them for misleading coolies, and thought that men in good positions with anti-foreign proclivities ought to be deported.[134] When Ho Amei offered to arrange for the shipment of patients to Canton, there was strong opposition to the 'self-styled Chinese Committee running a British Colony'.[135]

Inevitably, they closed in on the Tung Wah Hospital. When cargo boats went on strike on 23 May it was held responsible. In an editorial entitled 'The Hong Kong Government and Chinese Traitors', the *Hong Kong Telegraph* called the Committee members of the Hospital and the Po Leung Kuk 'would be satraps' who believed that Hong Kong was a Chinese city and they its dictators, and accused them point-blank of encouraging the lower classes to break out into open rebellion. The newspaper was delighted that the *Tweed* was stationed opposite the Hospital since 'the belligerent Tung Wah autocrats and their miserable coolie dupes will now doubtless find it convenient to abandon the rather desperate attack on the recognized authority of this colony'.[136] The Hospital Committee's efforts to keep Chinese patients in Chinese-run hospitals were interpreted as attempts to get power and practical government into their hands — 'to make the government their tool. . . and to turn the ignorance, apathy and weakness of the officials to their own ends', one journalist wrote.[137] The image of the Tung Wah Directors as power grabbers mobilizing a rebellious mob against the colonial government was projected with zeal.

That hackneyed rhetorical question of whether the Tung Wah Hospital or the government ruled the colony was repeatedly raised. The Committee was accused of having arrogated an intolerable and illegitimate dictatorship while making a mess of the Hospital. The government was urged to end the *imperium in imperio* and place the whole institution under the Colonial Surgeon.[138]

In fact the *imperium in imperio* imagery was rather anachronistic by then, since the Hospital Committee's political influence had been in abeyance since the late 1880s. True, the plague did catapult the Hospital Committee into the limelight again, and it was even possible that some of the Directors saw this as an opportunity to re-establish their former status. But the Governor, arrogant and egotistical, refused to let this happen. Even when making concessions he took care not to give the impression that he was giving in to *their* demands. He did not seek their advice. Instead, a gunboat, that symbol of imperialist power, was ordered to remind it of the government's displeasure and determination to put it in its place.

When the Directors appealed to Canton, exercizing their option to seek protection from an alternative authority, they also failed to gain ground. Despite winning the sympathy of the Tsungli Yamen, the Governor-General at Canton, and even British diplomats, they could not change the Governor's attitude. Instead, Robinson turned that occasion to his own advantage. At the expense of issuing a worthless proclamation, he embarrassed and humiliated the Hospital Committee and the proclamation became a public declaration of its political decline.

When the plague subsided, the Governor called a special meeting to thank those who had helped fight the epidemic. The military and the navy were profusely thanked; so was F. H. May and even J. J. Francis.[139] The Tung Wah Hospital Committee, despite its relentless efforts, was not. The omission was conspicuous and ominous.

Ironically, there was no gratitude either from the people whom it purported to champion. The Chinese petitioning for the Hospital's protection turned into violent mobs. The assault on the Chairman was the ultimate act, annulling the Hospital's years of service as leaders of the Chinese community. Between accusations that they had sold out to the government on the one hand, and that they were establishing an *imperium in imperio* on the other, the Hospital Committee found itself in a no-win position. The plague must have made it clear that theirs was a thankless job.

Ironically, too, the plague provided the occasion for sectors of the Chinese community to publicly disassociate themselves from the Tung Wah. There were Chinese, well-educated and writing fluently in the English language, keen to detach themselves from the ignorance and prejudice associated with it. Though their number might be small, their very existence was significant. By denying that the Hospital Committee represented them they called into question its long-established claim to represent the whole Chinese community and challenged the very nature of its leadership. In this respect, the plague signalled a new era not only in the Hospital's history but also in the history of the Chinese community in Hong Kong as well.

7

A New Crisis: Toward Integration

THE plague had led to confrontation between the Tung Wah Hospital and the government; at the same time, it also led to a confrontation between Western medical doctors and the Hospital authorities which was in every way as bitter and far-reaching in its consequences.

Medical Confrontation

Contagious disease, it is claimed, has historically been the spur to public health reforms.[1] In Britain, the tendency towards centralization and standardization in the administration of public health began in the 1840s and gained momentum during the 1870s, urged on by growing faith in the supremacy of sanitation in maintaining health. The plague allowed this tendency to gain ground in Hong Kong and, soon, there was little room for institutions and practices which did not fall in line.

The epidemic started a routine by which Western doctors began inspecting the Tung Wah and interfering with its operations. Where, before, Chinese medicine had merely been despised and largely ignored as an unfortunate phenomenon, Western medical practitioners were now brought face to face with the issue. They might expound the superiority of Western medicine and try to enlighten the Chinese and win them over intellectually but, ultimately, they imposed their views with the support of the state's coercive power. In Britain, medical practitioners had educated the state to the need for public health measures[2] because it was impossible to implement the necessary centralization without it. In a colonial situation, the imposition of Western medicine on an institution dedicated to the practice of native medicine assumed the character of cultural imperialism. Government intervention on behalf of Western medicine, moreover, transformed a cultural and intellectual confrontation into a social and political one.

The Tung Wah Hospital had been subject to criticisms, but as a medical institution it had been less scrutinized. Its severest critic in this respect was one of the Colonial Surgeons, Dr Ayres, who soon grew complacent; otherwise, it was treated mostly as a curiosity. By and large, it retained the autonomy for which it had fought so fiercely from the start. The plague had now brought it into direct contact with Western doctors whose attention went from its administration to its sanitation and, finally, to its medical proficiency. In the end, the jealously-guarded autonomy was lost for ever, ending another phase of the Hospital's history.

Soon after plague broke out, J. J. Francis asked at a Sanitary Board meeting why there was no proper registration of patients and of causes of death at the Tung Wah.[3] In fact, the latter were recorded in Chinese medical terms while, at the Government and other European-run hospitals, Western medical terms were used. Francis's point was significant for revealing the absence of a uniform system for registering causes of death, which in turn precluded any systematic medical statistics for the colony as a whole. To answer this criticism, the Tung Wah Committee immediately employed U I-kai (Hu Erjie),[4] a Chinese doctor trained at the College of Medicine for Chinese and at the Civil Hospital, as visiting surgeon to register deaths in Western medical terms.[5]

Other critics were more difficult to answer. The most zealous of these was Dr Lowson of the Civil Hospital. He had visited the Hospital before 1894 largely out of curiosity, but his visit, on instructions, on 10 May 1894 produced very different reactions. The emergency had changed his relations with the Hospital, and his opinions could have crucial bearings on its development. His visits became frequent; sometimes he had to be there twice a day, and only a week after his first official visit, he reported on it in the strongest terms:

The question of dealing with the Tung Wa [sic] Hospital must now be seriously considered. I cannot denounce this hot-bed of medical and sanitary vice in sufficiently strong terms. I venture to say that if the question of allowing this to remain was to be submitted to the Public Health Authorities at home they would order its immediate abolition. Here I know that a political element enters into the question, but I doubt if those who have supported it most would do so now if they knew what a Disgrace and Danger to the Public Health of Hong Kong it is.[6]

These initial impressions were reinforced during the plague.

His infringement on the Hospital grew. The 'Glass Works'

Hospital which opened on 21 May was supposedly operated by Tung Wah doctors, but not for long. There was much wrangling over sanitation; conflicting views naturally caused ill-feelings. For instance, one can imagine the reaction of the Chinese, who considered open windows and draughts as anathema, especially during times of illness, when the windowpanes of the 'Glass Works' were removed by the medical authorities to improve ventilation![7] There were conflicting views regarding health care, too. One of the Chinese patients' main complaints was that they were given ice water to drink[8] — another Chinese anathema. No wonder, to maintain their standard, the medical authorities found it necessary to use 'extreme measures'.[9] Discovering the incompetence of Tung Wah doctors and administrators, Lowson and his staff gradually took over the 'Glass Works' Hospital.[10]

Lowson found sanitary conditions at the Tung Wah equally appalling. In his opinion, Surgeon-Major James's duties there were more revolting than the dirty work that sanitary officers had to do in clearing the slum areas.[11] The medical practice there was even worse; indeed, it was nothing short of quackery and *malpraxis*. He believed that the non-segregation of patients by different classes of diseases, the non-use of antiseptics, and the unscientific classification of causes of death actually endangered patients.[12] He was convinced that authorities in Britain would find it incredible that such medical and surgical atrocities were allowed to take place.[13]

Clashes with the Chinese hospital management sharpened. Where once segregation had made each other's prejudices tolerable, they were now too close for comfort. With the press ready to reproduce every report of dysfunction at the Hospital in the most malicious and sensational terms, such as calling it the 'Chamber of Death',[14] the situation was exacerbated.

The end of the plague brought no relief. Lowson's feelings remained as intense as ever. In his report on the bubonic plague written in February 1895, he concluded with this damning indictment: 'Conducted as it is at present, under the patronage and protection of the local government, a certain amount of countenance is...lent to what I can only describe as medical and surgical atrocities.... I believe that it constitutes a serious menace to the health of the community.'[15] Conceding the need to show deference to Chinese prejudices, he suggested 'a scheme might be devised that would satisfy the wishes of the Chinese without sacrificing the sanitary well-being of the colony'.[16]

Of course he was aware of the politics involved. He saw the influential Chinese as trouble-makers, responsible for bullying plague patients into going to Canton and for the public disturbances.[17] He also felt government tolerance had allowed the medical atrocities to persist. Despite this, as a professional, he could not remain silent.[18] His reaction is reminiscent of the young Dr Ayres but, unlike him, he pursued his persecution and, by not letting his case rest, he was able to get his message across to London.

Parts of his report were so vituperative that the Hong Kong government thought that 'no useful purpose would be served by their publication', and forwarded only an edited version to London;[19] but even then, it caused concern at the Colonial Office. The Secretary of State, especially interested in Lowson's scheme to improve the medical service of the colony without upsetting the Chinese, asked the Governor's opinion on the scheme.[20] It was this report of Lowson's which partly led the Commission to enquire into the working of the Hospital in February 1896.

More Intervention

That was in the future. One immediate effect of Lowson's report was that the Sanitary Board's secretary, Hugh McCallum, was instructed to pay the Hospital a surprise visit.[21] His report was significantly different from Lowson's. He pointed out certain shortcomings with the lighting, the drainage, and the conservancy arrangements, but in general he found conditions reasonable.[22] Part of the reason for his comparative leniency was the way he conceived of the Hospital. To him, it was a place where very poor people were taken to die, not to be cured, and for that purpose things were adequate. He was also aware that the expenses of the Hospital were borne by charitable persons rather than by the rate-payers,[23] the implication being that one should not make extravagant demands. His attitude could also be explained by his 17 years in the colony and the general inertia of the sanitary administration. His report also underlines the fact that any report on the Hospital conditions was likely to be largely subjective.

However, one thing was clear. Interference with the Hospital, whether sympathetic or otherwise, was growing. Some time after August 1895, Justices of the Peace, at Lowson's request, began to inspect the Tung Wah Hospital as they did other public institutions.[24] Moreover, Dr J. M. Atkinson,[25] who inspected the Hospital as acting Colonial Surgeon from April 1895, was far less complacent than Ayres had been.

Atkinson's impressions of the Hospital were typically unfavourable. He found the place 'grossly mismanaged'[26] and dirty. He could see no organization: for all the months he had been there, he could not tell if any doctor was regularly on duty, or who had authority; he had not even been able to get a list of the staff.[27] It soon became clear that he would change things. He began meeting the Hospital Committee with the Registrar General, presenting his views on how improvements should be made. These covered many items, from new buildings, lavatories, receptacles for clothes, to the type of buckets for night soil. Some of the recommendations were carried out, others not, or not satisfactorily,[28] but, to the extent that they were considered at all, they indicated that the medical authorities were exerting unprecedented influence on the running of the Hospital.

Atkinson's power was manifest in his direct interference with the treatment of diseases. He had been authorized by the 1894 Committee not only to see patients at the receiving wards but also to screen them before discharge. This in fact gave his judgement precedence over that of Chinese doctors, and gave him effective control over medical administration.[29] However, the new Committee for 1895, elected into office in October, was unwilling to accept this. It began by rejecting some of Atkinson's proposals for change and, toward the end of the year, it allowed patients to be discharged without his knowledge or approval. Atkinson was appalled.[30] If patients were discharged before full recovery, this could have serious consequences, especially in infectious cases. In fact, he thought the Tung Wah was not equipped to deal with these cases at all.[31] Like Lowson, he had a sense of mission to introduce Western medical science to the ignorant, and the authority he relied upon was not only the state's but also his own idea of what was right — that same sense of cultural and intellectual superiority that had played such a central role in the history of the British Empire.

This became evident in his dispute with the Committee over the treatment of surgical cases. Chinese medicine in general he found useless, but Chinese treatment of surgical cases he found dangerous and abominable. Chinese doctors did not perform amputations; Chinese patients were dead set against them. But Atkinson, so certain that surgical patients would have a better chance at the Government Civil Hospital, began transferring them from the Tung Wah, sometimes even against their wishes.[32] Objecting strongly to this, the Hospital Committee protested to Lockhart, the Registrar General, who was sympathetic, and who urged Atkinson that compulsion must not be used. Not knowing what to do, Atkinson asked Governor Robinson for advice, and was instructed that in cases where the patients objected, he should report to the Governor, who would consider the case. Subsequently, four cases reported by Atkinson were sent to the Civil Hospital under the Governor's order.[33]

Resisting Intervention

When the new Committee came into office in November, things took a new turn. On 6 November one Chan Kam Shing was admitted to the Tung Wah with a compound fracture of the left wrist and a fracture of the right fore-arm. Atkinson felt he should be transferred to the Civil Hospital, but when Chan refused, an order from the Governor was applied for and granted.[34] At the Tung Wah, an emergency meeting was held with all the Directors present, and it was unanimously agreed to take legal action.[35] Clearly the Hospital was striking back. The Governor, with a reputation for riding roughshod over the Chinese, had gone too far.

That evening, before Chan could be removed, Atkinson received a letter from the Hospital's solicitor, Vincent Deacon, who, instructed by the Tung Wah Directors, asked that no steps be taken toward removing the patient. He reminded Atkinson that under the Chinese Hospital Ordinance, the only power given to the Colonial Surgeon was that of *inspecting* the Hospital, and that the Board of Directors had full power to manage and direct

Hospital matters.[36] In brief, the compulsory removal of patients was illegal.

What the Committee objected to was not so much that patients were being removed; in the past, cases had been sent from the Tung Wah to the Alice Memorial Hospital and the Civil Hospital.[37] What they objected to was that it was done against the patients' wishes, and the Committee members knew that no government had the power to order anyone to go to hospital except in infectious cases. On another level, the Hospital's ability to protect its own patients had been challenged, and the Committee could not take it lightly. As a last resort, it sought redress in English law.

Chan was not transferred. After that, despite Atkinson's continued appeal to Robinson, no orders for removal came. Deacon's letter must have made the Governor realize that he had overstepped the law, and the Tung Wah Committee was not letting him get away with it. He therefore left Atkinson to fight his own battle. Some of the untransferred cases died, and Atkinson's bitter verdict was that 'they lost their lives by being treated in the Tung Wah Hospital'.[38] He became even more bitter when the Committee refused even to let him dress wounds.[39] Most frustrating for him, Chinese patients simply would not go voluntarily to the Civil Hospital. He could only explain this by alleging that the Hospital Committee was using its influence to prevent them.[40] This reflects his ignorance of the deep-seated prejudice of the ordinary Chinese and, by blaming the Tung Wah, he was simply being unrealistic.

He changed his tactics. He tried to make himself more acceptable at the Tung Wah by taking U I-kai with him as interpreter on his visits. When appropriate, U would explain to the patients why it would be better for them to go to the Civil Hospital, and ask whether they would be willing.[41] This, however, made very little difference and Atkinson became more convinced that only drastic changes could improve matters — the abolition of the Hospital being one of the possibilities.

Chinese resentment against interference in any form deepened as the interference multiplied. The presence of a European doctor created much tension, making the Committee worried that Western medicine would somehow be introduced through the back door. The Governor's support for Atkinson had caused much annoyance. On the other hand, since the plague, a European — probably a policeman or sailor from the Sailors' Home — had been stationed at the Hospital by the medical authorities to ensure that plague patients reported their addresses correctly. However, he seems to have exceeded both his powers and his duties, and was clearly making a nuisance of himself. When Dr Eitel, the Inspector of Schools, visited the Hospital, the man would not even let him see the registration books.[42] The significance was pointed out by Wei Yuk — if he could be so arrogant toward a European, how much more so would he be toward the Chinese?[43]

In resistance, the new Committee turned down some of the recommended changes in building structure and sanitation arrangements, ostensibly because of a shortge of funds.[44] Perhaps it did not agree that such changes were necessary. Perhaps it feared that if it gave in on one point, a flood of other demands would follow. Above all, it resented the loss of autonomy, the most jealously guarded asset of the institution. It was an honoured tradition, and no Committee wished to go down in history as being responsible for losing it. As individuals, some of the members might admire Western medicine and consult Western doctors, but as members of an institution, the majority felt a strong obligation to uphold its principles. Moreover, its autonomy was the basis of its claim to community leadership.

Loss of autonomy could erode the Committee's standing in society; one sign of this was that since 1894 it had been difficult getting men to serve on the Committee. As Dr Ayres observed, this was in great contrast to the days when men sought election eagerly.[45] The subscription fund was another useful indicator: the presence of a European doctor 'who goes about the Hospital and makes a noise' had led to the decline of subscriptions, the Chairman reported, predicting that if a European doctor were installed, they would fall off altogether.[46]

Even as the Tung Wah Committee was fighting to preserve its autonomy, the Hospital's influence was clearly being challenged. In decline since the late 1880s, its prestige suffered severely from the Governor's humiliation of it during the plague. Sectors of the Chinese community also queried its effectiveness and scorned its ignorance and stubborn resistance against change. More clearly than ever, the need for a body constituted specifically to speak for the Chinese community and to overcome the anomaly of a hospital — in brief, an entirely new institution to mark a fresh start — was manifest. In these circumstances, plans for the Chinese Chamber of Commerce gathered momentum in late 1895. Its main promoters were Tung Wah men, notably Ho Amei, Li Sing, and Wei Yuk, Chairman of 1880 and 1887. The frustration they experienced as Tung Wah Committee members might have prompted them once and for all to resolve the unsatisfactory situation by founding an alternative organization. In January 1896 the Chamber was opened with great fanfare and prominent display of Mandarin robes.[47] In many ways, it was reminiscent of the Tung Wah's own opening some 30 years before.

In the meantime, in view of the pressures, the Committee made a last desperate attempt to rid itself of interference by petitioning the Governor on their objections to the presence of a European doctor and the infringement on its autonomy.[48] The matter remained in abeyance until 23 December 1895 when the newly elected Board was presented to the Governor. The meeting, which turned out to be a bitter encounter, deserves detailed treatment.

Robinson took the opportunity to answer the petition. He explained that the Colonial Surgeon, Atkinson, was an extremely capable and sincere doctor and that Western medicine was making great progress — even Li Hongzhang admitted to its superiority. On matters of principle, he was not prepared to compromise. He hit at the Hospital's claim to autonomy, reminding the Committee that the Chinese Hospital Ordinance, with built-in safeguards against mismanagement and other eventualities, had not given it a free hand.[49] It *did* provide for the Registrar General and the Colonial Surgeon to inspect the Hospital at any time; and though the latter's power was confined to inspection, he could consult the Governor when necessary. This was obviously a rebuttal to the solicitor's letter challenging the Governor's right to interfere.

The most telling point he made was that though the Hospital had been established for Chinese doctors using Chinese methods to serve the Chinese, they were all subject to the Governor's approval, and he was empowered not only to change the regulations but also to abolish the Hospital altogether.[50] This was his ultimate hold over the Committee. He assured his guests that at this point he had no intention of abolishing it, but almost in the same breath he said that Atkinson would continue visiting the Hospital, and he wanted them to co-operate with him. They were to stop sending petitions, instructing solicitors to write, and especially to stop listening to ill advice.[51]

He informed them of his decision to install a Chinese doctor trained in Western medicine to register causes of death, to see that lives were not endangered, and that infections were prevented.[52] The Committee members, however, would not commit themselves. They told him that as they had been elected by the Chinese community which objected to Western medical methods, his proposals were putting them in a difficult position, and they would have to consult the kaifongs before making a decision.[53] As the Governor's proposal was so radical, it is understandable that the Committee should wish to consult its 'constituency'. But it could also be using the 'Chinese community' as a subtle reminder that the feelings of the general public could not be completely discounted.

At this, Robinson broke into a tirade about a meeting at the Tung Wah Hospital the day before, held to discuss the Light and Pass system. On the surface, he seems to have gone off on a tangent, but careful examination shows that what he said was wholly relevant.

The Light and Pass system had long been a bone of contention, and the Tung Wah Hospital itself had protested against it in the past. Since Hennessy's governorship, this had largely fallen into abeyance. In late 1895, however, three daring robberies created so much outcry that the system was again vigorously enforced.[54] The Chinese protested vehemently as many were arrested and fined.[55] Some time in December 1895 Ho Tung (He Dong),[56] a wealthy Eurasian making his début as a public figure, submitted a petition against this system signed by most of the Chinese residents in Hong Kong, but the government did not respond. The next step was to hold a meeting at the Tung Wah Hospital on 22 December. Some 400 persons, including the most influential Chinese, attended, Ho Kai being the conspicuous exception.[57] It was doubtless an issue that deeply concerned the Chinese community.

Ho Amei started the meeting by condemning the Light and Pass system as 'class legislation'. Ho Tung agreed, but he took the issue further. 'We are the principal rate-payers in Hong Kong; we pay more taxes than the Europeans, and derive the least advantage', he cried, and suggested that 'If we have suffered any hardship before it is we who are to blame for being silent'.

He called upon the audience to unite and put pressure on the government, citing the example of the Chinese in America to illustrate that where there was no unity, injustice would prevail.[58] He also raised the issue to another level by putting the system in broader perspective — it was only *one* of the many injustices imposed on the Chinese, and it should be opposed not only because of practical inconvenience, economic losses, and its ineffectiveness in checking crime, but also as a matter of principle.[59] His attack on the system became a generalized attack on the government's discriminatory principle, hitting at the very basis of the colonial regime. The effect of his speech was far more devastating than Ho Amei's, and his call for solidarity among the Chinese must have appeared seditious.

Robinson certainly saw it as subversive, and this explains why at the meeting with the Tung Wah Committee a day later, he launched the bitter tirade about 'class legislation', an obvious reference to Ho Tung's speech. He called it a preposterous idea when the Chinese had the benefit of a well established government; they were more comfortable in Hong Kong than in their own country, and the treatment they received was in every way better than anywhere else. If they were dissatisfied, they ought to leave. He declared bluntly that if people began to stir up strife, he should have to take measures to suppress them.[60]

He might appear to have leapt from the Hospital to an unrelated topic, class legislation, but there was method in this apparent madness. To him, they were not separate issues. The meeting on the Light and Pass system had been held at the Tung Wah Hospital just the day before; it was attended by a large number of Chinese élite closely associated with the Hospital, and even though the issue was not presented to the government by the Hospital Committee as such this time, it could easily give the impression that the Hospital was behind Ho Tung's challenge to the colonial authorities.

Robinson obviously equated the resistance to the Light and Pass system with the Hospital's resistance against government interference, seeing both as mutinous attempts. Thus the Committee's reference to the need to consult the Chinese community might have conjured up in his mind visions of insurgent masses and triggered off his outburst. Although the Committee's political influence had declined since the late 1880s, he still saw it as a potentially dangerous and ambitious political force. Only this could explain his almost paranoid reaction to all its requests during the plague in 1894, and his determination to humiliate and embarrass it.

In the next few days, however, the tension eased. This was partly due to Ho Tung declaring in the *Daily Press* that he had no intention to stir up strife in the colony. Instead he argued convincingly that the Light and Pass system was ineffective in fighting crime.[61] The District Watch Committee concurred with his views, and this also made the government reconsider the matter.[62]

Another reason was that the Chinese community reacted much more calmly to the Governor's recommendations than the Committee had feared. Within a few days, the *Huazi ribao* published an article entitled '*Shen shi du shi lun*'[63] ('Judging the times and assessing the circumstances') persuading the Hospital Committee to consider the proposals rationally. After all, it pointed out, the doctor Robinson suggested was merely there to prevent plague, not to treat patients; more pragmatically, it thought that it would be a pity to see the Hospital abolished simply because the Directors refused to give in on a small point. Clearly there were Chinese individuals who disagreed that the Hospital Committee should resist change for its own sake. To them, the situation was not irreconcilable, nor were the Hospital's interests necessarily diametrically opposed to the government's. The key word was compromise.[64]

As the atmosphere became more conciliatory, Robinson conceded to the Chinese community by relaxing the Light and Pass Ordinance.[65] As for the Hospital, despite his bullying words, he decided to avoid a head-on clash. While aware that its abolition or any unilaterally imposed change 'would be very unpopular with the Chinese', he also knew that it would be very expensive to replace the services the Hospital was providing. Abolition would not be seriously considered as long as there was a chance to improve its administration and sanitary arrangements.[66] For the moment, he took the more circuitous step of appointing a Commission to enquire into the working of the Hospital. This would allow a cooling off period, if nothing else; but, hopefully, it could also allow a number of experienced men to work out a solution to a difficult and highly sensitive problem. Any conclusion and proposal it arrived at would appear more fair and objective.

The Tung Wah Commission

The Governor appointed a Commission on 5 February 1896 to 'enquire into the working and organization of Tung Wah Hospital' with special reference to the following points:
(a) whether the Hospital was fulfilling the object and purpose of its incorporation;
(b) if yes, whether the Commission could suggest or recommend any matter or thing by which the Hospital's present organization and administration could be improved or carried on more effectively; and
(c) if no, whether its object and purpose could be fulfilled by any other organization.[67]

The Commission consisted of five Legislative Councillors. They were James Stewart Lockhart, concurrently Colonial Secretary and Registrar General, one of the most sympathetic government officials to the Chinese; Paul Chater,[68] a prominent Armenian business man; Thomas Whitehead of the Chartered Bank, one of the sharpest and most outspoken critics of the government; A. M. Thomson, acting Colonial Secretary; and Ho Kai. In other words, it consisted of two government officials, two business men, and one professional; three Britons, one Chinese, and one Armenian. They were all senior in terms of their experience as public figures and social standing, and influential in their own professional fields. The three unofficial Councillors had frequently shown themselves independent-minded. Such a Commission was perhaps the most senior and high-powered one possible at the time and shows that the government was taking this business very seriously.

Interestingly, the Colonial Surgeon, so centrally involved in the matter, was not appointed to the Commission, making one suspect that the government considered it not a medical but a political enquiry. Perhaps one might also say that the Commission was set up to preside over this great quarrel between the Western doctors and the Tung Wah, so that the government's own confrontation with the Hospital could be downplayed.

The enquiry took place between 14 February and 2 July, interviewing 13 witnesses at nine meetings. They fell into four main groups — three past Chairmen of the Hospital, the current Chairman, and one of the Hospital's clerks; five European doctors; two Sanitary Board members; and an architect. At the same time, since the enquiry touched upon the original intentions of the Hospital's establishment, a large volume of materials pertaining to its foundation were produced and printed for the Commissioners' reference. The Commission Report, appending all the reference materials and later presented as a Sessional Paper, is one of the most comprehensive sources of information on the Hospital's history.

Each witness was asked his experience with the Hospital, his opinion as to whether Western medicine should be introduced, and how the Hospital needed to be reformed. Opinions, of course, differed widely. At one extreme were Doctors Lowson and Atkinson, who believed that having failed to fulfil the object and purposes of the Ordinance, namely, the proper treatment of the Chinese indigent sick, it should be abolished. In its stead, they proposed a pauper hospital where Western medicine would be practised, and if the Tung Wah had to be retained at all, it should serve only as a death house for moribund cases.[69] Lowson thought that nothing short of this was sufficient. He even objected to having a Chinese doctor trained in Western medicine there because he would be unable to hold out against the other Chinese — presumably a reference to the Directors.[70] Lowson was only too aware of the Committee's power and influence from his dealings with it in 1894. Neither would employing a student from the College of Medicine for Chinese improve things, because his inexperience would only give a false sense of security.[71]

At the other extreme were the opinions of the Chinese witnesses, with Ho Amei's being the most radical. Ho, one of the most dynamic of the Tung Wah Chairmen (1882), had always taken a strong line in all things relating to the Hospital and the Chinese community at large. At the enquiry, he spoke with his usual eloquence and simple logic. To him, installing a Western doctor was out of the question because it was 'purely a Chinese Hospital' founded with the principle that 'everything in the Hospital should be Chinese, that the Chinese would be treated by Chinese doctors and Chinese medicines, and that no interference was to take place by the government except to look after the cleanliness'.[72] Nor did he see any necessity to have a Chinese doctor trained in Western medicine there — not even for recording causes of death. As he put it, it should be 'very queer for one man to treat a patient and another man to report upon the cause of death'. He also foresaw controversy if the doctors disagreed on the causes. His strongest argument was that the Hospital had given satisfaction to the Chinese public for 25 years, and his simple solution was that Chinese who wanted Western treatment could go to the Civil Hospital.[73]

Opinions among the Chinese witnesses differed, but they all showed an unmistakable sense of annoyance at being subjected to the enquiry. There was, it seems, something humiliating about being summoned before a panel and asked searching questions about an institution of which one was a part. In addition, they knew that the government was under pressure to introduce changes and, regardless of how they felt, it would be done. As Ku Fai-shan (Gu Huishan),[74] the current Chairman, said repeatedly, it was not up to them to accept or refuse the government's recommendations because 'we should not like to disobey any instructions',[75] but the government should make it clear to the Chinese public that *it* was imposing the changes. This was their way of disclaiming responsibility. He also mentioned the attack on Lau Wai Chuen during the plague,[76] apparently to warn others against the wrath of the mob.

There were moderate views too. Some of the European witnesses realized that introducing Western elements into the Hospital might lead to a decline of the subscriptions, even to its closing altogether. Despite its shortcomings, almost everyone agreed that the Hospital was providing an important service. Even Ayres, who doubted its value as a medical institution, believed that if the Hospital were abolished, people would simply die at home, making it even more difficult to trace cases of infectious diseases.[77] Most felt that some changes were mandatory. Certain problems such as insanitary conditions, improper use of space, and proper segregation of patients must be resolved without undue interference.

The dilemma was clear. The Chinese involved with the Hospital were prepared to accept some changes so long as they remained autonomous, and free from the interference of European doctors and the imposition of Western medicine. The European doctors, however, could not trust the Chinese to manage their own affairs. Apart from distrusting Chinese medicine itself, they were even more contemptuous of the Hospital Committee's amateurishness in running the institution. The ultimate dilemma was that if the Hospital were abolished, what would take its place? The government would either have to establish a pauper hospital — by levying a special rate on the Chinese, Lowson suggested[78] — or face a worse situation, as Ayres foresaw.

These deep-seated conflicts are reflected in the Commission Report submitted in September. There were in fact three reports, as no consensus could be reached, and Chater and Whitehead felt strongly enough to insist on separate reports. Interestingly, the diversity of opinion was echoed by the Colonial Office staff.

The majority report emphasized the fact that the Tung Wah was a Chinese hospital, as had been intended from the beginning.[79] It was exactly because Western principles of medicine had been rejected that it was necessary to found a separate hospital. The report pointed out the wide range of good work the Tung Wah had performed. Though sanitary conditions were not perfect, neither were they irreparable. It went on to make several recommendations, the main ones being:

(a) a Chinese trained in Western medicine appointed and paid by government to reside at the Tung Wah chiefly to give correct death returns, and to act as interpreter for the Colonial Surgeon and Justices of the Peace. It should be made very clear that he was not to treat patients unless requested.

(b) a Chinese of good standing to be steward to overlook the sanitary maintenance of the buildings, drainage, cleanliness of patients, and so on.

(c) the appointment of some Chinese residents of long standing and experienced with the Hospital to be associated with it. This would compensate for the lack of continuity and experience of the Board, which was elected every year, in dealing with the government and in running the Hospital.[80]

Throughout the investigation, it is obvious that Lockhart and Ho Kai were sympathetic to the Hospital and played a significant role in drawing out positive views from witnesses whenever possible. It is perhaps due to them that the Hospital survived.

Chater, while admitting that the Hospital had done admirable work as a charitable institution, had grave reservations regarding its medical work. He questioned the qualification of doctors there and was convinced by Atkinson's startling accounts of their practices. Though he realized the practical difficulties of introducing Western medicine, he still believed that Lockhart's recommendations could be carried slightly further. The Chinese trained in Western medicine, he felt, should 'quietly and gradually' introduce the Western system. If natives in India, where religious scruples and racial hatreds presented so much impediment, could come to appreciate Western medicine, then it should be possible, he believed, to similarly persuade the Chinese in Hong Kong.[81]

Analytical and detailed, Whitehead's report stressed the Hospital's original incorporation and the regulations governing it. Although the Ordinance had provided for effective supervision by the Colonial Surgeon and Registrar General, these officers, in his opinion, had failed in their duties.[82] This we may take as his almost habitual swiping at the government, but he did raise a fundamental issue which had been largely overlooked, or condoned, by the others. Where others had argued from the premise that the Hospital Committee was to be autonomous, he highlighted how the ordinance sought to check its autonomy. To forestall a repeat of the I-ts'z scandal, MacDonnell had recommended government supervision as a safeguard against abuse. Whitehead's point was that the Hospital had fallen into such an appalling state partly due to government negligence; but, more consequently, he asserted, the Chinese had fallaciously claimed complete autonomy when it was never intended in the Ordinance in the first place.[83] In other words, they had misinterpreted the Ordinance in their own favour all along.

Whitehead also touched another raw nerve by criticizing the Registrars General. Problems arose, he claimed, 'mainly owing to the lack of intelligent firmness in dealing with the Chinese on the part of the successive Registrar Generals [sic] and their failure to exercise any effective control over the working of the establishment'.[84] Perpetuating the illusion that it was doing good work would only impede the gradual introduction of Western medicine and true advancement. More importantly, the Registrars' General failure signified the basic problem in the management of the Chinese community in Hong Kong. In short, Whitehead was re-establising a point he had put forward vigorously during the enquiry into the Po Leung Kuk in 1893 — that an emergent Chinese élite might create an *imperium in imperio* by exploiting its special relationship with the Registrar General.[85]

He recommended that the Hospital premises be enlarged, that a European steward be installed to oversee general cleanliness, and that medical officers should exercise effective and continuous control. Distrusting the Tung Wah's doctors for their lack of formal qualifications, he hoped that over a number of years they would be slowly replaced by Chinese with some training in Western medicine, so that while practising Chinese medicine they could provide Western treatment when patients required it.[86]

The Settlement

Robinson took some time considering the reports, and when he eventually presented his proposal to the new Hospital Committee on 29 December 1896 it is evident that he had planned his tactics well.

The mood now was far more conciliatory than the previous December. One reason was that the government had handled the 1896 plague much more tactfully. As soon as it broke out, Robinson gave orders that sick people might be removed to Canton and sanitary measures were carried out with greater care and consideration. Although there was still resentment, no violence erupted. For Robinson it was especially gratifying that rich Chinese business men had not started an exodus as in 1894 and business suffered much less.[87] These could be signs that the Chinese population was accepting plague measures as inevitable, even if undesirable, and that the government had learnt a lesson from bitter experience.

The atmosphere was more harmonious also because a second Chinese Legislative Councillor had been appointed in July.[88] Demands for constitutional changes were renewed in 1894, mainly by European residents. Besides, the sanitary problems, especially during the plague, made Lord Ripon, the Secretary of State for the Colonies, realize that it might be useful to have a Chinese on the Executive Council. Robinson disagreed, doubting whether any Chinese could be really independent. As a compromise, he appointed Wei Yuk the junior Chinese representative on the Legislative Council. Wei, educated in England and Scotland, was compradore of the Mercantile Bank. Twice Chairman of the Tung Wah Hospital (1880, 1887), he was an accepted leader of the Chinese community and his appointment must have pacified it to some extent. A Justice of the Peace since 1883 and a member of the District Watch Committee, his association with the government was also of long standing.[89] Wei was energetic and a man of action, apparently without Ho Kai's arrogance and abrasiveness, and was more inclined to solve problems by compromise and manipulation than by confrontation. His appointment at this juncture was propitious, with important ramifications for the Hospital's future.

Thirdly, though the Commission itself might have aroused the Hospital people's resentment at first, its verdict on the whole was favourable. All the Commissioners, despite their divergent views, expressed appreciation for its good work. For the Governor this could be a source of strength against die-hards such as Lowson. For the Chinese, it dispelled their worst fears.

Robinson was also encouraged that the Hospital's three new Principal Directors were men who knew English, two being compradores, and long connected with the colony; this he hoped was a sign that the Hospital was ready for change.[90] At the meeting he persuaded the Committee to accept three main changes of personnel: the appointment of a steward to oversee the Hospital's sanitary conditions, a Chinese doctor trained in Western medicine, and a visiting surgeon.[91] The steward, he pointed out, would be able to relieve some of the duties of the Directors who were all so busy with their own businesses. The Chinese doctor would offer Western medicine to patients who asked for it, not supplant Chinese methods, and he assured them there would not be compulsion. As for the visiting surgeon, Robinson pacified the Committee by saying that this would no longer be Atkinson, the Colonial Surgeon, but Dr John C. Thomson[92] of the Alice Memorial Hospital, who had worked for years among the Chinese, and was notably more sympathetic and tactful.

While Robinson still threatened to deal with people trying to stir up strife, he was much more conciliatory, stressing his hopes to create harmony and to advance the Hospital's welfare. He pleaded for the Committee to co-operate with him. He must have realized that there was no room for failure. The matter had been dragged out long enough. He had bullied and threatened; he had gone through the motion of appointing a Commission. Now he resorted to persuasion. The ball was back in the Tung Wah Committee's court.

A meeting was held at the Hospital on the 13 December with present and past Directors.[93] There was no longer fierce opposition and the only hesitation was over how the kaifongs might react to these proposals. We can detect changes in the composition of the kaifong leadership between the early 1870s and 1896. In the earlier period, the most prominent merchants were kaifong leaders, and it was from them that the Tung Wah Committee itself had emerged. In the later period, however, things had changed. The wealthiest merchants still provided Directors to the Tung Wah Board through the mechanism of guild representation, but as this meeting indicates, they were no longer serving as kaifong leaders. Instead, kaifong leaders tended to come from among shopkeepers, a situation that lasted into the post Second World War period.[94] In other words, as the Chinese community grew more heterogeneous and stratified, it made room for more levels of social leadership. The kaifongs, who had once been relatively high-powered, had declined as new organizations such as the Tung Wah Hospital and the Po Leung Kuk Committees were added at the top of the hierarchy. If we take into account institutions created by the government by which Chinese individuals could now attain political and social status, the relative status of kaifong leaders must have been significantly reduced.

The man who pushed the Governor's proposals most vigorously at this meeting turned out not to be any of the new Directors but Fung Wa Chuen (Feng Huachuan),[95] a Tung Wah Director of 1892, a Po Leung Kuk Director of 1894, and compradore of the National Bank. He pointed out that it would be much better to have a Chinese doctor trained in Western medicine than a European doctor. It was also a good idea to let the Governor make the appointment so that he could be asked to pay for the new doctor who would be under the Committee's direction. He claimed that the Governor was not seeking to diminish the Committee's power. Neither was Fung too worried about the kaifongs' opinion. After all, he added dismissively, they had been sent for and it was their own fault if they had not turned up. If the Committee was worried about them complaining, all it had to do was to ask Lockhart to issue a notice telling them that the doctor 'must be appointed'.[96] In other words, he invoked the government's power to crush any prospective opposition, and if the kaifongs' approval was needed at all, it could be frightened out of them.

The Chairman, more cautious, resolved that no decision be taken until the kaifongs had been consulted. (It is worth noting that, even up to the present, it is usually the current Directors who are most circumspect, because whatever happens within their term of office will forever be associated with them. The past Directors can afford to be more cavalier.)

Before a second meeting was held for the benefit of the

kaifongs, the Governor had made further concessions. He reconfirmed that government would pay for the Chinese doctor, aware that, otherwise, the Directors would never consent. He also dropped the proposal for a steward, explaining rather unconvincingly to London that such an appointment might retard the progress resulting from the other appointment.[97] In fact, this looks more like a further concession to appease the Chinese. At the same time, Lockhart told the Directors that the decision could be delayed no longer, leaving them to present the *fait accompli* to the kaifongs as best they could.[98]

A week later, the kaifongs were finally assembled. The Directors in effect told them that all they could do was to make the best of a bad job — to accept the government proposals while trying to get as many safeguards as possible; to make sure that government would pay for the new Chinese doctor and that it would grant a site to build a new wing for the additional patients coming to consult him.[99] Fung Wa Chuen repeated the Governor's warning against trouble makers. Wei Yuk, on the other hand, reminded them more subtly of the Governor's power to abolish the Hospital. Between Fung and Wei, there was no room for hesitation or opposition. No one present objected to the changes. Subsequently Dr Chung Boon-chor (Zhong Penchu), the House Surgeon at the Alice Memorial Hospital, was appointed.[100]

The 'Chinese Hospital' offering 'purely' Chinese treatment was no more.

The Conversion

The struggle to convert the Tung Wah Hospital into a partly Western medical institution begun during the plague in 1894 was a long drawn out one, marked by bitter cultural, social, and political contentions. During the gruelling two years, pressure from the medical authorities had locked the Hospital Committee and the government in battle, each going through a series of attitudes. The Governor threatened, intimidated, persuaded, and compromised. The Hospital people, on the other hand, must have been holding their breath since May 1894, waiting for some calamity to befall it. Though some were originally prepared to resist to the hilt, they too finally yielded to pre-empt complete abolition.

Several factors made conversion possible. The Western medical doctors involved, particularly Lowson and Atkinson, insisted on the more centralized and uniform medical administration currently popular in Britain with unusual tenacity. The almost religious faith in public health reforms would not tolerate deviation. With their interference the segregated medical systems in Hong Kong were finally forced to move toward integration.

In addition, behind the Governor's apparent tactlessness was a shrewd awareness that concessions needed to be made, the Hospital's abolition being quite out of the question. Though he might be unsympathetic towards the Chinese community, and hostile towards 'trouble makers', he had nothing to gain from antagonizing them to the point of revolt. To neutralize Robinson's belligerence was James Stewart Lockhart, whose good will toward the Chinese inspired trust and who convinced them of the advantages of the reform and of compromise.

On the Chinese side, there was also an interesting interplay of personalities. To begin with, Ho Amei was absent at the December meetings. He seems to have kept a low profile after mid-1896 — he might have left town or may have been suffering from ill health; at least some very good reason must have kept him away from these meetings which decided the fate of the 'Chinese Hospital'. As the inimitable champion of the 'old guards', his absence might have been crucial. With no one to lead the oppositions began to decline.[4] At the same time the Committee's autonomy was curtailed. The appointment in 1896 of Wei Yuk, definitely a 'new man', to the Legislative Council, certainly strengthened the so-called 'progressive' party. Wei was instrumental in conciliating the views of the government and the Chinese community and in making them yield for the sake of harmony. Fung Wa Chuen, whose contribution to the settlement was no less decisive, also shows how the 'progressive' party was important in demonstrating to the Chinese public that change was not necessarily an evil thing to be totally rejected as a matter of principle.

The reforms introduced in late 1896 marked the beginning of the Tung Wah Hospital as a modern medical institution. Before long a number of other reforms were introduced, confirming predictions and fears that the early reforms, however minor, would invariably lead to further intrusion. From 1897 patients were segregated in different wards according to their illnesses and rooms were put aside for surgery.[101] Various changes, including structural ones, recommended by Dr Thomson, were adopted to bring sanitary conditions closer to those expected of a Western hospital.[102] Though the vast majority of patients still opted for Chinese treatment, it was nevertheless modified. For instance, Thomson and Chung insisted on using quinine for *all* cases of malaria, thus breaking Robinson's promise of no compulsion. This caused bad feelings among Chinese doctors and patients, many of whom left.[103] By the end of 1897 a Chinese steward was appointed to supervise the sanitary maintenence of the buildings,[104] and so removed this central aspect of administration from the amateurish direction of the Board.

The steadily increasing influence of Western medicine is also seen in the appointment of a young assistant to Dr Chung, who was given permission to study at the College of Medicine for Chinese. In 1898, when the Tung Wah set up branch hospitals to receive plague patients, Dr Thomson engaged two students of the College to keep the necessary records, prepare returns, maintain sanitary conditions, and when called upon to assist Chinese doctors, and though the patients made little demand on them, they did, to some extent, introduce Western treatment.[105] In 1899 surgery was performed for the first time at the Tung Wah by Dr Chung, who, by keeping in touch with the community of Western doctors, also kept the Hospital in line with modern medical progress.[106]

Many of the reforms introduced after 1896 were possible due to the energetic promotion of Fung Wa Chuen,[107] who, not surprisingly, was identified by government as representing the 'progressive party'.[108] Thus, the Hospital's medical work, hardly developed since 1869, embarked on a more dynamic course after 1896. One could say that as a 'Chinese' hospital in this period, it was almost impossible by definition to grow. As a partly Western hospital however, there was much room for improvement and plenty of examples to follow.

Conclusion

The plague was a landmark in the Hospital's history in more than the medical sense. Instead of allowing the Hospital Committee to make a political comeback, it witnessed its further decline. Although the enquiry into the Tung Wah's working was ostensibly a medical one, the social-political ramifications were much more far-reaching. That an enquiry was instituted at all was a blatant loss of face for the Hospital. Some of the Commission's recommendations, which the Government forced on the Hospital, struck at the very basis of its autonomy. The fundamental issue was not whether a Western-trained doctor should be recruited but whether the Hospital Committee was able, as an independent informal power group, to resist the change, and whether, as defenders of the Chinese community, to keep it 'Chinese'. This ability, as we have pointed out, was one of the prerequisites of leadership.

The confrontation in 1896 was also significant in enabling new men to come forward to make their marks. They might be a small minority in the 1890s, but they were strategically placed. This was partly the result of the government's policy toward the Chinese, which began to gain coherence in the mid-1880s. It departed from segregationism typical of the first four decades of British rule in Hong Kong based on leaving the social control of the Chinese community with its own leaders but without giving them official recognition. From the mid-1880s onwards there was more direct rule partly through the re-organization of the Registrar General's office, and partly through the integration of Chinese individuals into the official power structure. In short, there was a move toward political integration.

The Tung Wah Hospital Committee, as the congregating point of the Chinese élite, was partially overshadowed. Of course it did not lose its standing or attraction over night, and as Lethbridge claims, it became a channel for advancement into the official bodies:[109] the Directors' performance was judged for advancement. They could prove themselves competent as well as receptive to government policies. While championing the Chinese community's interests they could also influence the community to see the government's point of view, highlighting common grounds and common interests. Where once the Hospital Committee members had insisted that their 'legitimacy' was derived from the kaifongs, Fung Wa Chuen's attitude reveals that perhaps this source was no longer so vital. Government patronage was at least equally important for legitimizing and establishing their position in the Chinese community.

At first the new situation created polarized feelings and the stoning of Lau Wai Chuen demonstrates the extent of alienation.

But that was at the height of a crisis. When the dust had finally settled, Wei Yuk and Fung again tried to show that there was room for compromise. Fung's re-election to the Tung Wah Board in 1897, and appointment to the Sanitary Board in 1899, indeed show that one could serve the Chinese community and the government at the same time. Significantly, conservatives blocked him from being elected as one of the Principal Directors in 1897, showing that their influence was still considerable.[110] Yet he succeeded in being elected in 1901, an indication that the strength of the 'progressives' was equally formidable. New men and new political norms transformed the former confrontational situation, and the former image of the Tung Wah Hospital as being independent and in opposition to the government was modified. The bitter struggle between the government and the Hospital between 1894 and 1896 never occurred again, as their relationship and the government's management tactics changed.

The reforms at the Hospital in 1896 marked the beginning of a gradual process toward integration in Hong Kong in medical administration as well as in politics and society. While the introduction of Western medicine was a significant step in the history of the Hospital as a medical institution, the circumstances enabling the conversion and the subsequent change in its relations with government have even greater ramifications for the Hospital as a social and political institution, and for Hong Kong society as a whole.

Epilogue

THE Tung Wah Hospital of the nineteenth century defies simple classification and its story up to 1896 shows that it was indeed many things to many people. But the Tung Wah story does not stop in 1896. As a hospital, it went on to expand in terms of space, service, and facilities. In 1931 the Kwong Wah (Guanghua) Hospital, founded in 1911, and the Eastern Hospital, founded in 1929, were amalgamated with it under a single management to form the Tung Wah Group of Hospitals. Even when the part Western medicine played grew and Chinese medicine became subsidiary, it continued to provide much-needed medical service to the Chinese community. Its philanthropic activities persisted, as did its close connections with Overseas Chinese. It raised funds for China for many years, and in 1926 it was said to be 'probably one of the largest philanthropic institutions in existence'.[1]

In the twentieth century its Chairmanship remained a coveted post,[2] and its Board of Directors remained the avenue for ambitious Chinese on their way up the social and political ladder in Hong Kong. As late as 1933, Sir Lo Man-kam (Luo Wenjian), Chairman of 1929, likened its Chairman to the 'unofficial mayor of the Chinese community'.[3] Together with the Chinese Chamber of Commerce and the Po Leung Kuk, it continued to speak and act on community issues. Government continued to pay it great deference and to see it as a major stabilizing force.

Important changes, however, did take place. Its dependence on government increased. From 1903 a government grant of $6,000 was made annually, a welcome addition as guild subscriptions began to decline.[4] At the same time the Committee's autonomy was curtailed. The 1896 Hospital Commission had criticized its lack of continuity, resulting from the annual change of the Committee. This became unusually obvious in 1904, with misunderstanding among the Directors of different years over the construction of the Smallpox Hospital and, in 1906, with trouble over funds.[5] The Registrar General, W. A. Brewin, reviving the Commission's recommendation, invited 16 gentlemen, all past Directors of the Hospital, to assist him as an Advisory Board.

This later developed into the Tung Wah Hospital Advisory Board, with the Registrar General (after 1913, the Secretary for Chinese Affairs) as *ex officio* Chairman. In 1908 the Advisory Board included eight members who had not been Directors of the Hospital, and the two Chinese Legislative Councillors became *ex officio* members. This was not provided for in the Hospital's Constitution, and though intended as a purely consultative body, by playing an active role in the Hospital's planning and development, its influence was considerable.[6] This, like the Permanent Board of the Po Leung Kuk, institutionalized government interference and eroded the Hospital Committee's autonomy.

The Hospital's position in the Chinese community was also conditioned by the nature of the community. By the end of the nineteenth century the emergence of 'new' men who modified some of the Hospital Committee's most conservative attitudes and ideas is notable. But more important changes were taking place in society in Hong Kong and China which outpaced transformations at the Hospital.

The early decades of twentieth-century China were predominated by the growth of two closely related ideologies, modern nationalism and labour consciousness, both with strong anti-imperialist overtones.[7] For British Hong Kong and for the Tung Wah these ideological changes had far-reaching ramifications. By 1911 labour organizations in Hong Kong had developed sufficiently to alert the government into passing Ordinance 47 of 1911, 'for a more effective control over Societies and Clubs'.[8] Practically and emotionally, the new labour consciousness sharply divided the community, and for the Tung Wah, which had long claimed to represent the 'entire Chinese community', the effect was overwhelming. The 1922 Seamen's Strike[9] illustrates this best. The Hospital Committee, asked by government to arbitrate, failed, partly because the workers preferred the services of another arbitration delegation composed of 'all the labour unions' in Hong Kong.[10] Not surprisingly, the workers felt no rapport with the Hospital. As a union leader later wrote, although the Tung Wah was nominally a hospital, it was actually an association of Chinese *shenshang*, a *yangnu* ('slave to foreigners') organization at the beck and call of imperialism, which accounted for its influence in Hong Kong.[11]

The Tung Wah became the target of anti-imperialism again during the 1925 Hong Kong strike which evolved into a boycott by the Canton government against Hong Kong.[12] As the Directors tried to assist the colonial government in maintaining law and order, they were charged with being 'English dog' [sic], caring only to keep their property and disregarding the 'loss of national prestige'.[13] Abusive letters and telegrams poured in from many parts of the world denouncing its imperialist nature. Its position became even clearer when $50,000 of its funds were lent to finance the warlord Chen Jiongming against the leftist Guangdong government.[14] In the meantime, the anti-*muitsai* struggle, carried out throughout the 1920s by different sectors of the Chinese and European communities, brought into contrast the paternalistic and conservative, even anachronistic, character of the Tung Wah Hospital and the Po Leung Kuk.[15]

We can see the Hospital Committee losing touch with sectors of the Chinese community and in so far as government depended on it, however secondarily, to communicate with the community, the policy was unsatisfactory and unrealistic. This can also be seen in the political structure. Though there was gradual desegregation as government brought certain Chinese individuals into its scheme of things, the fact that they were mostly wealthy, English-educated, and élitist[16] created alienation. In the late nineteenth century they were alienated from the Chinese adhering to traditional Chinese customs and moral principles. In the twentieth century their alienation from the advocates of Chinese nationalism and the 'proletariat' became even more irreconcilable. Likewise, the Registrar General's office, which conceived of 'Chinese' in mainly traditionalist terms, was unable to reach the entire Chinese community as it grew ever more heterogeneous. This meant that despite government's more coherent policy toward the Chinese, it was not always dynamic enough to cope with the fast-changing circumstances or to contain the anti-colonial challenge. As an effective means of communicating with the different sectors of the Chinese community failed to develop, the scope and degree of social and political integration was limited. That Hong Kong society was not less stable was due to reasons other than the government's efforts.

Government policy toward the Chinese, generally passive and unimaginative, changed slowly. As late as 1969 the Secretary for Chinese Affairs admitted that his staff depended very much on contact with organizations such as the Tung Wah Hospital Group to reach the public — even while aware that these contacts did not necessarily reach the poorer people or the well-to-do who were not interested in public activities or public life.[17] Fortunately this realization prompted the government to implement the City District Office and other schemes to reach the people in the late 1960s, but its basic inertia up to this point is manifest. If the Hospital Committee after 1896 had evolved slowly compared to the rapid changes in society, the government's policy and administration was as hopelessly out of step with the real world. The integration of medical administration remained incomplete. Captain Elliot's 1841 proclamation had permitted Chinese to be governed according to Chinese laws and customs, but over the decades the scope of this freedom has been vastly reduced. Yet the freedom to practise Chinese medicine beyond government control remains largely intact to this day.[18] Today, besides Western medicine, the Tung Wah Group of Hospitals offers free Chinese medicine, which still proliferates in its many forms in Hong Kong, and in recent years there has been a revitalization of Chinese medical science. It would be interesting to see whether the government, in view of this phenomenon, would intervene in this last stronghold of 'Chinese customs' protected by the proclamation. The drama of Hong Kong's medical history, much of it embodied by the Tung Wah story, is still unfolding.

Notes

Note to Preface

1. H. J. Lethbridge, 'A Chinese Association in Hong Kong: the Tung Wah', *Contributions to Asian Studies* (Toronto) 1 (1971), pp. 144–58; reprinted in his *Hong Kong: Stability and Change, A Collection of Essays* (Hong Kong: Oxford University Press, 1978), pp. 52–70; Carl T. Smith, 'Visit to Tung Wah Group of Hospitals' Museum, 2nd October, 1976' (Notes and Queries), *Journal of the Hong Kong Branch of the Royal Asiatic Society* (hereafter *JHKBRAS*) 16 (1976), pp. 262–80.

Notes to Introduction

1. Elliot to Palmerston, 25 March 1841: Great Britain, Foreign Office, General Correspondence: China 1815–1905, Series 17 (hereafter FO 17)/48. Captain Charles Elliot, R. N. (1801–75) became Chief Superintendent of Trade to China in 1837 and Plenipotentiary in 1840. During the Opium War he negotiated with China for the cession of Hong Kong, and he occupied the island in January 1841; he was dismissed for going against London's instructions. For a biographical sketch, see G. B. Endacott, *A Biographical Sketchbook of Early Hong Kong* (Hong Kong: Eastern Universities Press, 1962).

2. Pottinger to Aberdeen, 29 August 1842: Great Britain, Colonial Office, Original Correspondence: Hong Kong, 1841–1951, Series 129 (hereafter CO 129)/1. Sir Henry Pottinger (1789–1856) was appointed to succeed Charles Elliot as Plenipotentiary to China. After administering Hong Kong for two years, he was appointed its first Governor in 1843. See Endacott, *Sketchbook*, pp. 13–22.

3. James Stephen to H. U. Addington, 3 June 1843, quoted in Gerald Graham, *The China Station, War and Diplomacy 1830–1860* (Oxford: Oxford University Press, 1978), p. 234. Stephen was Under-Secretary for the Colonies 1836–47.

4. Stanley Lane-Poole, *Thirty Years of Colonial Government, Selections from the Despatches and Letters of the Right Honourable Sir George Ferguson Bowen G.C.M.G.*, 2 volumes (London: Longmans, Green, 1887), Vol. I, p. 13.

5. G. B. Endacott, *A History of Hong Kong* (Hong Kong: Oxford University Press, 1983; first published 1958), p. vii. In fact J. S. Furnivall argues that since all colonies served economic reasons, the prime concern of all colonial powers was to maintain order as essential for deriving economic advantages. See J. S. Furnivall, *Colonial Policy and Practice, A Comparative Study of Burma and Netherlands India* (New York: New York University Press, 1956; first published 1948), p. 8. It seems, however, that in colonies designed for settlement, this might not be absolutely correct. Furnivall's view might be compared to W. M. Morrell, *British Colonial Policy in the Age of Peel and Russell* (Oxford: Clarendon Press, 1930), which claims that other principles were at work in colonial policy, for example, humanitarianism.

6. Harold Ingrams, quoted by Robert Huessler, *Yesterday's Rulers, The Making of the British Colonial Service* (New York: Syracuse University Press, 1963), p. 6.

7. Robert V. Kubicek, *The Administration of Imperialism — Joseph Chamberlain at the Colonial Office* (Durham, N.C.: Duke University Press, 1969), p. 43; John W. Cell, *British Colonial Administration in the Mid-nineteenth Century:*

the Policy Making Process (New Haven and London: Yale University Press, 1970), pp. 45–6.

8. E. J. Eitel, *Europe in China* (Hong Kong: Oxford University Press, 1983; first published 1895), with an Introduction by H. J. Lethbridge, p. *i*. Having lived 35 years in Hong Kong and having been much involved with Chinese matters, Eitel ought to be a reliable judge. For a biographical sketch of Eitel, see Lethbridge's Introduction; G. B. Endacott, 'A Hong Kong History: *Europe in China* by E. J. Eitel: The Man and the Book', *Journal of Oriental Studies* 4 (1957/58), pp. 41–65.

9. William H. Liu, 'The Legal Person of Hong Kong Chinese in British Law', *Asian Profile* 4:3 (June 1976), pp. 195–202.

Notes to Chapter 1

1. D. K. Fieldhouse, *The Colonial Empires, A Comparative Study from the Eighteenth Century* (London: Weidenfeld & Nicolson, 1966; first published 1965), p. 246. See also John W. Cell, *British Colonial Administration in the Mid-nineteenth Century: the Policy Making Process* (New Haven and London: Yale University Press, 1970), especially pp. 3–44, 'The Colonial Office'; Brian L. Blakeley, *The Colonial Office 1868–1892* (Durham, N. C.: Duke University Press, 1972); Helen Taft Manning, 'Who Ran the Empire — 1830–1850?', *Journal of British Studies* 5 (1965), pp. 88–121.

2. Fieldhouse, *The Colonial Empires*, p. 247.

3. Singapore, Penang, and Malacca had Chinese residents but these places did not become Crown Colonies until 1867.

4. James William Norton-Kyshe, *The History of the Laws and Courts of Hong Kong*, 2 volumes (Hong Kong: Vetch & Lee, 1971; first published 1898), Vol. I, pp. 4–6.

5. Fieldhouse, *The Colonial Empires*, pp. 278, 283.

6. John King Fairbank, *Trade and Diplomacy on the China Coast* (Stanford: Stanford University Press, 1968; first published 1953), p. 128. For early negotiations see J. Y. Wong, 'The Cession of Hong Kong: A Chapter of Imperial History', *Journal of Oriental Society of Australia* 2 (1976), pp. 49–61. For a research guide to the documents on the subject, see J. Y. Wong, *Anglo-Chinese Relations 1839–1860* (London: The British Academy, 1983).

7. F. O. to C. O., 6 April 1843: CO 129/3.

8. Pottinger to Stanley, 9 December 1843: CO 129/2.

9. John Davis (1795–1890) had had long experience with China before serving as Governor of Hong Kong. He had spent many years in the East India Company in South China before becoming Chief Superintendent of Trade in 1835. He was author of a two-volume work on China, *The Chinese: A General Description of the Empire of China, and its Inhabitants*, published in 1836. See E. J. Eitel, *Europe in China* (Hong Kong: Oxford University Press, 1983), p. 211; G. B. Endacott, *A Biographical Sketchbook of Early Hong Kong* (Hong Kong: Eastern Universities Press Limited, 1962), pp. 23–9.

10. Qiying (耆英) (1790–1858) was commissioned to negotiate with the British in 1842, and later with the Americans and the French. See Arthur W. Hummel (ed.), *Eminent Chinese of the Ch'ing Period (1644–1912)*, 2 volumes (Washington: Government Printing Office, 1943–4), Vol. I, pp. 130–4; *Zhongguo shixue hui* (中國史學會) (Chinese History Society) (ed.), *(The Opium War)*, 6 volumes (Shanghai: 1954), Vol. VI, pp. 418–24; Cai Guanlo (蔡冠洛) (ed.), *Qingdai qibai mingren zhuan* (清代七百名人傳) (*Biographies of 700*

Prominent Qing Personalities), 3 volumes (Hong Kong: 1963; preface dated 1936), Vol. III, pp. 1350-6.

11. Fairbank, *Trade and Diplomacy*, p. 129.

12. G. B. Endacott, *Government and People in Hong Kong* (Hong Kong: Hong Kong University Press, 1964), p. 32.

13. Eitel, *Europe in China*, p. 134.

14. See Carl T. Smith, 'The Chinese Settlement of British Hong Kong', *Chung Chi Bulletin* 48 (May 1970), pp. 26-32.

15. *Chouban yiwu shimo* (籌辦夷務始末) (*The complete account of the management of barbarian affairs*), *juan* 52:3, quoted by Ding You (丁又), *Xianggang chuqi shihua (1841-1907)* (香港初期史話) (*Early History of Hong Kong*) (Peking: 1983; first published 1958), p. 76. See also Robert Montgmery Martin, 'Report on the Island of Hong Kong' in his *Reports, Minutes and Despatches on the British Position and Prospects in China* (London [1846]), pp. 2-32.

16. For Chinese Imperial policy towards Overseas Chinese, see Yen Ching-Hwang, 'Changing Images of the Overseas Chinese (1644-1912)', *Modern Asian Studies* (hereafter *MAS*) 15:2 (1981), pp. 261-85.

17. Yen, 'Changing Images', pp. 267-76; *Chouban yiwu shimo*, *juan* 50:39, quoted in Ding, *Xianggang*, p. 76. Article IX of the Nanking Treaty provided for amnesty to all subjects of China who might have been guilty of 'residing under, or had dealings and intercourse with, or having entered the service of Her Britannic Majesty, or Her Majesty's officers'.

18. Davis to Stanley, 1 June 1844, #10: CO 129/6.

19. Norton-Kyshe, *Laws and Courts*, Vol. I, pp. 29.

20. Endacott, *Government and People*, pp. 36-7; Ding, *Xianggang*, pp. 87-8.

21. Endacott, *Government and People*, p. 36; see also Paul Knaplund, *James Stephen and the British Colonial System 1813-1847* (Madison: University of Wisconsin Press, 1933).

22. Davis to Stanley, 21 January 1845, #5: CO 129/11.

23. 'Translations from the *Lü-li* or General Code of Laws of the Chinese Empire', *China Review* 8 (1879-1880), pp. 259-61; for an analysis of its working, see Ch'ü T'ung-tsu, *Local Government in China under the Ch'ing* (Cambridge, Mass.: Harvard University Press, 1962), pp. 150-4; Hsiao Kung-chuan, *Rural China: Imperial Control in the Nineteenth Century* (Seattle: University of Washington Press, 1960).

24. Davis to Stanley, 28 January 1845, #9: CO 129/11.

25. Eitel, *Europe in China*, p. 222; Norton-Kyshe, *Laws and Courts*, Vol. I, p. 338.

26. Eitel, *Europe in China*, pp. 222-6.

27. Eitel, *Europe in China*, pp. 222-6; Great Britain, Foreign Office, Miscellanea 1759-1935. Series 233 (hereafter FO 233)/185, Records of letters between the Plenipotentiary and High Provincial Authorities, notifications 29/1844; 32/1844.

28. Eitel, *Europe in China*, p. 226; Norton-Kyshe, *Laws and Courts*, Vol. I, p. 73.

29. Norton-Kyshe, *Laws and Courts*, Vol. I, p. 93.

30. See 'Civil Establishment', *Hong Kong Blue Book*, 1844 to 1855; Norton-Kyshe, *Laws and Courts*, Vol. I, p. 284.

31. See especially Maurice Freedman, 'Immigrants and Associations: Chinese in 19th Century Singapore', *Comparative Studies in Social History* 3 (1961), pp. 25-48; G. W. Skinner, *Chinese Society in Thailand; An Analytical History* (Ithaca, N. Y.: Cornell University Press, 1957) and *Leadership and Power in the Chinese Community of Thailand* (Ithaca, N. Y.: Cornell University Press, 1958); Lawrence W. Crissman, 'The Segmentary Structure of Urban Overseas Chinese

Communities', *Man* 2:2 (June 1967), pp. 185-204; W. E. Willmott, *The Politic Structure of the Chinese Community in Cambodia* (London: London School Economics Monographs on Social Anthropology, no. 42, 1970), Chapter 1 There are also scholars who consider this view too limited. See Donald R. Glopper, 'City on the Sands: Social Structure in a Nineteenth Century Chine: City' (Ph. D. thesis, Cornell University, 1973).

32. Dafydd E. Evans, 'Chinatown in Hong Kong: The Beginnings of Taipin shan', *JHKBRAS* 10 (1970), pp. 69-78; the petitions relating to the move are 5, 7, and 8 of 1844: FO 233/185.

33. J. Chesneaux, 'Secret Societies in China's Historical Evolution' in Chesneaux (ed.), *Popular Movements and Secret Societies in China, 1840-19!* (Stanford: Stanford University Press, 1972), pp. 1-21; for a contemporai account, see Charles Gutzlaff, 'On the Secret Triad Society of China, Chief from Papers Belonging to the Society found at Hong Kong', *Journal of the Roy Asiatic Society* 8 (1846), pp. 361-7.

34. W. P. Morgan, *Triad Societies in Hong Kong* (Hong Kong: Governmei Printer, 1982; first published 1960), p. 60.

35. Davis to Stanley, 21 January 1845, #5 and 4 March 1845, #20: C(129/11; 11 September 1845, #127: CO 129/13.

36. 2/1846: FO 233/186; 20/1847: FO 233/187.

37. Ch'ü T'ung-tsu, *Law and Society in Traditional China* (Paris: Moutoi 1965).

38. In fact the lack of understanding of the workings of Chinese guilds was long-standing problem among foreigners in China. See Hosea Ballou Morse, *Tl Gilds of China with an Account of the Gild Merchants or Co-hong of Canton* (Ne York: Russell & Russell, 1967; first published 1932); Daniel Jerome McGowai 'Chinese Guilds or Chambers of Commerce and Trade Unions', *Journal of tl Royal Asiatic Society, China Branch new (2nd) series* 21, 3 (1886), pp. 133-9. Peter J. Golas, 'Early Ch'ing Guilds' in G. W. Skinner, *The City in Late Imperi China* (Stanford: Stanford University Press, 1977), pp. 581-608; Quan Hansher (全漢昇), *Zhongguo hanghui zhidu shi* (中國行會制度史) (*The Guild System China*) (Taipei: 1978; first published 1935).

39. Joe England and John Rear, *Chinese Labour under British Rule* (Hor Kong: Oxford University Press, 1975), pp. 74, 207; Norton-Kyshe, *Laws an Courts*, Vol. I, pp. 437.

40. Norton-Kyshe, *Laws and Courts*, Vol. I, p. 436.

41. Norton-Kyshe, *Laws and Courts*, Vol. I, pp. 436-7.

42. G. W. Skinner, 'Introduction: Urban Social Structure in Ch'ing China' i Skinner, *The City in Late Imperial China*, pp. 521-54; Sybille van der Sprenke 'Urban Social Control' in Skinner, *The City in Late Imperial China*, pp. 609-3. Donald R. de Glopper, 'Temple, Faction and Loan Club: Voluntary Associatior in a Taiwanese Town', paper prepared for 23rd Annual Meeting, Association fc Asian Studies, Washington, D. C., March, 1971; *Huaqiao zhi zongzuan weiyua hui* (華僑誌總纂委員會) (ed.), *Huaqiao zhi zongzhi* (華僑誌總誌) (Records of Ovei seas Chinese: a summary) (Taipei: 1964; 1st published 1956), pp. 383-4. This is compendium of information on Overseas Chinese all over the world; there ar separate volumes for each country.

43. For records relating to the origins of the Man Mo Temple, see 11/184(10, 11, 22, 23, 24/1847: FO 233/186; Carl T. Smith, 'Notes on Chinese Temples i Hong Kong', *JHKBRAS* 13 (1973), pp. 133-9; '*Yingyi ru Yue jilue*' (英夷入粵紀略 ('A record of the British entry into Canton') in *Zhongguo shixue hui* (ed.; *Yapian zhanzheng*, Vol. III, pp. 1-27.

44. Smith, 'Notes on Chinese Temples', p. 135; Carl T. Smith, 'The Emerg ence of a Chinese Élite in Hong Kong', *JHKBRAS* 11 (1971), pp. 74-11!

reprinted in his *Chinese Christians: Élites, Middlemen and the Church in Hong Kong* (Hong Kong: Oxford University Press, 1985), pp. 103-38.

45. 'The Districts of Hong Kong and the name Kwan Tai'Lo', *China Review* 1 (1872-73), pp. 333-4.

46. William Tarrant, 'History of Hong Kong' in *The Friend of China*, 1860-1861, 23 November 1860; and see also Smith, *Chinese Christians*, pp. 114-15, 123-4.

47. 'Hong Kong and Kwan Tai Lo'.

48. 'Hong Kong and Kwan Tai Lo'.

49. See the *'He Gang Wenwu Miao jishi lu'* (闔港文武廟紀事錄) ('A record of the Man Mo Temple of the whole Hong Kong'), *Wenwu Miao zhengxinlu* (文武廟徵信錄) (*Annual report of the Man Mo Temple*) 1911, pp. 1a-2a.

50. Tam Achoy was from Kaiping (開平), Loo was Tanka. Several people from Panyu (番禺) donated a couplet and the stone columns at the main entrance were donated by a mason surnamed Zeng (曾), probably a Hakka. Ho Asik (He Axi) (何錫) was from Shunde (順德). The stone lions in the yard were given by the Pork Dealer's Guild. There are still several tablets presented by various guilds, including the Shoe Makers' Guild and Washermen's Guild.

51. Quoted in Smith, 'Notes on Chinese Temples', p. 135.

52. *The Friend of China*, quoted in Smith, *Chinese Christians*, pp. 114-15.

53. *'He Gang Wenwu Miao jishi lu'*. For Ho Asik, see Smith, *Chinese Christians*, pp. 122-3, 225-6, n. 43.

54. *Wenwu Miao zhengxinlu* 1911: accounts.

55. 'Hong Kong and Kwan Tai Lo'. In 1858, for example, a meeting was held at the 'Joss House' to discuss the formation of a fire brigade; see Vincent H. G. Jarrett, 'Old Hong Kong', p. 306. This is a series of articles on the history of Hong Kong taken from the *South China Morning Post* between 17 June 1933 and 13 April 1935 and re-organized alphabetically by subject. The copy used for this book is a photographic copy of a copy typed from the original articles deposited at the Hong Kong University Library, in four volumes.

56. Quoted from a post-war Hong Kong government department report by James Hayes, *The Hong Kong Region 1850-1911: Institutes and Leadership in Town and Countryside* (Hamden, Connecticut: Archon Books, Dawson, 1977), p. 65.

57. H. J. Lethbridge, *Stability and Change*, pp. 58-9; Aline K. Wong, 'Chinese Voluntary Associations in Southeast Asian Cities and the Kaifongs in Hong Kong', *JHKBRAS* 11 (1971), pp. 62-73 and her *The Kaifong Associations and the Society of Hong Kong*, Asian Folklore and Social Life Monographs, Vol. 43 (Taipei: Overseas Cultural Service, 1973) discusses the post-war situation.

58. Smith, *Chinese Christians*, pp. 90-2.

59. 'The Districts of Hong Kong', *China Directory 1874* (Hong Kong: China Mail Office, 1874), pp. 47-8.

60. The couplet reads:

公爾忘私入斯門貴無偏袒
所欲與聚到此地切莫糊塗

They can still be seen at the kung-so today. A photograph of what appears to be a pre-1862 version of the kung-so is in the possession of the Stockhouse Co. The kung-so was referred to as the kaifong kung-so in 'The Districts of Hong Kong', p. 48.

61. *Hong Kong Daily Press* (hereafter *DP*), 23 September 1870.

62. Eitel, *Europe in China*, p. 282.

63. 'Petition by Lu A-ling, Tam A-tsoi, Cheung Sau, T'ong Chiu, Wang Ho

Un, Wong Ping and 8 others, 1st October, 1851' in Hong Kong, *Report of the Commission appointed by H. E. Sir William Robinson K.C.M.G. . . . to enquire into the Working and Organization of the Tung Wa Hospital, 1896*, published as a Sessional Paper (hereafter *TWR*), p. XVII; W. Caine to Surveyor General, 17 January 1851, *TWR*, p. XVIII.

64. C. S. Wong, *A Gallery of Chinese Kapitans* (Singapore: Ministry of Culture, 1963), p. 8; an examination of the *huiguan* will show that this was one of their major functions, see Quan, *Zhongguo hanghui*, p. 98; Dou Jiliang' (竇季良), *Tongxiang zuzhi zhi yanjiu* (同鄉組織之研究) (*The Study of Regional Organizations*) (Chungking: 1943), pp. 70–1.

65. Caldwell's evidence at the I-ts'z inquest, *TWR*, p. XXX.

66. Caldwell's evidence, *TWR*, pp. XXIV–XXXI.

67. Caldwell's evidence, *TWR*, p. XXX.

68. Caldwell's evidence, *TWR*, p. XXIV.

69. Eitel, *Europe in China*, p. 462.

70. *TWR*, pp. XXV–XXVI.

71. *TWR*, p. XXX.

72. *TWR*, p. XXX.

73. Eitel, *Europe in China*, p. 189. For a history of medicine in Hong Kong, see G. H. Choa, 'A History of Medicine of Hong Kong', *Medical Directory of Hong Kong* 1970, pp. 12–26.

74. *Blue Book* 1864, pp. 350–1; MacDonnell to Granville, 21 June 1869, #726: CO 129/138.

75. Harold Balme, in *China and Modern Medicine, A Study in Medical Mission Development* (London: United Council for Missionary Education, 1921), pp. 82–3, argues that the Chinese had no hospital. There was no Chinese institution to receive and treat the sick poor. In many of the works on the history of Chinese medicine there is no mention of hospitals except the *Yu yiyuan* (御醫院) or Imperial medical institute, which catered to the court. See Chen Bangxian (陳邦賢), *Zhongguo yixue shi* (中國醫學史) (*History of Medicine in China*) (Shanghai: 1955; 1st published 1936); Yu Shenchu (俞慎初), *Zhongguo yixue jianshi* (中國醫學簡史) (*Brief History of Medicine in China*) (Fuzhou: 1983); Chen Yongliang (陳永亮), *Zhongguo yixueshi gangyao* (中國醫學史綱要) (*An Outline History of Medicine in China*) (Canton: 1947); Jia Dedao (賈得道), *Zhongguo yixue shilue* (中國醫學史略) (*Brief History of Medicine in China*) (Taiyuan: 1979). One work, however, argues that hospitals did exist in ancient China, but the author fails to show that they were permanent or specialized institutions, and for the Qing period the author gives no example. See Ren Yingqiu (任應秋), '*Yiyuan de jianli–bingfang*' (醫院的建立－病坊) ('The establishment of hospitals') reprinted in *Ming bao yuekan* (明報月刊) (*Ming Pao Monthly*) 57 (September 1970), p. 19.

76. William Lockhart, *The Medical Missionary in China* (London: Hurst & Blackett, 1861), pp. 23–9, describes these institutions in Shanghai; John Kerr, 'The Native Benevolent Institutions of Canton', part 1: *China Review* 2 (1873), pp. 88–95, and part 2:3 (1874–5), pp. 108–14. See also John Henry Gray, *China, A History of the Law, Manners and Customs of the People*, 2 volumes (London: Macmillan, 1878), Vol. II, Chapter XVIII, 'Benevolent Institutions and Beggars'.

77. Kerr, 'The Native Benevolent Institutions of Canton', part 2, p. 112; Ren, '*Bingfang*'.

78. For medical efforts of Westerners, see K. C. Wong, *The Lancet and the Cross* (Shanghai: Council of Christian Medical Work, 1950), which gives biographical sketches of 50 medical missionaries in China; K. C. Wong and Wu Lien-teh, *History of Chinese Medicine* (Tientsin: the Tientsin Press, 1932); Lockhart, *Medical Missionary*. There is a wealth of literature on the subject, especially

biographical and autobiographical works on doctors who practised in China.
79. Marjorie Topley, 'Chinese Traditional Etiology and Methods of Cure in Hong Kong' in Charles Leslie (ed.), *Asian Medical Systems* (Berkeley: University of California Press, 1976), pp. 243-65; Wong and Wu, *History of Chinese Medicine*, Book I; S. H. Chuan, 'Chinese Patients and their Prejudices', *China Medical Journal*, Vol. XXXI:5 (October 1917), pp. 504-10, gives a good analysis of how Chinese patients insisted on using the Chinese medical system as the frame of reference even in the twentieth century.
80. *Xunhuan ribao* (循環日報) (*Universal Circulating Herald*) (hereafter *XH*), 21 July 1874.
81. For the introduction and acceptance of Jennerian vaccination, see Wong and Wu, *History of Chinese Medicine*, Book II, pp. 139-65; Peter Parker's Report, *China Repository* 17 (1848), p. 133.
82. Dr Benjamin Hobson wrote in 1844 that dissection of the body, even *sectio cadavers*, is utterly discountenanced as a breach of filial piety. See Dr Hobson's Report, June 1844, *China Repository* 13 (1844), pp. 377-82.
83. Eitel, *Europe in China*, p. 462. Thus Dr Patrick Manson commented, 'The Civil Hospital, besides having association of a kind not pleasing or attractive to the native mind, is too rigidly foreign in its ways and discipline to suit the great majority of the sick Chinese.' Inauguration speech at the College of Medicine, 1887, quoted in G. H. Choa, *The Life and Times of Sir Kai Ho Kai* (Hong Kong: Chinese University Press, 1981), p. 56.
84. A. R. Hall, 'The Scientific Movement and its Influence on Thought and Material Development' in *New Cambridge Modern History*, Vol. X, *The Zenith of European Power, 1830-70* (Cambridge: Cambridge University Press, 1967; first published 1960), pp. 49-75, 71-3.
85. Lockhart, *Medical Missionary*, pp. 202-9; Hobson's Report, *China Repository* 13 (1844), pp. 377-82, 18 (1847), pp. 254-9; Eitel, *Europe in China*, pp. 191, 281. There is some confusion over when the hospital closed. Eitel claimed it did in 1850 while Lockhart wrote that work was still carried on in 1853. For Benjamin Hobson, see Wong, *The Lancet and the Cross*, pp. 12-14.
86. Hobson's Report, *China Repository* 13 (1844), p. 377.
87. Hobson's Report, *China Repository* 13 (1844), p. 377.
88. Eitel, *Europe in China*, p. 281.
89. Sergio Ticozzi, *Xianggang Tianzhujiao zhanggu* (香港天主教掌故) (*Stories of the Catholic Church in Hong Kong*) translated by You Liqing (游麗清) (Hong Kong: 1983), pp. 52-3; '*Diyi jian Tianzhujiao yiyuan*' (第一間天主教醫院) ('The first Catholic hospital'); Hong Kong, 'Assessment of Police and Lighting Rates, 1871', p. 187.
90. Jervois to Newcastle, 5 December 1854, #94: CO 129/43.
91. Major-General William Jervois, Lieutenant-Governor and Commander of the Forces, arrived in Hong Kong on 14 April 1851, and was sworn in as a member of the Executive Council the following day. When Governor Bonham left in 1852 he took over the government and acted as British Superintendent of Trade in China until 1854.
92. Jervois to Newcastle, 5 December 1854, #94: CO 129/43.
93. Jervois to Newcastle, 5 December 1854, #94. For a discussion of the *dibao*, see Hsiao, *Rural China*, pp. 64-6.
94. James Legge's 'Lecture on Reminiscences of a Long Residence in the East, delivered in the City Hall, 5th November, 1872', in *China Review* 1 (1872), pp. 163-76, 171. The improvement in business and quality of Chinese settlers was also noted by the officiating Registrar General, C. May, in his report to the Colonial Secretary, enclosed in Bowring to Russell, 4 July 1855, #99: CO 129/51.

95. 'Population', *Blue Book* 1858, 1859.
96. Sir John Bowring (1792–1897), see Endacott, *Sketchbook*, pp. 36–44; *Autobiographical Recollections of Sir John Bowring with a Memoir by Lewin B. Bowring* (London: 1877).
97. Endacott, *Government and People*, p. 51.
98. Endacott, *Government and People*, pp. 51–2.
99. Endacott, *Government and People*, p. 53.
100. John Pope Hennessy (1834–91). Born in County Kerry, Ireland, Member of Parliament 1859, the first Roman Catholic Conservative to sit in Parliament. He was called to the Bar, Inner Temple, in 1861. He became Governor of Labuan in 1867, the Gold Coast in 1872, the Bahamas in 1875, Hong Kong from 1877–82, and Governor of Mauritius, 1883–89. See Endacott, *Government and People*, p. 89, n. 2. His biography is in James Pope-Hennessy, *Verandah: Some Episodes in the Crown Colonies, 1867–1889* (London: George Allen & Unwin, 1964).
101. Caine to Labouchere, 22 November 1856, #196: CO 129/59.
102. D. R. Caldwell was one of the most dramatic characters in Hong Kong history and deserves more scholarly attention. As yet, only a brief account of his life is given in Endacott, *Sketchbook*, pp. 95–9.
103. Bowring to Labouchere, 9 December 1856, #198: CO 129/59.
104. Government notification of 4 December 1856, enclosed in Bowring to Labouchere, 9 December 1856, #198.
105. Government notification of 4 December 1856.
106. For a narrative account of the event, see James Pope-Hennessy, *Half-Crown Colony: A Hong Kong Note Book* (London: Jonathan Cape, 1969), pp. 55–8; 'Papers Respecting the Confinement and Trial of Chinese Prisoners in Hong Kong 1857' (155, Session 2) XLIII, Great Britain, *Parliamentary Papers: China* (Shannon: Irish University Press, 1971–) (hereafter *BPP*), Vol. XXIV, pp. 151–88; Norton-Kyshe, *Laws and Courts*, Vol. I, pp. 414–24.
107. Norton-Kyshe, *Laws and Courts*, Vol. I, pp. 412–13.
108. Petition 1, enclosed in Bowring to Lytton, 22 February 1859, #39: CO 129/73.
109. 'Civil Establishment', *Blue Book* 1858, p. 112.
110. See 'Civil Service Abuses', 1860 (C. 161) XLVIII, *BPP*, Vol. XXIV.
111. Hercules Robinson (1824–97) left the army in 1846 for a post in the Irish government. In 1854 he became President of Monserrat in the West Indies, Lieutenant-Governor of St Christopher in 1855, and Governor of Hong Kong in 1859–65. Afterwards he served as Governor of Ceylon, New South Wales, New Zealand, and the Cape. In 1896 he was made Lord Rosemead. See Endacott, *Government and People*, p. 81, n. 1; see also Endacott, *Sketchbook*, pp. 45–51.
112. Robinson to Newcastle, 23 March 1861, #39: CO 129/80. H. J. Lethbridge, 'Hong Kong Cadets, 1862–1941', *JHKBRAS* 10 (1970), pp. 36–56, reprinted in his *Stability and Change*, pp. 31–51.
113. H. J. Lethbridge, *Stability and Change*, p. 48; C. M. Turnbull, *A History of Singapore* (Kuala Lumpur: Oxford University Press, 1977), pp. 89–90.
114. 'Civil Establishment', *Blue Book* 1864, p. 150.
115. 'Civil Establishment', *Blue Book* 1865–69.
116. *DP*, 22 October 1869; 22 August 1870.
117. Robinson to Newcastle, 28 March 1862, #57: CO 129/85.
118. Robinson to Newcastle, 28 March 1862, #57.
119. *XH*, 7 and 12 July 1880.
120. Davis to Stanley, 1 June 1844, #10: CO 129/6; see also Norton-Kyshe, *Laws and Courts*, Vol. I, pp. 254–5, 279 for the constitution of the police.
121. The Colonial Surgeon wrote in his Report for 1856, 'I regret that I can say

nothing in favour of this force', 'Colonial Surgeon's Report', *Blue Book* 1856, p. 232. See also 'Colonial Surgeon's Report' in 1855, p. 243.

122. H. J. Lethbridge, 'The District Watch Committee', *JHKBRAS* 11 (1971), pp. 116–41, reprinted in his *Stability and Change*, pp. 104–29. See also 'Reports of the Registrar General, 1867', in *Blue Book* 1867, pp. 247–9; and Norton-Kyshe, *Laws and Courts*, Vol. II, p. 86.

123. 'Report of the Registrar General', *Blue Book* 1867, p. 248.

124. 'Report of the Registrar General', 1867, p. 248.

125. 'Registrar General's Report for 1868', *Hong Kong Government Gazette* (hereafter *HKGG*) 1869, pp. 127–9.

126. Endacott, *Government and People*, p. 51. In 1856 persons paying rates of £10 a year numbered 1,999 of whom 1,637 were Chinese. See also Smith, *Chinese Christians*.

127. See the Nam Pak Hong Association's history in *Nanbei hang gongsuo* (南北行公所) (ed.), *Xinsha luocheng ji chengli bashiliu zhounian jinian tekan* (新厦落成暨成立八十六周年紀念特刊) (*Special Publication to Commemorate Its 86th Anniversary and the Completion of the New Building*) (Hong Kong: 1954) and *Chengli yibai zhounian jinian tekan* (成立壹佰周年紀念特刊) (*Centenary Publication of the Nam Pak Hong*) (Hong Kong: 1968); also 'The Nam Pak Hong Commercial Association in Hong Kong' (Notes & Queries), *JHKBRAS* 19 (1979), pp. 216–26.

128. Compare Turnbull, *A History of Singapore*, p. 50; Victor Purcell, *The Chinese in Malaya* (Kuala Lumpur, Hong Kong, and London: Oxford University Press, 1967; first published 1948), p. 145.

Notes to Chapter 2

1. 'Petition of U Chuk Pan, Wong Yau Ho, Wong Fun Wan, Fan Wai and Im A Chak, 23 May 1866, Hong Kong': *Report of the Commission appointed by H. E. Sir William Robinson, K.C.M.G. . . . to enquire into the working and Organization of the Tung Wa [sic] Hospital together with the Evidence taken before the Commission and other Appendices (1896)* (hereafter *TWR*), p. XV. Fan A-wye (Fan Awei) (范阿爲) was a student at the Anglo-Chinese College and was sent to Melbourne after his studies. Returning to Hong Kong, he was appointed Chinese clerk and interpreter in the office of the Colonial Secretary in 1862. In 1867 he was transferred to the Registrar General's office and stayed until 1873. See Carl T. Smith, 'The English-educated Élite in 19th century Hong Kong', *Symposium Paper*, Royal Asiatic Society, Hong Kong Branch, November 1972, pp. 65–96; reprinted in his *Chinese Christians: Élites, Middlemen and the Church in Hong Kong* (Hong Kong: Oxford University Press, 1985), pp. 139–71.

2. Malcolm Struan Tonnochy (1840–82) arrived in Hong Kong in 1862 as one of the first cadets. See H. J. Lethbridge, 'Hong Kong Cadets' in his *Hong Kong: Stability and Change, A Collection of Essays* (Hong Kong: Oxford University Press, 1978), pp. 34–5, 46–7, n. 12.

3. Tonnochy's minute, 22 [sic] May 1866 on 'Petition of U Chuk Pan and others', *TWR*, p. XV.

4. Richard Graves MacDonnell (1814–81). Called to the Bar at Lincoln's Inn, 1838; Chief Justice of the Gambia, 1843; Governor of British Settlements on the Gambia, 1847; Governor of St Lucia, 1852; of South Australia, 1855; Lieutenant-Governor of Nova Scotia, 1864, and Governor of Hong Kong, 1866–72. See G. B. Endacott, *Government and People in Hong Kong* (Hong Kong: Hong Kong University Press, 1964), p. 81, n. 2.

222 NOTES TO PAGES 31–38

5. E. J. Eitel, *Europe in China* (Hong Kong: Oxford University Press, 1983), pp. 413–14.

6. Surveyor General's minute, 25 May 1866 on 'Petition of U Chak Pan and others', *TWR*, p. XVI.

7. MacDonnell's minute, 26 May 1866 on 'Petition of U Chak Pan and others', *TWR*, p. XVI.

8. Surveyor General's minute, 7 June 1866 on 'Petition of U Chak Pan and others', *TWR*, p. XVI.

9. MacDonnell's minute, 29 June 1866 on 'Petition of U Chak Pan and others', *TWR*, p. XVII.

10. Surveyor General to acting Colonial Secretary, 8 June 1866, *TWR*, p. XVIII.

11. Minute by I. Murray, Colonial Surgeon, 9 June 1866, *TWR*, p. XIX.

12. Cecil C. Smith to Colonial Secretary, 19 February 1867, *TWR*, p. XIV.

13. MacDonnell's minute, 19 February 1867, *TWR*, p. XIV.

14. Report by Alfred Lister, 24 April 1869, *TWR*, pp. IX–X.

15. Alfred Lister (1843–90). See H. J. Lethbridge, *Stability and Change*, pp. 34–5, 47, n. 15.

16. Lister to Colonial Secretary, 22 April 1869, *TWR*, pp. VI–VII.

17. MacDonnell to Granville, 21 June 1869, #726: CO 129/138.

18. National Association for Promotion of Social Science to C.O., 17 July 1869: CO 129/142.

19. MacDonnell's minute on Mr Willcocks's memorandum, 23 April 1869, *TWR*, pp. VIII–IX, p. IX.

20. *TWR*, pp. VIII–IX.

21. Report by Alfred Lister, 24 April 1869, *TWR*, pp. IX–X.

22. Report by Lister, 24 April 1869, *TWR*, pp. IX–X.

23. Report by the Harbour Master, H. G. Thomsett, 27 April 1869, *TWR*, pp. XI–XIII.

24. MacDonnell to Austin, 28 April, *TWR*, p. XIII.

25. Report by the Colonial Surgeon, 30 April 1869, *TWR*, p. XIV.

26. MacDonnell to Austin, 5 May 1869, *TWR*, pp. V–VI.

27. MacDonnell to Austin, 5 May 1869, *TWR*, pp. V–VI, and Report by Alfred Lister, 24 April, 1869, *TWR*, pp. IX–X.

28. MacDonnell to Granville, 21 June 1869, #726: CO 129/138.

29. Report by Alfred Lister, 24 April 1869, *TWR*, pp. IX–X.

30. MacDonnell to Austin, 5 May 1869, *TWR*, pp. V–VI.

31. MacDonnell to Austin, 5 May 1869, *TWR*, pp. V–VI.

32. MacDonnell to Granville, 21 June 1869, #726: CO 129/138.

33. MacDonnell to Austin, 5 May 1869, *TWR*, p. V.

34. MacDonnell to Austin, 5 May 1869, *TWR*, p. V.

35. MacDonnell to Granville, 21 June 1869, #726: CO 129/138.

36. MacDonnell to Granville, 21 June 1869, #726: CO 129/138.

37. MacDonnell to Granville, 8 June 1869, #714: CO 129/138.

38. G. B. Endacott, *A History of Hong Kong* (Hong Kong: Oxford University Press, 1983), p. 150.

39. Endacott, *History of Hong Kong*, p. 150.

40. MacDonnell to Granville, 8 June 1869, #714: CO 129/138.

41. MacDonnell to Granville, 8 June 1869, #714:CO 129/138.

42. MacDonnell to Granville, 8 June 1869, #714.

43. MacDonnell to Austin, 2 June 1869, enclosed in MacDonnell to Granville, 8 June 1869, #714.

44. MacDonnell to Granville, 21 June 1869, #726: CO 129/138.

45. MacDonnell to Granville, 18 August 1869, #775: CO 129/138.

46. Granville's minute on MacDonnell to Granville, 8 June, #714: CO 129/138.

47. National Association for the Promotion of Social Science to C.O., 17 July 1869: CO 129/142.

48. Frederick Rogers to MacDonnell, 1 July 1869, #94, *TWR*, p. XXXII; Granville to MacDonnell, 30 July 1869, #112, *TWR*, p. XXXVI.

49. Granville to MacDonnell, 7 October 1869, #158: CO 129/138.

50. Granville to MacDonnell, 7 October 1869, #158.

51. *China Mail* (hereafter *CM*), 1 June 1869.

52. Leung On (梁安) was one of the most aggressive of the Chinese community leaders in nineteenth-century Hong Kong. He was Chairman of the Founding Committee (1869–71) and of the Board of Directors in 1877. See Carl T. Smith, 'The Emergence of a Chinese Elite in Hong Kong', in *Chinese Christians: Élites, Middlemen and the Church in Hong Kong* (Hong Kong: Oxford University Press, 1985), pp. 125–6.

53. *CM*, 1 June 1869; 'Registrar General's Report, 1869', *Hong Kong Blue Book* 1969, pp. 275–6.

54. MacDonnell to Granville, 21 June 1869, #726: CO 129/138; *CM*, 1 June 1869.

55. Petition by Leung On and others on the Committee of the 'I-ts'z' hospital, 30 July 1869, enclosed in MacDonnell to Granville, 18 August 1869, #775: CO 129/138.

56. Petition by Leung On and others, 30 July 1869.

57. Petition by Leung On and others, 30 July 1869.

58. Petition by Leung On and others, 30 July 1869.

59. MacDonnell to Granville, 18 August 1869, #775: CO 129/138.

60. MacDonnell to Granville, 18 August 1869, #775.

61. MacDonnell to Granville, 18 August 1869, #775.

62. MacDonnell to Granville, 18 Angust 1869, #775; MacDonnell to Granville, 19 February 1872, #947: CO 129/156.

63. MacDonnell to Granville, 21 June 1869, #726: CO 129/138.

64. The Victoria Registration Ordinance was introduced in 1866 soon after MacDonnell arrived in Hong Kong. Among other things, there was the application of the principle of vicarious responsibility making registered householders responsible for residents and lodgers. See Eitel, *Europe in China*, p. 429. It gave the police undue power to interfere with Chinese life. See 'Report by the Registrar General', *Blue Book* 1866, p. 241 and *Blue Book* 1867, p. 248.

65. MacDonnell to Granville, 18 August 1869, #775: CO 129/138.

66. A cumulative membership list was printed in the Hospital's *Zhengxinlu* (徵信錄) (Annual Reports) until 1907. MacDonnell headed the list.

67. Report by the Attorney General upon Ordinance no. 3 of 1870, entitled 'An Ordinance enacted by the Governor of Hong Kong with the Advice of the Legislative Council thereof for establishing a Chinese Hospital to be supported by Voluntary Contributions, for erecting the same into an Eleemosynary Corporation', enclosed in MacDonnell to Granville, 9 April 1870, #903: CO 129/144.

68. Report by the Attorney General upon Ordinance no. 3 of 1870.

69. Julian Pauncefote (1828–1902), Attorney General, Hong Kong, 1866; Chief Justice of Leeward Islands, 1874; Assistant Under-secretary of State for the Colonies, 1874; Assistant Under-secretary of State for the Foreign Office, 1876; Permanent Under-secretary of State for Foreign Affairs, 1882. He later became British Ambassador to Washington.

70. *DP*, 25 May 1872.

71. Report by the Attorney General upon Ordinance no. 3 of 1870.

72. Report by the Attorney General upon Ordinance no. 3 of 1870.

73. Report by the Attorney General upon Ordinance no. 3 of 1870.
74. Report by the Attorney General upon Ordinance no. 3 of 1870. A 13th Director was added afterwards and listed in the Committee list in the *Zhengxinlu.*
75. See Hao Yen-p'ing, *The Comprador in Nineteenth-Century China — Bridge between East and West* (Cambridge, Mass.: Harvard University Press, 1970).
76. See the description of the Hospital's opening in Chapter 3; unfortunately the newspaper reports are not specific about which of the Directors were wearing peacock feathers. See Chapter 3, note 1. The pursuit of Chinese honours is discussed in Chapter 4.
77. 'Surveyor General's Report', *Blue Book* 1856, pp. 65–91.
78. Notification of 9 October 1869, *HKGG* 1869, p. 477.

Notes to Chapter 3

1. *CM,* 14 February 1872; *DP* and *Daily Advertizer,* 15 February 1872; *Zhongwai xinwen qiri bao* (中外新聞七日報) (*China and World News Weekly*) (hereafter *ZW*), 17 February 1872. This last journal was published and appended to the *China Mail* from March 1871 to March 1872 when the *Huazi ribao* (華字日報) (*Chinese Mail*) was published separately. Unfortunately the *Huazi ribao* is only extant from 1895.
2. K. C. Wong and Wu Lien-teh, *History of Chinese Medicine* (Tientsin: The Tientsin Press, 1932), Book I, p. 5.
3. Governor's speech, extracted in *DP,* 15 February 1872.
4. *Daily Advertizer,* 15 February 1872.
5. Isabella Bird, *The Golden Chersonese* (Kuala Lumpur: Oxford University Press, 1967; first published 1883), pp. 87–8. Isabella Bird visited the Hospital with Sir John Pope Hennessy in January 1879.
6. Some of the plaques will be discussed below. Many can still be found at the Tung Wah Hospital, the Group's Museum at Kwong Wah Hospital, and the Man Mo Temple. See Plates.
7. *Daily Advertizer,* 15 February 1872.
8. '*Donghua yiyuan guitiao*' (東華醫院規條) ('Regulations of the Tung Wah Hospital') (hereafter '*Guitiao*'), p. 21a. These are included in the *Zhengxinlu* 1874, and reprinted each year, with additional regulations in subsequent years. This was confirmed by Bird, *Golden Chersonese,* p. 89.
9. Bird, *Golden Chersonese,* p. 90; see rules regarding this in '*Guitiao*', pp. 31a–33a.
10. Dr John Kerr ran the Canton Medical Missionary Society Hospital. See Wong and Wu, *History of Chinese Medicine*; and William Lockhart, *The Medical Missionary in China* (London: Hurst & Blackett, 1861). Kerr was the author of 'Chinese Medicine', *China Review* 1, (1872), pp. 176–81.
11. John Kerr, 'Native Benevolent Institutions of Canton', part 2, *China Review* 3 (1874–5), p. 112. Although Lawrence W. Crissman in 'The Segmentary Structure of Overseas Chinese Communities', *Man* 2:2 (June, 1967), p. 197, claims that Chinese Hospital Committees were common, he gives no example of any operating in the nineteenth century; in fact, his time scope is unclear. This author argues that the Tung Wah Hospital was the first 'Chinese hospital', and the discussion will be taken up at the end of this chapter.
12. Report by the Attorney General upon Ordinance no. 3 of 1870 entitled 'An Ordinance enacted by the Governor of Hong Kong with the Advice of the Legislative Council thereof for establishing a Chinese Hospital to be supported by Voluntary Contributions, for erecting the same into an Eleemosynary Corporation', enclosed in MacDonnell to Granville, 9 April 1870, #903: CO 129/144.

13. Guo Songdao (郭嵩燾), *Guo Songdao riji* (郭嵩燾日記) (*The Diary of Guo Songdao*), 4 volumes (Zhangsha: 1981–), Vol. III [1875–1879] (1982), p. 817. Guo (1818–91) became China's first Minister to London in 1877, and later also to Paris, but he served only two years before returning to China in 1879. As one of the early reformist officials he was censured by his peers, but has won acclaim in modern times. See Guo Tingyi (郭廷以), *Guo Songdao xiansheng nianpu* (郭嵩燾先生年譜) (*Chronological Biography of Guo Songdao*) (Taipei: 1971). For his own works see *Yangzhi shuwu yiji* (養知書屋遺集) (*Works from the Yangzhi studio*) (Taipei: photographic reprint, 1964). There are also a number of articles on his thought, for example, Wu Pangyi (吳鵬翼) '*Zhongguo xiandaihua yundong di yishi — Guo Songdao di yangwu guan*' (中國現代化運動的異士：一郭嵩燾的洋務觀) ('An eccentric in China's modernization: Guo Songdao's concept of *yangwu*') in Chang Hao (張灝) and others, *Wan Qing sixiang* (晚清思想) (*Thought in the Late Qing Period*) (Taipei: 1971), pp. 271–88.
14. Wong and Wu, *History of Chinese Medicine*, pp. 208–10; Lockhart, *Medical Missionary*.
15. Report of the Attorney General upon Ordinance no. 3 of 1870.
16. '*Guitiao*', p. 2b.
17. *TWR*, p. 3.
18. '*Guitiao*', p. 8a.
19. '*Guitiao*', p. 2b.
20. '*Guitiao*', p. 8b. In 1903 the number of Directors was increased to 16, with representatives from three additional guilds, the Chinese Bankers' Guild, the Insurance Guild, and the Foreign Goods Importers and Exporters' Guild. Another change took place in 1916 when opium became a government monopoly and for the first time in 54 years there was no representative from the Opium Guild. The guild-based selection largely remained until the mid-1920s when the number of *yinhu* started to grow, and in the 1930s guilds ceased to send representatives.
21. The procedure of elections is described by Sir M. K. Lo, Tung Wah Chairman of 1929. See Vincent H. G. Jarrett, 'Old Hong Kong', articles on Hong Kong history taken from the *South China Morning Post* from 17 June 1933 to 13 April 1935, Vol. II, pp. 534–5. Although he was speaking in the 1930s, there is reason to believe the descriptions were applicable to the nineteenth century as well. One reason is the consistency of the guild and *yinhu* representation. Secondly, a number of invitations to guilds and their nominees are found in the Tung Wah archives which testify to this procedure. (See below.) Thirdly the largely ritualistic show of hands by the kaifongs representing 'elections' was carried out until 1967, according to Mr Leo Lee, Chairman of 1960. See Tung Wah to Compradores' Guild, 20 November 1900 asking it to make nominations (Tung Wah Hospital, '*Fachu xinbu*' (發出信簿) ('Outward Letters') 1900–1907' (hereafter '*Xinbu*' I), p. 253); Tung Wah to Wei Yuk, 20 November 1900, inviting him to be Director (Tung Wah '*Xinbu*' I), p. 154; Tung Wah to Fung Wa Chuen, 31 October 1901, insisting that he accept the invitation to serve (Tung Wah '*Xinbu*' I), p. 432; see also '*Xinbu*' I, pp. 270, 273 for similar letters.
22. 'Registrar General's Report, 1905', *Hong Kong Sessional Papers* (hereafter *HKSP*) 1906, pp. 225–54.
23. H. J. Lethbridge, 'A Chinese Association in Hong Kong: the Tung Wah', in his *Hong Kong: Stability and Change, A Collection of Essays* (Hong Kong: Oxford University Press, 1978), pp. 52–70, pp. 58, 60.
24. Letter signed 'A member of the Chinese community' to the *China Mail*, 13 November 1875.
25. Crissman, 'The Segmentary Structure'. For more concrete examples, see *Huaqiao zhi zongzuan weiyuan hui* (ed.), *Huaqiao zhi zongzhi* ('Records of Overseas Chinese, a Summary') (Taipei: 1964), *passim*, which provides informa-

tion on the composition of various organizations. Gary G. Hamilton, 'Ethnicity and Regionalism: Some Factors Influencing Chinese Identities in Southeast Asia', *Ethnicity* 4 (1977), pp. 337–51 and 'Regional Associations and the Chinese City: A Comparative Perspective', *Comparative Studies in Society and History* 21 (1979), pp. 346–61. Eve Armentrout-Ma, 'Urban Chinese at the Sinitic Frontier: Social Organization in United States's Chinatowns 1849–1898', *MAS* 17:1 (1983), pp. 107–35 and 'Fellow Regional Associations in the Ch'ing Dynasty: Organization in the Flux for Mobile People: A Preliminary Survey', *MAS* 18 (1984), pp. 307–30.

26. Ho Ping-ti, *Zhongguo huiguan shilun (A Historical Survey of Landsmannschaften in China)* (Taipei: 1966).

27. By studying the places of origin of guild representatives on the Tung Wah Hospital Boards, one can see that each of the guilds was represented by persons from more than one region, showing that the guilds, at least the ones represented, were cross-regional in nature. See Elizabeth Sinn, 'A Preliminary History of Regional Associations in Pre-War Hong Kong', conference paper presented at the Centre of Asian Studies, December 1986, to be published by the Centre. This subject deserves much more research.

28. Wu Tingfang (伍廷芳) (1842–1922) was born in Singapore and graduated at the St Paul's College in Hong Kong. Having studied law in England, he became the first Chinese barrister in Hong Kong, and then its first Chinese Legislative Councillor in 1880. He left in 1882 to join Li Hongzhang's staff. From 1896 he was Chinese Minister to Washington, Madrid, and Lima. After the 1911 revolution, he worked in the Judiciary Department of the Chinese Republic, but later joined Sun Yat-sen against the Peking government. There are many works on him, the major ones being, Linda Pomerantz Shin, 'China in Transition: The Role of Wu Ting-fang (1842–1922)' (Ph.D. thesis, University of California, Los Angeles, 1970); Yu Ch'i-hsing (余啓興), '*Wu Tingfang yu Xianggang zhi guanxi*' (伍廷芳與香港之關係) ('Wu Tingfang and Hong Kong') in *Shou Luo Xianglin jiaoshou lunwen ji* (壽羅香林教授論文集) (*Essays in Chinese Studies presented to Professor Lo Hsiang-lin*) (Hong Kong: 1970), pp. 255–78; Chang Yun-chao, 'Wu T'ing-fang's Contribution towards Political Reforms in late Ch'ing period' (Ph.D. thesis, University of Hong Kong, 1982).

29. Wang Tao (王韜) (1828–97) was a first degree holder, who during the Taiping rebellion was implicated as a collaborator and escaped to Hong Kong. He helped James Legge translate the Chinese Classics, and travelled with him to Britain and parts of Europe. Returning to Hong Kong, he wrote frequently in the newspapers and to Chinese officials on the need for China to reform and was considered an authority on foreign matters. In 1874 he founded the *Xunhuan ribao* (循環日報) (*Universal Circulating Herald*), making him an important contributor to the development of modern Chinese journalism. Many works have been written about him, the major ones being Paul A. Cohen, 'Wang T'ao and Incipient Chinese Nationalism', *Journal of Asian Studies* XXVI:4 (August 1967), pp. 557–74 and *Between Tradition and Modernity: Wang T'ao and Reform in Late Ch'ing China* (Cambridge, Mass.: Harvard University Press, 1974); Lai Guanglin (賴光臨), '*Wang Tao yu Xunhuan ribao*' (王韜與循環日報) ('Wang Tao and *Xunhuan ribao*'), *Baoxue* (報學) (*Journalism*) 3:9 (Taipei: December, 1967), pp. 52–64; Lee Chi-fang, 'Wang T'ao: His Life, Thought and Scholarship and Literary Achievement' (Ph.D. thesis, University of Wisconsin, 1973); Henry McAleavy, *Wang T'ao: Life and Writings of a Displaced Person* (London: China Society, 1953); Nishisato Yoshiyuki (西里喜行), '*Ō Tō to Junken nippo ni tsuide*' (王韜と循環日報について) ('Wang Tao and the *Xunhuan ribao*'), *Tōyōshi kenkiū* (東洋史研究) (*Chinese Historical Studies*) 43:3 (December 1985), pp. 508–47. Wang was a most prolific writer but his thoughts are best revealed in his *Taoyuan*

wenlu waibian (弢園文錄外編) (*Additional essays of Wang Tao*), 12 *juan* (Peking: 1959; first published Hong Kong, 1883). For the *Xunhuan ribao, see Xunhuan ribao liushi zhounian jinian tekan* (循環日報六十周年紀念特刊) (*Special Publication to Commemorate the 60th Anniversary of the 'Xunhuan ribao'*) (Hong Kong: 1932). He was an Assistant Director of the 1872 Committee.

30. Chan Ayin, also known as Chen Aiting (陳靄亭), was an Assistant Director of the 1873 Committee. See Smith, 'The Emergence of a Chinese Élite' in his *Chinese Christians: Élites, Middlemen and the Church in Hong Kong* (Hong Kong: Oxford University Press, 1985), p. 133; Lin Youlan (林友蘭), '*Chen Aiting yu Xianggang Huazi ribao*' (陳靄亭與香港華字日報) ('Chen Aiting and the *Chinese Mail* of Hong Kong'), *Baoxue* 5:10 (June 1978), pp. 131–3. His appointment to the Chinese mission is given in *DP*, 1 April 1878. The *Huazi ribao* was started in 1872 by Chen with Ng Choy's assistance; see *Huazi ribao qishiyi zhounian jinian tekan* (華字日報七十一周年紀念特刊) (*Publication to commemorate the 71st Anniversary of the Huazi ribao*) (Hong Kong: 1934). Though according to many sources the *Huazi ribao* was started in 1864, there is evidence that it did not begin until 1872. See *ZW*, 30 March 1872. See also Chapter 4 for his diplomatic career; Chapter 4, Note 158.

31. Ho Fuk Tong (何福堂) was an Ordinary Committee member of the Founding Committee. See Smith, *Chinese Christians*, pp. 129–33; G. H. Chao, *The Life and Times of Sir Kai Ho Kai* (Hong Kong: Chinese University Press, 1981), pp. 9–13.

32. Ho Kai (何啓) (1859–1914) was born in Hong Kong and educated in the United Kingdom both as a lawyer and a doctor. There are a large number of works on him, especially as a reform thinker. The major ones are Chiu Ling-yeong, 'The Life and Thought of Sir Kai Ho Kai' (Ph.D. thesis, University of Sydney, 1968); Ts'ai Jung-fang, 'Comprador Ideologists in Modern China: Ho Kai (He Ch'i) (1859–1914) and Hu Li-yuan (1847–1916)' (Ph.D. thesis, University of California, Los Angeles, 1975). A more general work is Choa, *Sir Kai Ho Kai*.

33. There was some confusion over the term 'Committee'. Sometimes it was used to denote the Board of Directors, and sometimes the whole General Committee. In Chinese, there was the same confusion over the word *zhishi* (值事) which referred to Directors, to the Ordinary Committee, and sometimes to the whole General Committee. The names of the Board of Directors were published in the *HKGG* from 1880. The General Committees of previous years were listed cumulatively in the *Zhengxinlu*.

34. 'Guitiao', p. 4a.

35. 'Guitiao', p. 11a.

36. Smith, *Chinese Christians*, p. 130. Smith deals with Ho Amei in great detail in 'A Sense of History', a long series of articles in the *South China Morning Post* appearing each Wednesday between January 1978 and May 1979. The first part of the series is reprinted in *JHKBRAS* 26 (1986), pp. 144–264.

37. See Epilogue.

38. In 1873 the members numbered 870, in 1885 1,278, and in 1896, 2,345. These figures are not precise since there were some 'double entries'. It can be seen that the growth in membership was slow.

39. 'Guitiao', pp. 4a–5b; 8b–9a.

40. Meetings were sometimes attended by hundreds of people and all present voted. A clear picture of how meetings went can be seen from the '*Dongshiju huiyi lu*' (董事局會議錄) ('Minutes of Board Meetings') of the Hospital which are extant from 1904; to a large extent these later meetings were similar to the nineteenth century ones.

41. 'Guitiao', p. 3a. For a later example of notices in the newspapers, see *Huazi ribao*, 4 January 1906.

42. 'Guitiao', p. 3a.

43. 'Guitiao', p. 5b.

44. 'Guitiao', p. 2b.

45. Donald R. de Glopper, 'Temple, Faction and Loan Club', quoted in Steven P. Sangren, 'Traditional Chinese Corporations: Beyond Kinship', *Journal of Asian Studies* XLIII:3 (May 1984), pp. 391–415, p. 406.

46. 'Guitiao', p. 15b.

47. 'Colonial Surgeon's Report of 1869', *HKGG* 1870, pp. 240–52, p. 240.

48. *Daily Advertizer*, 15 February 1872.

49. 'Guitiao', pp. 1a–ab, 18b; '*Xuzheng guitiao*', pp. 38a–38b. The '*Xuzheng guitiao*' (續增規條) ('Additional Regulations') were added in 1872 and are found in the *Zhengxinlu* 1874, pp. 26a–40a, after the 'Guitiao'.

50. 'Guitiao', p. 13b.

51. Ayres' evidence, *TWR*, pp. 60–5, p. 63; Lockhart, *Medical Missionary*, pp. 112–13.

52. *TWR*, p. 26.

53. Au Ki-nam's (Ou jinan) (區建南) evidence, *TWR*, pp. 30–1. Au had been one of the vaccinators before he became a clerk at the Hospital.

54. Au Ki-nam's evidence, *TWR*, pp. 30–1.

55. For example when Zheng Xinhu (曾心壺), a former doctor at the Tung Wah wrote '*Jiaoqi chuyan*' (腳氣芻言) ('Notes on beri beri'), enclosed in *Changyan ji* (昌言集) (*Collection of Brilliant Statements*) (no publisher; no date), pp. 307–58, he took care to include letters of recommendation from the Tung Wah Hospital's chairmen (pp. 332–4). A dentist who had given free consultation at the Tung Wah also advertized the fact in the papers, showing that evidently this added to his credibility (*XH*, 11 February 1874). Later it became the practice of other hospitals to send their treatises to be assessed by Tung Wah doctors. See Tung Wah to Nanhua (南華) Hospital, 6 September 1900, in Tung Wah '*Xinbu*' I, p. 219; Tung Wah to Tongji (同濟) Hospital, 6 July 1901, '*Xinbu*' I, p. 375.

56. Guo, *Riji*, Vol. III, p. 817.

57. *XH*, 11 February 1874; see also Note 55.

58. Many works claim that formal medical training had existed. See Chen Bangxian, *Zhongguo yixue shi* (*History of Medicine in China*) (Shanghai: 1955). More recent debates centre on when medical education was revived in modern times: see Lin Qianliang (林乾艮), '*Wo guo jindai caoji de Zhongyi xuexiao*' (我國近代早期的中醫學校) ('Early Chinese medical schools in modern times'), *Zhonghua yishi zazhi* (中華醫學雜誌) (*Chinese Journal of Medical History*) 10:2 (February 1980), pp. 90–1; Jin Rihong (金日紅), '*Liji Yixuetang shimo ji jiaoxue gaikuang*' (利濟醫學堂始末及教學概況) ('A brief account of the Liji medical school'), *Zhonghua yishi zazhi* 12:2 (February 1982), pp. 90–2; Liu Xiaobin (劉小斌), '*Guangdong jindai de Zhongyi jiaoyu — tiyao*' (廣東近代的中醫教育－提要) ('Chinese medical education in modern Guangdong — abstract'), *Zhonghua yishi zazhi* 12:3 (March 1982), pp. 133–7; Fu Weikang (傅維康) and others, *Yiyao shihua* (醫藥史話) (*History of Medicine*) (Shanghai: 1982), pp. 135–40. But it seems that the Tung Wah's was the earliest effort.

59. 'Supplement to Annual Report on Government Education' — speech by the Governor at Central School, 25 January 1878 at annual distribution of prizes, *HKGG* 1878, pp. 311–21.

60. Frederick Stewart began his career in Hong Kong as Headmaster of the Central School in 1862, and was concurrently Inspector of Schools. He also acted as police magistrate and coroner. He became Registrar General and Treasurer in 1883. In 1887 he became Colonial Secretary and Auditor General. He died in Hong Kong in 1889. See Jarrett, 'Old Hong Kong', Vol. IV, p. 1011.

61. Guo, '*Riji*', Vol. III, p. 817; '*Simao nian yi xiyi guitiao*' (己卯年擬習醫規條)

('Regulations regarding medical training, 1879') were included in subsequent *Zhengxinlu*. Here, the reference is taken from *Zhengxinlu* 1885, pp. 35a–36b.

62. Guo, '*Riji*', Vol. III, p. 817; *DP*, 30 June 1880.

63. *Zhengxinlu* 1885, p. 36b.

64. *TWR*, p. 31; *XH*, 12 July 1880.

65. *TWR*, p. 31. The Po Leung Kuk (*baoliangju*) (保良局) is discussed in Chapter 4.

66. Bird, *Golden Chersonese*, pp. 88–9.

67. *DP*, 15 May 1873.

. 68. 'Colonial Surgeon's Report for 1872', *HKGG* 1873, pp. 228–38. This compared with 4.86% for European patients and 2.39% for coloured patients and an overall average of 6.82% for all admissions.

69. For the death rates of each year, see Colonial Surgeon's Reports.

70. 'Registrar General's Report, 1893', *HKGG*, pp. 157–83.

71. 'Guitiao', pp. 1b–2a.

72. ·*DP*, 21 March 1874.

73. *DP*, 21 March 1874; 'Guitiao', pp. 1b–2a.

74. '*Xuzheng guitiao*', pp. 32a–32b, 37a–37b; the death figures are taken from *Zhengxinlu* 1893, Part 6: pp. 1b–15b; 'Registrar General's Report for 1891' *HKGG* 1892, pp. 357–487.

75. 'Registrar General's Report, 1895', *HKSP* 1896, pp. 389–416, p. 391.

76. For James H. Stewart Lockhart (1858–1937) see H. J. Lethbridge, 'Sir James H. Stewart Lockhart: Colonial Civil Servant and Scholar', in his *Stability and Change*, pp. 130–62; for his career in Weihaiwei, see Pamela Atwell, *British Mandarins and Chinese Reformers: the British Administration of Weihaiwei, 1898–1930 and the Territory's Return to Chinese Rule* (Hong Kong: Oxford University Press, 1985). His personal papers are deposited at the University of Edinburgh in the custody of George Watsons College. A biography is being prepared by Ms Shiona Airlie.

77. 'Registrar General's Report, 1891', p. 362.

78. 'Colonial Surgeon's Report, 1877', *HKGG* 1878, pp. 321–58.

79. The Alice Memorial Hospital was established in 1887 in memory of Ho Kai's English wife Alice who died in 1884. It was run by the London Missionary Society. See Carl T. Smith, 'Sun Yat-sen's School Days in Hong Kong: The Establishment of the Alice Memorial Hospital', *Ching Feng*, XXI:2 (1978), pp. 78–94; Choa, *Sir Kai Ho Kai*, pp. 55–7; *Alice Ho Mui Ling Nethersole Hospital 1887–1967* ([Hong Kong: the Hospital, 1967]); E. H. Paterson, *A Hospital for Hong Kong 1887–1987* (Hong Kong: the Nethersole Hospital, 1987).

80. The Nethersole Hospital was founded in 1893 for treatment of women and children. It was also run by the London Missionary Society; see Paterson, *A Hospital for Hong Kong*.

81. *TWR*, p. 62. For instance, the number of in-patients at the Alice Memorial Hospital were 872, 722, and 614 (1892–4) compared to 2,455, 2,857, and 2,359 for the same years at the Tung Wah. Statistics for the Alice Memorial Hospital for 1887 to 1891 can be found in the 'Registrar General's Report for 1892', *HKGG* 1893, pp. 439–66, p. 464. See also Dr Thomson's evidence, *TWR*, pp. 55–9, p. 57.

82. See Joseph Needham, *China and the Origins of Immunology* (Hong Kong: Centre of Asian Studies, University of Hong Kong, 1980).

83. Wong and Wu, *History of Chinese Medicine*, Book II, Chapter III, 'Introduction of Jennerian Vaccination against Small-pox in China and its Future Progress in the Country'.

84. 'Colonial Surgeon's Report', *Blue Book* 1852, pp. 139–63, p. 143; the merits of vaccination were extolled by Chinese in *XH*, 18 May 1874.

85. 'Colonial Surgeon's Report for 1882', *HKGG* 1883, pp. 637–60, p. 643; '*Guitiao*', p. 25b; 'Registrar General's Report for 1869', *HKGG* 1870, pp. 127–9.

86. 'Statement of H. E. Governor Sir John Pope Hennessy, KCMG, on the Census Returns and the Progress of the Colony' in *HKGG* 1881, pp. 415–30, p. 421.

87. 'Colonial Surgeon's Report, 1892', p. 594; Barker to Knutsford, 30 September 1891, #321: CO 129/251.

88. 'Statement of Hennessy', p. 420.

89. Ayres was Colonial Surgeon from 1873 to 1897. See Jarrett, 'Old Hong Kong', Vol. I, p. 31.

90. 'Colonial Surgeon's Report, 1874', *HKGG* 1875, pp. 170–8, p. 172.

91. 'Colonial Surgeon's Report, 1876', *HKGG* 1877, p. 206.

92. *Zhengxinlu*, 1878, p. 116a for 1876 accounts; 'Statement of Hennessy', p. 420. The governor claimed the Hospital's vaccination on the Mainland started in 1878; in fact the *Zhengxinlu* shows that it had started in 1876.

93. George Bowen (1821–99) was born in County Donegal and was Fellow of Braesenose College, 1844, and President of the University of Corfu, 1847. He was Chief Secretary of the Government in the Ionian Islands, 1854; Governor of Queensland, 1859; New Zealand, 1867; Victoria, 1872; Mauritius, 1879; and Hong Kong, 1883–5. See Endacott, *Government and People*, p. 97, n. 1; Stanley Lane-Poole, *Thirty Years of Colonial Government: Selections from the Despatches and Letters of the Right Honourable Sir George Ferguson Bowen*, G.C.M.G., 2 volumes (London: Longmans, Green, 1887).

94. Bowen to Derby, 25 August 1884 #298: CO 129/217; Bowen to Derby, 29 April 1885, #199: CO 129/221.

95. 'Colonial Surgeon's Report, 1871', *HKGG* 1872, pp. 128–41, p. 129.

96. Arthur Kennedy (1810–83) had an army career before serving in the Irish Government. He was Governor of the Gambia, 1851; Sierra Leone, 1852; Western Australia, 1854; Vancouver Island, 1863; and West African Settlements, 1867 before becoming Governor of Hong Kong, 1872–7. After that, he served as Governor of Queensland, 1878. See Endacott, *Government and People*, p. 81, n. 3.

97. '*Xuzheng guitiao*', pp. 38b–40a; *DP*, 12 July 1873.

98. Bowen to Derby, 25 August 1884, #298: CO 129/217.

99. Minute on Bowen to Derby, 25 August 1884, #298.

100. 'Smallpox Epidemic Report', *HKGG* 1888, pp. 79–82, p. 81.

101. 'Smallpox Epidemic Report', p. 80; 'Colonial Surgeon's Report for 1888', *HKGG* 1889, pp. 573–616, p. 587.

102. Bird, *Golden Chersonese*, p. 87; compare Governor Sir G. William des Voeux's impression in *My Colonial Service*, 2 volumes (London: 1903), Vol. II, pp. 199–201.

103. For Manson, see Philip H. Manson-Bahr and A. Alcock, *The Life and Work of Sir Patrick Manson* (London: Cassell, 1927).

104. The College of Medicine was founded by the London Missionary Society in 1887 for the training of young Chinese men. Classes took place at the Alice Memorial Hospital. See Choa, *Sir Kai Ho Kai*, pp. 57–69; Lo Hsiang-lin, *Xianggang yu Zhong Xi wenhua zhi jiaoliu* (香港與中西文化之交流) (*Hong Kong and East-West Cultural Exchange*) (Hong Kong: 1961), pp. 135–77. The most recent work on the College is D. M. Emrys Evans, *Constancy of Purpose* (Hong Kong: Hong Kong University Press, 1987) which gives an account of the College as the forerunner of the University of Hong Kong's Medical Faculty.

105. Dr Patrick Manson's address to mark the inauguration of the Hong Kong College of Medicine, quoted in Choa, *Sir Kai Ho Kai*, p. 56.

106. F. H. Hineley, 'Introduction' to *New Cambridge Modern History*, Vol.

XI, *Material Progress and World Wide Problems 1870-1898* (Cambridge: Cambridge University Press, 1967; first edition 1962), pp. 1-48; Trevor I. Williams, 'Science and Technology', *New Cambridge Modern History*, Vol. XI, pp. 76-100, pp. 82-4; R. Bledstein, *The Culture of Professionalism* (New York: W. W. Norton, 1976); E. Friedson (ed.), *Profession of Medicine* (New York: Dodd Mead, 1970); D. Hamilton, 'The Nineteenth Century Surgical Revolution — Antisepsis or Better Nutrition?', *Bulletin of History of Medicine* 56 (1982), pp. 30-40.

107. See Note 105. The development of hospitals can be seen in E. Friedson (ed.), *The Hospital in Modern Society* (New York: Free Press, 1963); I. Waddington, 'The Role of the Hospital in the Development of Modern Medicine', *Sociology* 7 (1973), pp. 211-24; M. J. Vogel, 'The Transformation of the American Hospital', in S. Reverby and D. Rosner (eds.), *Health Care in America* (Philadelphia: Temple University Press, 1979).

108. 'Colonial Surgeon's Report for 1872', p. 229.

109. 'Colonial Surgeon's Report for 1872', p. 229.

110. 'Colonial Surgeon's Report for 1872', p. 228.

111. Ayres to Lockhart, 9 June 1896, *TWR*, pp. LXXV-VI.

112. 'Colonial Surgeon's Report for 1873', p. 158.

113. 'Colonial Surgeon's Report, 1874', enclosed in Hennessy to Kimberley, 15 July 1880, in 'Papers on Restrictions upon Chinese in Hong Kong', (426) 1881, *BPP*, XXV, pp. 641-760, p. 690.

114. 'Colonial Surgeon's Report for 1876', p. 206.

115. 'Colonial Surgeon's Report for 1876', p. 206.

116. Eitel's Report on Paupers, enclosed in Hennessy to Kimberley, 26 May 1881, #73: CO 129/193.

117. Sergei Ticozzi, *Xianggang Tianzhujiao zhanggu* (香港天主教学故) (Stories of the Catholic Church in Hong Kong (Hong Kong: 1983); Liu Yuesheng (劉粵聲), *Xianggang Jidujiao huishi* (香港基督教會史) (*A History of the Protestant Church in Hong Kong*) (Hong Kong: 1941); E. J. Eitel, *Europe in China* (Hong Kong: Oxford University Press, 1983), pp. 391-3. It seems that the churches were more successful providing education than other forms of welfare.

118. *Zhengxinlu* 1893, Part 6: pp. 15a-20b.

119. For coffin-home rules, see '*Xuzheng guitiao*' pp. 37a-37b; the earliest evidence of such service was in January 1874 when the Hospital issued a notice calling upon residents to take away a number of dead bodies which had been forwarded to it from Shanghai and elsewhere, to be returned to native places, *DP*, 12 January 1874; in that year it also repatriated coffins from Japan, *XH*, 8 April 1874; there were trans-shipments of human remains from Annam in 1878, *Zhengxinlu* 1878, p. 56b, and 1887 (*Guangzhao gungsuo* (廣肇公所) (Regional association of the Guangzhou and Zhaoqing prefectures) of Cholon to Tung Wah, 10 May 1887, in Po Leung Kuk, '*Dinghai nian gebu laiwang xin chaoteng bu*' (丁亥年各埠來往信抄謄簿) ('Copy of letters to and from abroad, 1887') (hereafter, '*Xinbu*' III); from the USA, see *XH*, 21 April 1882 and 1 June 1883; from Canada, after 1883, Edgar Wickberg, *From China to Canada, A History of the Chinese Communities in Canada* (Toronto: Minister of Supply and Services, Canada, 1982), p. 66; from Sydney, *Zhengxinlu* 1887, Part 4: p. 30b; in 1887, it also buried 95 coffins from overseas, *Zhengxinlu* 1878, pp. 19b-21a. Coffins from Annam and California were often buried in Hong Kong when they were unclaimed, *XH*, 1 June 1883; Liu Pei-ch'i (劉伯驥), *Meiguo Huaqiao shi* (美國華僑史) ('*A History of the Chinese in the United States of America*') (Taipei: 1976), p. 164.

120. Tung Wah to the Hall of Sustaining Love, 20 March 1899, Tung Wah '*Xinbu*' I, p. 6.

121. *Zhengxinlu* 1874, Preface and p. 85b.

122. See Tung Wah to Lockhart, 28 July 1899 on the removal of old graves near Tokwawan (Tung Wah '*Xinbu*' I, p. 58); Tung Wah to May, 11 April 1900 on the removal of graves from Aberdeen (Tung Wah 'Xinbu' I, p. 146); Tung Wah to Brewin, ? February 1901 on the removal of graves from Matauwei to make room for a church (Tung Wah 'Xinbu' I, p. 312); Tung Wah to Brewin, 28 March 1901 on the removal of graves from Mount Davis (Tung Wah 'Xinbu' I, p. 313); Tung Wah to Brewin, 18 April, 1901 (Tung Wah 'Xinbu' I, p. 324) on the removal of graves from Wongneichung; Tung Wah to Brewin, 20 May 1901 (Tung Wah 'Xinbu' I, p. 340) on the moving of graves from Mount Davis; Tung Wah to Brewin, 8 October 1901 (Tung Wah 'Xinbu' I, p. 414), asking him to clear accounts for the removing of graves each month, and on problems over the claim of ownership of land; Tung Wah to Brewin, 14 October 1901, (Tung Wah 'Xinbu' I, p. 419) on negotiation between government and owners over grave land; Tung Wah to Brewin, 31 October 1901 (Tung Wah 'Xinbu' I, p. 431) on the need to pay workers and on the above negotiation; Tung Wah to Brewin, 6 August (Tung Wah 'Xinbu' I, p. 381): the Tung Wah had been asked to remove certain graves, and it advised the government to put notices in newspapers and in street posters to allow relatives to come and claim the bones, and tell them where the new locations would be; Tung Wah to Brewin, 16 October 1901 (Tung Wah 'Xinbu' I, p. 421) on the removal of graves from Kennedy Town. These letters give us some idea of the extensive work the Tung Wah did regarding graves and the government's heavy dependence on it. Another interesting series of letters was from the Tung Wah to the Dunshantang (敦善堂) in Kobe which shows the Hospital sending workers to help exhume bones in Kobe, placing bones in the coffin-home and then advertising them and receiving coffins from Kobe. (Tung Wah to Dunshantang, 18 September 1899, 'Xinbu' I, p. 69; 13 October 1899, 'Xinbu' I, p. 91; 14 March 1900, 'Xinbu' I, p. 139; 21 April 1901, 'Xinbu' I, p. 325).

123. 'Registrar General's Report, 1895', *HKSP* 1896, pp. 389–416, p. 391.

124. *Zhengxinlu* 1873, pp. 30b–32b; 61a–61b; 1893; Part 4, pp. 10b–12b, 28a–32a; Part 5, pp. 16a–26a; also see *Zhengxinlu* 1878, p. 113b for repatriation of destitutes from Annam; 'Tung Wah Hospital Report for 1877', *HKGG* 1878, pp. 351–2, p. 351. Unfortunately, this report was the only one of its kind. An early example of repatriation was that of the emigrants on the *Dolores Uqarte* in 1871 (see Chapter 4); it also repatriated prostitutes from America (*DP*, 20 October 1873); a case of blind men repatriated from Australia through the Tung Wah can be seen in correspondence between the Immigration Office at Perth and the Colonial Secretary in Hong Kong: Documents at C. S. Office, File no. 183 at Battye Library, Perth, Western Australia. I am grateful to Ms Anne Atkinson for this information. See also Police Magistrate to Tung Wah, 18 June 1884, in Po Leung Kuk, 'Jiashen nian laiwang xinbu' (甲申年來往信簿) ('Records of correspondence, 1884') (hereafter, Po Leung Kuk '*Xinbu*' I) asking the Tung Wah to allow three boys waiting for shipment to Amoy to stay at the Hospital; Tung Wah and Po Leung Kuk to Hall of Sustaining Love (see Note 161), 19 August 1884, (Po Leung Kuk 'Xinbu' I) about sending four kidnapped men to it; Jinghu (鏡湖) Hospital, Macao to Tung Wah, 30 June 1887 (Po Leung Kuk '*Xinbu*' III) on repatriating girls to Yangjiang (陽江); Hall of Sustaining Love to Tung Wah, 15 July 1887, (Po Leung Kuk '*Xinbu*' I) on repatriating kidnapped girls to Hanoi; Jinghu Hospital to Tung Wah, 22 July 1887 (Po Leung Kuk '*Xinbu*' I) on repatriating Annamese women; Liang Tingcan (梁廷贊), Chinese Consul at San Francisco to Tung Wah, 19 December 1887, (Po Leung Kuk '*Xinbu*' I) on sending kidnapped women to Canton via the Tung Wah; Guangzhao gongsuo (廣肇公所) of Saigon to Tung Wah, 17 October 1888 (Po Leung Kuk, '*Wuzinian gebu laiwang dibu*' (戊子年各埠來往信底簿) ('Copies of letters to and from abroad, 1888) (hereafter '*Xinbu*' IV) on kidnapped women returned to Hong Kong for repatria-

tion; Taihe (太和) Hospital at Beihai to Tung Wah and Po Leung Kuk, 24 October 1891 (Po Leung Kuk, '*Xinmao nian gebu laiwang xinbu*' (辛卯年各埠來往信簿) ('Copies of letters to and from abroad, 1891') (hereafter '*Xinbu*' X) on a couple to be repatriated to Canton; Guanghe zhacan (廣和茶棧) (Guanghe tea house, Amoy), 18 October 1891 '*Xinbu*' X) asking help for the repatriation of a boy returning from Amoy to Canton via Hong Kong; Hall of Sustaining Love, 23 October 1891 ('*Xinbu*' X) on two kidnapped women to be repatriated on Qiongzhou (瓊州); Po Leung Kuk to Guangren (廣仁) Hospital, 17 November 1898 (Po Leung Kuk, '*Wuxu nian ji gebu xinbu*' (戊戌年寄各埠信簿) ('Letters going abroad, 1898') (hereafter '*Xinbu*' XIX) on the repatriation of women from Singapore, request made to Tung Wah from the Chinese Consul at Singapore; Liang Bingqiu (梁炳球) to Tung Wah, 23 August 1902 (Po Leung Kuk, '*Renyin nian jie gebu xinbu*' (壬寅年接各埠信簿) ('Incoming letters from abroad, 1902') (hereafter '*Xinbu*' XXVIII) requests it to repatriate a maid sold by her husband to Singapore. The Tung Wah Hospital's fight against emigration abuses is discussed in the next chapter. See also Hennessy's praise for its work in sending poor people home in Hennessy to Kimberley, 26 May 1881, #73: CO 129/193.

125. *XH*, 4 August 1882; Chen Lanbin (陳蘭彬) was appointed Chinese Minister to Washington in 1875 but he did not actually leave China till 1878. See his '*Shi Mei jilue*' (使美紀略) ('A brief account of my ministry in America') in Wang Xiji (王錫祺), *Xiao fanghu cai yudi zong cao* (小方壺齋輿地叢鈔) (*Collected Texts on Geography from the Xiao fanghu cai Study*) (Shanghai: preface 1877; second supplement 1897); 2nd supplement, *ji* 12. See Tan Qianchu (譚乾初), '*Guba zaji*' (左巴雜記) ('Miscellaneous writings from Cuba'), in Wang, *Xiao fanghu cai yudi zong cao*, *ji* 12, p. 4b on the distribution of letters from Cuba by the Tung Wah. Tan was interpreter on Chen Lanbin's mission to Cuba in 1878. Hall of Sustaining Love to Tung Wah, 23 October 1891 (Po Leung Kuk '*Xinbu*' X) on the distribution of letters from Peru and San Francisco.

Later correspondence gives us some idea of the scale of its work. Each year, the Tonghui Zongju (通惠總局), a Chinese association founded in Peru in 1884 with close ties with the Tung Wah, sent letters and money for it to distribute and, in turn, the Tung Wah sent letters to the Zongju for distribution. See Tung Wah to Tonghui Zongju, 6 June 1899 (Tung Wah '*Xinbu*' I, p. 50): the Tung Wah had received a batch of 110 letters and Peruvian money which was converted to HK$2,945 which it would distribute with the letters. In return, the Tung Wah sent 131 letters to Peru; Tung Wah to Tonghui, 11 December 1900 (Tung Wah '*Xinbu*' I, p. 271) acknowledged receipt of 141 letters and Peruvian money approximately equivalent to HK$11,314. Unfortunately, it is impossible to collect statistics systematically. However these letters give some idea of the hundreds of letters and tens of thousands of dollars which went through the Tung Wah each year. One must also bear in mind that each letter and remittance must be individually handled to ensure safety in order to appreciate the amount of work involved.

See also Tung Wah to Guangzhao shanzhuang (廣肇山莊), 10 November 1900 (Tung Wah '*Xinbu*' I, p. 250) about money remitted, part of which was distributed, and the rest paid to the Tung Wah to offset expenses; Tung Wah to Guangdong gongsi (廣東公司) (Guangdong regional association, Rangoon), 7 October 1901 (Tung Wah '*Xinbu*' I, p. 412) on receiving money, letters, and human remains; Tung Wah to Mr [?] Choqing (焯卿仁翁) (month and day missing) 1906 (Tung Wah '*Xinbu*' I [P. 3]) on the personal belongings of a man who had died on board a ship from San Francisco to be collected; Tung Wah to Guangzhao gongsuo, Shanghai, 18 July 1906 (Tung Wah '*Xinbu*' I [P. 4]) on the personal belongings of workers who had died in South Africa. For the repatriation of bones and coffins, see Note 119.

126. For the development of Chinese newspapers in Hong Kong, see *Huazi*

ribao qishiyi zhounian jinian kan, especially see Mai Siyuan (麥思源), 'Qishinian lai zhi Xianggang baoye' (七十年來之香港報業) ('The development of journalism in Hong Kong in the last 70 years') in it; *Xunhuan ribao liushi zhounian jinian tekan*; Go Gongzhen (戈公振), *Zhongguo baoye shi* (中國報業史) (*The History of Chinese Journalism*) (Hong Kong: 1964); Zeng Xubai (曾虛白), *Zhongguo xinwen shi* (中國新聞史) (*History of Chinese Journalism*) (Taipei: 1967); Yuan Changchao (袁昶超), *Zhongguo baoye xiaoshi* (中國報業小史) (*A Brief history of Chinese Journalism*) (Hong Kong: [1957]), and Lin Youlan, '*Xianggang baoye fazhan shilue*' (香港報業發展史略) ('A brief history of the development of journalism in Hong Kong'), *Baoxue* 2:10 (August 1962), pp. 100–115.

Expenses for advertisement were entered into the *Zhengxinlu* under miscellaneous items; for example, in 1878, it paid for advertisements about coffins returning to Hong Kong from Annam (*Zhengxinlu* 1878, p. 56b) and about human remains from Sydney (*Zhengxinlu* 1887, Part 4:30b).

127. 'Registrar General's Report for 1892', *HKGG* 1893, p. 440.

128. 'Colonial Surgeon's Report, 1876', p. 206.

129. For instance, in 1873, 17 women were married off, three girls were adopted (*Zhengxinlu* 1873, pp. 61a–61b); in 1887, 49 were married off and nine adopted (*Zhengxinlu* 1887, p. 85a). See *XH*, 25 September 1882 for advertisement putting up two girls and one boy for adoption and two women for marriage offers. Thereafter, these responsibilities were devolved on the Po Leung Kuk, leaving only the repatriation work to the Tung Wah.

130. Hugh McCallum, 'Memorandum having reference to certain matters in connection with the Tung Wah Hospital', *TWR*, pp. LXI–LXII, p. LXI.

131. 'Colonial Surgeon's Report for 1877', p. 323.

132. Bird, *Golden Chersonese*, p. 87.

133. *Hong Kong Telegraph*, quoted in *TWR*, p. LXXVIII. 'Colonial Surgeon's Report for 1891', *HKGG* 1892, pp. 909–60, p. 914.

134. The Hospital's accounts were published in the *Zhengxinlu* in great detail; from 1880 a summary appeared in the *HKGG*.

135. MacDonnell to Kimberley, 19 February 1872, #947: CO 129/156.

136. *Zhengxinlu* 1873, pp. 6a–6b.

137. *DP*, 1 May 1872.

138. Phineas Ryrie of Turner & Co. arrived in the colony in 1854 and resided until his death in 1892. He was a member of the Legislative Council for some 25 years (1867–92) and was chairman of the General Chamber of Commerce 1867–68, 1871–76, 1886–89. See Endacott, *Government and People*, p. 88.

139. *DP*, 1 May 1872.

140. *DP*, 9 May 1872.

141. W. S. K. Waung, *The Controversy: Opium and Sino-British Relations 1858–1887* (Hong Kong: Lungmen Press, [1977]). In this work Dr Waung gives a very detailed description of the smuggling of opium, the customs blockade, and the subsequent Opium Convention of 1887 aimed at solving the situation.

142. 'The Piece Goods Tax', *North China Daily News*, reprinted in *DP*, 25 May 1872.

143. *DP*, 9 May 1872.

144. The *North China Daily News*, Shanghai, 1864–1911, was often extracted in the *Hong Kong Daily Press*.

145. 'The Piece Good Tax', *DP*, 25 May 1872.

146. Quan, *Zhongguo hanghui*, pp. 116, 156.

147. *XH*, 7 December 1885; 15 January 1886.

148. *Zhengxinlu* 1873, pp. 81–12a; *Zhengxinlu* 1887, Part 3:32b.

149. *Zhengxinlu* 1877, pp. 22a–23a.

150. *Zhengxinlu* 1886, Part 3:23a; *Zhengxinlu* 1895, Part 3:43a–47b.

151. *Zhengxinlu* 1873, pp. 12b, 46a. The 1870 Ordinance had not empowered the Hospital to purchase or own property. This was not discovered until 1899 when one of the tenants refused to pay rent. This urged the Directors to take steps to safeguard their interests, and in 1904, 'An Ordinance for enabling the Tung Wah Hospital to acquire, hold, mortgage and sell land and hereditaments, in the colony of Hong Kong' was passed. In 1908 the 'Man Mo Temple Ordinance' also transferred the management of the Temple and all its property to the Tung Wah under separate books of account. (Tung Wah, Board of Directors, 1970–1971, *One Hundred Years of the Tung Wah Group of Hospitals, 1870–1970,* I, [Hong Kong: The Hospital, (1970)] pp. 209–15.) For a complete list of the Tung Wah's own properties, see *One Hundred Years of the Tung Wah Group of Hospitals,* pp. 258–268.

152. Particulars relating to Tung Wah Hospital Property, *TWR*, p. LXXXVI.

153. *DP*, 23 October 1875.

154. Letters in 1899–1900 on these subjects can be found in Tung Wah *'Xinbu'* I, which give some idea of the burden of the work.

155. 'Statement of the Receipts — Disbursements of the Tung Wah Hospital, for the Kap Ng (*jiawu* 甲午) year (1894)', *TWR*, p. LXXII.

156. 'In a medical point of view, it is almost a mere nothing', *DP*, 13 April 1874.

157. Dr. Clark's evidence, *TWR*, pp. 50–4; Dr Thomson's evidence *TWR*, pp. 55–9.

158. According to Au Ki-nam, there were accommodations for 112 patients in 1896, but there were sometimes as many as 160 people (*TWR*, p. 31); Lowson's evidence, *TWR*, pp. 38–48, pp. 38–9; according to Dr Clark, verandahs were used as sleeping places (*TWR*, p. 52.)

159. The lunatic ward was added in early 1879. See Bird, *Golden Chersonese*, p. 87.

160. Dr Ayres's evidence, *TWR*, pp. 60–5, p. 65.

161. Kerr, 'Benevolent Institutions of Canton', part 2, describes its establishment and operations; *Nanhai xianzhi* (南海縣志) (*Nanhai gazetteer*) (1901) *juan* 6:10b.

162. *Jinghu Yiyuan jiushi zhouji jinian tekan* (鏡湖醫院九十周季紀念特刊), (*Special 90th anniversary memorial magazine of the Jinghu Hospital*) (Macao: [1961]), p. 17; Wang Tao, 'Changjian Aomen Jinghu yiyuan xu' (倡建澳門鏡湖醫院) ('On the proposed establishment of the Jinghu Hospital in Macao') in his *Taoyuan wenlu waibian,* pp. 241–2; according to the *Zhongwai xinwen qiri bao,* the Jinghu Hospital had been planned for two years before it was finished in May 1871, that is, 1870. See *ZW*, 27 May 1871.

163. *Chengxi Fangbian yiyuan zhengxinlu* (城西方便醫院徵信錄) (*Annual Report of the Fangbian Hospital, Western Canton*) 1916, shows the Tung Wah Hospital heading the list of founding directors. The Fangbian (方便) and Guangji (廣濟) Hospitals were among the nine benevolent institutions in Canton in the late nineteenth century. See Edward J. Rhoads, 'Merchant Associations in Canton, 1895–1911' in Mark Elvin and G. W. Skinner (eds.), *The Chinese City Between Two Worlds* (Stanford: Stanford University Press, 1974), pp. 97–118, p. 104.

164. There is some dispute concerning the date of its origin. In its Centenary Commemorative publication, it claimed to have started in 1867, but then it was only a dispensary. See *Tongji yiyuan yibai zhounian jinian tekan* (同濟醫院壹佰周年紀念特刊) (*Centenary publication of the Thong Chai Medical Institution*) (Singapore: [1968]); in 1885 the promoters petitioned the government to build a Chinese hospital and it was completed in 1892. See *Thong Chai Medical Institution Opening Ceremony Souvenir Magazine* (同濟醫院大廈落成紀念特刊) (bilingual) (Singapore: [1979]), pp. 95–102. It had 12 directors, six of Fujian origin and six of

Guangdong origin. Strangely enough, the Principal Civil Medical Officer of Singapore reported in 1895 that there was no Chinese Hospital using native treatment and that although there had been a scheme for one for some years, it had come to nothing. See J. A. Swettenham, Colonial Secretary, Straits Settlements to the Colonial Secretary, Hong Kong, 17 September 1895, *TWR*, pp. LXVI–LXVII.

165. *A History of the Sam Yup Benevolent Association in the United States 1850–1975* (旅美三邑總會館簡史) (bilingual) (San Francisco: Sam Yup Benevolent Association, 1975), pp. 132–5. It was an aborted effort because the American government would not accept the medical qualification of Chinese doctors.

166. The Tianhua (天華) Hospital was organized between 1904–06, representing all five speech groups. At first it used Chinese medicine, but changed to Western medicine in the 1930s. See G. W. Skinner, *Chinese Society in Thailand*, (Ithaca, New York: Cornell University Press, 1957) pp. 170, 257–8.

167. There were the Zhonghua (中華) Hospital in Pnom Penh, and the Nanhua (南華) at Penang.

168. In Hawaii there was also an attempt in 1886 to build a hospital modelled on the Tung Wah, but it failed. See Zhang Yinhuan (張蔭桓), *Sanzhou riji* (三洲日記) (*Diary of Three Continents*) 8 *juan*, (no publisher, no date), *juan* 2:24a.

169. This is clearly shown in the Fangbian Hospital's *Zhengxinlu*: This was specifically stated in the petition for the establishment of the Thong Chai. See petition printed in fascimile in *Thong Chai Medical Institution Opening Ceremony Souvenir Magazine*, p. 96. There is a letter in the Tung Wah Archives addressed to a Tongji (同濟) Hospital, place unknown, 25 November 1900 (Tung Wah 'Xinbu' I, p. 257) showing that when this Tongji was established, it had written to the Tung Wah for its *Zhengxinlu* and the 1870 Ordinance for reference. It would be interesting to know if this was the Singapore hospital. In any case, it shows that the Tung Wah had become the model of 'Chinese hospitals'. See also *XH*, 11 and 26 May, 8 December 1885.

170. Crissman, 'The Segmentary Structure', p. 197.

Notes to Chapter 4

1. John King Fairbank, *The United States and China* (Cambridge, Mass.: Harvard University Press, 1971; 1st edition 1949), pp. 29, 103; Ch'ü T'ung-tsu, *Local Government in China under the Ch'ing* (Cambridge Mass.: Harvard University Press, 1962), p. 168.

2. Ch'ü, *Local Government*, p. 175.

3. Ch'ü, *Local Government*, p. 168; Hsiao Kung-Chuan, *Rural China: Imperial Control in the Nineteenth-Century* (Seattle: University of Washington Press, 1960), pp. 316–17, 321; Chang Chungli, *The Chinese Gentry, Studies in Their Role in Nineteenth-century Chinese Society* (Seattle and London: University of Washington Press, 1955), Chapter 1; compare Ho Ping-ti, *The Ladder of Success in Imperial China: Aspects of Social Mobility, 1368–1911* (New York: Columbia University Press, 1962). There is a debate on the definition of *shen* among scholars; see below.

4. James Hayes, *The Hong Kong Region 1850–1911: Institutions and Leadership in Town and Countryside* (Hamden, Conn.: Archon Books, Dawson, 1977), describes life in traditional China under local leadership without the gentry; Donald Robert de Glopper, 'City on the Sands: Social Structure in a Nineteenth-century Chinese City (Ph. D. thesis, Cornell University, 1973), pp. 14–15.

5. de Glopper, 'City on the Sands', p. 15.

6. Ch'ü, *Local Government*, p. 170.

7. *ZW*, 17 February 1872; see also *XH*, 1 May 1874; Wang Tao, '*Chuangjian*

Donghua yiyuan xu' (創建東華醫院序) ('On the establishment of the Tung Wah Hospital'), in his *Taoyuan wenlu waibian* (*Additional Essays of Wang Tao*) 12 *juan* (Peking: 1959), pp. 239–40. It was written at Leung On's request, and might have been exaggerated. But his other writings also reveal that he did consider the establishment of the Tung Wah to be a momentous event transforming the nature of the Chinese community in Hong Kong, and marking a turning point in Hong Kong's history.

8. For the purchase of official titles, see Yen Ching-Hwang, 'Ch'ing's Sale of Honours and the Chinese Leadership in Singapore and Malaya, 1877–1912', *Journal of Southeast Asian Studies* 1:2 (September 1970), pp. 20–32.

9. *DP*, 7 October 1871.

10. *ZW*, 14 October 1871.

11. G. W. Skinner, 'Overseas Chinese Leadership: Paradigm for a Paradox' in Gehan Wijeyewardene, *Leadership and Authority: A Symposium* (Singapore: University of Malaya Press, 1968), pp. 191–207, and his *Leadership and Power in the Chinese Community of Thailand* (Ithaca, New York: Cornell University Press, 1958), pp. 80–3; Yen, 'Ch'ing's Sale of Honours'; C. M. Turnbull, *A History of Singapore* (Kuala Lumpur: Oxford University Press, 1977), p. 55.

12. G. B. Endacott, *Government and People in Hong Kong* (Hong Kong: Hong Kong University Press, 1964), pp. 90–1.

13. Hennessy to Carnavon, 27 September 1877, #123: CO 129/179.

14. 'Statement of Hennessy', *HKGG* 1881, p. 82. Hennessy further elaborated on the rate-payers in Hennessy to Kimberley, 31 August 1881, #140: CO 129/194.

15. Chinese petition for a Chinese Legislative Councillor enclosed in Hennessy to Hicks-Beach, 19 January 1880, 4: CO 129/187.

16. Yen, 'Ch'ing's Sale of Honours', p. 26.

17. Yen Ching-Hwang, 'Changing Images of the Overseas Chinese (1644–1912)', *MAS* 15:2 (1981), pp. 261–85.

18. Succesive Governors and Governors-General at Canton had complained about this. See *Zhouban Yiwu shimo* (籌辦夷務始末) (*The Complete Account of the Management of Barbarian Affairs*) 260 *juan* (Peiping: 1930), *juan* 41:36a; Guo Songdao, '*Fuchen Guangdong dagai qingxing shu*' (覆陳廣東大概情形疏) ('Memorial on conditions in Guangdon') in his *Yangzhi shuwu yiji* (*Works from the Yangzhi Studio*), *juan* 4:53a–59b; Liu Kunyi (劉坤一), '*Fuchen banli du'an qingxing zhe*' (覆陳辦理盜案情形摺) ('Reply on situation regarding robbery cases') in *Liu Kunyi yiji* (劉坤一遺集) (*Works of Liu Kunyi*), 6 volumes (Shanghai: 1959) (hereafter *LYJ*), Vol. I, pp. 432–6; Zhang Zhidong (張之洞) 'Qing cuishe Xianggang lingshi zhe' (請催設香港領事摺) ('Memorial urging the establishment of a Consul at Hong Kong'), 30 March 1886 in *Zhang Wenxiang Gong quanji* (張文襄公全集) (*Complete Works of Zhang Zhidong*) 228 *juan*, 6 volumes, photographic reprint (Taipei: 1963) (hereafter *ZQJ*), *juan* 15: 14a–17b. See also Wang Tao, '*Chuangjian Donghua yiyuan xu*'.

19. Guo Songdao, '*Na huo panju Xianggang zhaohuo jizei nishou shen ming zhengfa shu*' (拿獲盤據香港招夥濟賊逆首審明正法疏) ('Memorial on caputring bandit leader who had recruited men and aided robbers in Hong Kong, to investigate and punish him accordingly') in *Yangzhi shuwu yiji, juan* 6: 49a–51b.

20. Liu Kunyi, '*Fuchen Yuesheng shiyi chazhuo banli zhe*' (覆陳粵省事宜查酌辦理摺)('Reply on Guangdong investigations'), *LYJ*, Vol. I. pp. 389–94.

21. One was Gao Shunjin (高舜琴) who won a *juren* degree in 1888 and became a Director in 1882 and Chairman in 1892; see Gao Zhenbai (高貞白), '*Xianggang Donghua yiyuan yu Gao Manhe*' (香港東華醫院高滿和) ('The Tung Wah Hospital of Hong Kong and Gao Manhe'), *Da Hua* (大華) 1:4 (October 1970), pp.

2–6, p. 5. See also Note 21. Another was Liu Jinhua (劉金華), also a *juren*, who was Chairman in 1899. His porcelain photograph listing all his degrees and titles is in the Tung Wah Hospital.

22. Wang Tao, *Manyu suilu* (漫遊隨錄) (*A record of travels*) (Zhangsha, 1982; first published 1887), p. 60.

23. *XH*, 28 July 1874.

24. Yen, 'Ch'ing's Sale of Honours', pp. 22–4; Li Hongzhang, '*Waisheng juanju biantong zhengdun zhe*' (外省捐局變通整頓摺) ('Memorial on the reorganization of fund-raising bureaus in outer provinces'), 21 August 1878, in *Li Wenzhong Gong Quanji* (李文忠公全集) (*Complete Works of Li* Hongzhang), 7 volumes (Hong Kong: 1965) (hereafter *LQJ*), Vol. II, *zougao* (奏稿) (memorials), *juan* 32: 17a–19a; '*Jin zhen jiangzhang zhe*' (晉賑獎章摺) ('Awards for raising funds for Shanxi relief'), *LQJ*, *zougao*, *juan* 30: 48a–49a; Chang Chungli, *The Chinese Gentry*, Chapter 2.

25. *CM*, 23 March 1878; full price list is given in Li Hongzhang, '*Haifang juanshu biantong zhangzheng zhe*' (海防捐輸變通章程摺) ('Regulations on reorganization of coastal defence fund'), *LQJ*, Vol. II, *zougao*, juan 60: 13a–15a; in Hong Kong, the advertisement can be seen in *XH*, 30 September 1884 and on the subscription list in December that year; see also Yen, 'Ch'ing Sale of Honours'. A detailed description of the dress and insignia for each rank of office is given in John Henry Gray, *China, A History of the Law, Manners and Customs of the People* (London: Macmillan, 1878), Vol. 1, Chapter XIV.

26. Li Hongzhang, '*Chaozhou quanjuan Jin zhen pian*' (潮洲勸捐晉賑片) ('Memorial on raising funds for Shanxi at Chaozhou'), 18 December 1877 in *LQJ*, Vol. II, *zougao, juan* 30:28a–b; see Michael Godley, 'The Late Ch'ing's Courtship of the Chinese in Southeast Asia', *Journal of Asian Studies* XXXIV:2 (February 1975), pp. 311–85.

27. Wellington K. K. Chan, *Merchants, Mandarins and Modern Enterprise in Late Ch'ing China* (Cambridge, Mass.: Harvard University Press, 1977), Chapter 3; Ho Ping-ti, *The Ladder of Success*, Chapter 1, Section 3.

28. Chan, *Merchants, Chapter 3; see also* Michael Godley, *The Mandarin-Capitalists from Nanyang: Overseas Chinese Enterprise in the Modernization of China 1893–1911* (Cambridge, Mass.: Harvard University Press, 1981).

29. Examples can be found in *ZW*, 18 March 1871; 15 April 1871; *HKGG* 1880, p. 187; *HKGG* 1881, pp. 426, 654, 656.

30. Chan, *Merchants*, p. 58; Marianne Bastid, 'The Social Context of Reform', in Paul A. Cohen and John E. Schrecker (eds.), *Reforms in Nineteenth-Century China* (Cambridge, Mass.: Harvard University Press, 1976), pp. 117–27, p. 118.

31. Examples can be found in *ZW*, 27 May 1871, 17 February 1872; *XH*, 8, 9, 13 April 1874; *HKGG* 1880, p. 515; Wang Tao, '*Dai shang Guangzhou taishou Feng Zili douzhuan*' (代上廣州太守馮子立都轉) dated about 1874 ('Letter to the Prefect of Guangzhou on behalf of ——') in his *Taoyuan zhidu* (弢園尺牘) (*Letters of Wang Tao*), 12 *juan* (Shanghai: no date; 1st published 1893), *juan* 9:1a–8b. See *HKGG* 1880, p. 187.

32. Evidence of Sin Tak Fan (Xian Tefen) (冼德芬), Hong Kong, *Report of the Special Committee to Investigate and Report on Certain Points Connected with the Bill for the Inauguration of the Po Leung Kuk or Society for the Protection of Women and Girls* (Hong Kong: Noronha, Government Printer, 1893), pp. 113–30, p. 116. Sin was a Eurasian solicitor's clerk who became one of the few professionals who sat on the Tung Wah Board. He was a Committee member of the Tung Wah in 1878 and Chairman in 1908. See Arnold Wright (ed.), *Twentieth Century Impressions of Hong Kong, Shanghai and Other Treaty Ports* (London: Lloyd's Greater Britian Publishing, 1908), p. 187; W. Feldwick, *Present Day*

Impressions of the Far East and Prominent and Progressive Chinese at Home and Abroad: The History, People, Commerce, Industries and Resources of China, Hong Kong and Indo-China, Malaya and Netherlands Indies (London: 1917), p. 580.

33. The plaque, containing the words *'Jianyi yongwei'* (見義勇爲) was presented to the *'Xianggang Donghua Yiyuan xiezhen shendong'* (香港東華醫院協賑紳董) ('Fund-raising gentry-Directors of the Tung Wah Hospital of Hong Kong') by the Governor-General of Zhili, Li Hongzhang, and the Governor of Shandong, the Minister of the Board of Rites, and the acting Senior Vice-President of Board of Punishment, in 1884. (See Plate 7). For Li, see Note 74.

34. The Treasurer's letter is discussed in Chapter 5.

35. *CM*, 8 November 1875.

36. *London and China Express*, reprinted in *DP*, 15 February 1873.

37. See Additional List to Commission of the Peace, *HKGG* 1878, p. 599.; Endacott, *Government and People*, pp. 92–8; Hennessy to Kimberley, 19 January 1880, #4: CO 129/187.

38. E. J. Eitel, *Europe in China* (Hong Kong: Oxford University Press, 1983), p. 510. Also see *Daily Advertizer*, 22 August 1872.

39. Eitel, *Europe in China*, p. 543; *HKGG* 1879, pp. 229–33.

40. *CM*, 1 May 1879.

41. Tung Wah, *'Dongshiju huiyi lu'*, extant from 1904–41, give some idea of the form and content of the meetings.

42. *DP*, 2 June 1873. In fact, even before the Hospital building was officially opened, meetings were already being held under the Committee's auspices. See *ZW*, 25 March 1871. It does not say, however, where the meetings took place.

43. Minute by the Acting Colonial Secretary on the Secretary of State's Despatch #105 of 29 May 1882, dated 19 July 1882, enclosed in Marsh to Kimberley, 20 July 1882, #136: CO 129/202.

44. *DP*, 26 June 1872.

45. *DP*, 15 May, 12 July, 31 October 1873; 10 August 1874; *XH*, 8 April 1874; Bowen to Carnarvon, 6 August 1883, #175: CO 129/211; Marsh to Kimberley, 22 September 1882, #205: CO 129/202.

46. *DP*, 9 January, 15 February 1873.

47. *DP*, 18 May 1873.

48. *DP*, 18 May 1873.

49. Bowen to Kimberley, 6 August 1883, #175: CO 129/211.

50. Bowen to Kimberley, 6 August 1883, #175.

51. Letter from 'The Chinese', *CM*, 1 September 1870.

52. *DP*, 15 May 1873; See also James William Norton-Kyshe, *The History of the Laws and Courts of Hong Kong* (Hong Kong: Vetch & Lee, 1971), Vol. II, p. 473; Whitfield to Kimberley, 10 January 1871, #9: CO 129/149.

53. 'Memorandum on the Registration of Chinese Partners by J. H. Stewart Lockhart, CMG, Colonial Secretary', *HKGG* 1901, pp. 1883–1901.

54. 'Minutes of a meeting held at the Tung Wah Hospital on 16th August, 1874', Appendix I, to 'Memorandum on the Registration of Chinese Partners', pp. 1889–90.

55. 'Minutes of a meeting held at the Tung Wah Hospital'.

56. 'Memorandum on the Registration of Chinese Partners'.

57. *DP*, 7 October 1878.

58. *DP*, 7 October 1878.

59. *DP*, 7 October 1878.

60. *DP*, 9 October 1878; this episode is also described in Pope-Hennessy, *Verandah*, pp. 203–5. Hennessy defended himself in Hennessy to Hicks-Beach, 10 October 1878, #98: CO 129/98, and 31 May 1878, #77: CO 129/184.

61. *DP*, 9 October 1878.
62. *DP*, 15 November 1878.
63. *CM*, 29 September 1881.
64. Registrar General's Reports, 5 June and 7 June 1882, enclosed in Marsh to Kimberley, 20 June 1882, confidential: CO 129/201.
65. For the *muitsai (meizai)* (妹仔) system, see Wei Qingyuan (韋慶遠) and others, *Qingdai nubi zhidu* (清代奴婢制度) (*The Slavery System in Qing*) (Peking: 1984; first published 1982); Maria H. Jaschok, 'A Social History of the Mooi Jai Institution in Hong Kong, 1843–1939' (Ph. D. thesis, London University, 1981) and her *Concubines and Bondservants* (London: Zed Books, 1988).
66. For instance, Zhang Zhendong (張震東) to Tung Wah, 17 September 1889 (Po Leung Kuk, '*Jichou nian gebu laiwang xin di bu* (1)' (己丑年各埠來往信底簿(一)) ('Copies of letters to and from abroad, 1889') (hereafter '*Xinbu*' VI).
67. *DP*, 15 October 1873.
68. *DP*, 15 October 1873.
69. *DP*, 23 October 1875.
70. Registrar General to acting Colonial Secretary, 2 August 1882, enclosed in Marsh to Kimberley, 14 August 1882, #161: Co 129/202.
71. Registrar General's Report, 5 June 1882, enclosed in Marsh to Kimberley, 20 June 1882, confidential: CO 129/201.
72. Registrar General to acting Colonial Secretary, 2 August 1882, enclosed in Marsh to Kimberley, 14 August 1882, #161: CO 129/202.
73. *DP*, 6 January 1876; see also 23 October 1875.
74. Li Hongzhang (李鴻章) (1823–1901) was one of the most powerful officials of late Qing, having initially made his name fighting the Taipings. From 1870, he was Governor-General of Zhili and Superintendent of Trade for the Northern Ports in charge of diplomatic, military, and economic affairs. he was the leader of the so-called self-strengthening movement. For biographical accounts, see Wei Xiyu (韋息予), *Li Hongzhang* (李鴻章) (Shanghai: 1931); Lei Luqing (雷祿慶), *Li Hongzhang nianpu* (李鴻章年譜) (*Chronological Biography of Li Hongzhang*) (Taipei: 1977) and his *Li Hongzhang xinzhuan* (李鴻章新傳) (*New Biography of Li Hongzhang*) (Taipei: 1983); Li Shoukong (李守孔), *Li Hongzhang zhuan* (李鴻章傳) (Li Hongzhang) (Taipei: 1978); Stanley Spector, *Li Hung-chang and the Huai Army: A Study of 19th Century Chinese Regionalism* (Seattle: University of Washington Press, 1964).
75. Ding Richang (丁日昌) (1823–82), long an associate of Li Hongzhang in the self-strengthening movement, was a native of Chaozhou Prefecture which explains his familiarity with South China affairs and Overseas Chinese, many of whom had gone from that prefecture. See Lü Shiqiang (呂實強), *Ding Richang yu ziqiang yundong* (丁日昌與自強運動) (*Ding Richang and the Self-Strengthening Movement*) (Taipei: 1972); Arthur W. Hummel (ed.), *Eminent Chinese of the Ch'ing Period (1644–1912)* (Washington: Government Printing Office 1943–4), Vol. II, pp. 721–3.
76. Gao Zhenbai, '*Xianggang Donghua Yiyuan yu Gao Manhe*'; Lin Xi (林熙) (Gao Zhenbai), '*Cong Xianggang de Yuan Fa Hang tan qi*' (從香港的元發行談起) (Yuan Fa Hang of Hong Kong), *Da cheng* (大成) 117 (August 1983) pp. 47–52; 118 (September 1983), pp. 45–51, 119; (October 1983), pp. 34–9, 120; (November 1983) pp. 46–54. Gao Manhe (or Manhua), after making his fortunes in Hong Kong and Siam, returned to China around 1856 and found himself arrested for collaborating with barbarians. He subsequently bought a 5th rank official title to protect himself. The author is Gao Manhe's grandson.
77. Li Hongzhang, '*Chaozhou quanjuan Jin zhen pian*'.
78. The Xin'an (新安) Magistrate to the Tung Wah Hospital, (no date),

sub-enclosure in Marsh to O'Conor, 20 January 1886, enclosed in Marsh to Granville, 25 January 1886, confidential: CO 129/225. This dispatch also appears in Great Britain, Foreign Office, Embassy and Consular Archives: China Correspondence 1834–1930, series 228 (hereafter FO 228), Vol. 842, and the original Chinese documents appear here.

79. The plaque reads '*ke guang te xin*' (克廣德心), and is deposited in the Tung Wah Hospital at Po Yan Street. See Plate 8.

80. Xin'an Magistrate to the Tung Wah Hospital (no date).

81. Acknowledgement of receipt of the dispatch of instructions and the tablet scroll, extracted from the minutes of the Tung Wah Hospital of 1879, sub-enclosed in Marsh to O'Conor, 20 January 1886, enclosed in Marsh to Granville, 25 January 1886, confidential: CO 129/225.

82. The '*shen wei pu you*' (神威普佑) plaque is kept at the Man Mo Temple. The term 'by the imperial brush' is not literal — this only meant the Emperor personally instructed Hanlin scholars to write the characters.

83. Major fund-raising took place in 1885–6, see below, also in 1890, see Li Hongzhang, '*Ge sheng juanzhu Zhi zhen shumu zhe*' (各省捐助直賑數目摺) ('Memorial on relief funds for Zhili from other provinces'), 28 January 1891 in *LQJ*, Vol. II, *zougao, juan* 70:30a–32b. See Tung Wah Hospital, Board of Directors, 1960–1961, *Development of the Tung Wah Hospitals (1870–1960)*, Part 4, pp. 1–16, which gives a very interesting account of the Hospital's efforts to raise funds up to the 1950s.

84. Persia Crawford Campbell's *Chinese Coolie Emigration to Countries within the British Empire* (New York: Negro University Press, 1969; first published 1923) remains the classic work on Chinese emigration. More recently, there are Wang Sing-wu, *The Organization of Chinese Emigration, 1848–1888, with Special Reference to Chinese Emigration in Australia* (San Francisco: Chinese Materials Centre, Inc., 1978) and his 'The Attitude of the Ch'ing Court towards Chinese Emigration', *Chinese Culture 9:4 (December 1968), pp. 62–76; Elliott C. Arensmeyer, 'British Merchant Enterprise and the Chinese Coolie Labour Trade, 1850–1874*' (Ph.D. thesis, University of Hawaii, 1979). The most refreshing work is Robert Lee Irick, *Ch'ing Policy towards the Coolie Trade, 1847–1878* (Taipei: Chinese Materials Centre, 1980). Hiroaki Kani's (可兒明弘) *Kindai Chūgoku no kuri to choka* (近代中國の苦力と「豬花」) (*The Coolies and 'Slave Girls' of Modern China*) (Tokyo: 1979) also throws interesting light on the subject by using archival materials from the Po Leung Kuk. Useful material is also provided by Chen Hansheng (陳翰笙) (ed.), *Huagong chuguo shiliao huibian* (華工出國史料彙編) (*A Compilation of historical materials on the emigration of Chinese labourers*) volume 1 (Peking: 1980–   ). So far 10 volumes have been published. An older compilation is Zhu Shijia (朱士嘉), *Meiguo pohai Huagong shiliao* (美國迫害華工史料) (*Materials on American Persecution of Chinese Labour*) (Shanghai: 1958) which concentrates more on the abuses of the coolie trade. See also Wang Gungwu, *A Short History of the Chinese in Nanyang* (Singapore: Eastern Universities Press, 1959); 'Report accompanying the Blue Book', *Hong Kong Blue Book* 1852, pp. 130–9, 136–7.

85. See Irick, *Coolie Trade*, Chapter 2; 'Memorandum of the Coolie Ships on Board which Mutinies have occurred, or in Which the Vessels or Passengers have met with Disasters from the Year 1845 up to the Year 1872', enclosed in Sir B. Robertson to Lord Tenterden, 31 March 1874, in 'Correspondence respecting the Macao Coolie Trade 1874–75' [C.-1212] *BPP* IV, pp. 379–408, pp. 386–7 gives some idea of the hazards of emigrating. See also 'Harbour Master's Report for 1888', *HKGG* 1889, pp. 635–61 and 'Harbour Master's Report for 1889,' *HKGG* 1890, pp. 491–518 for emigration abuses. See Note 101.

86. Campbell, *Coolie Emigration*, pp. 100–3.

87. Campbell, *Coolie Emigration*, p. 150.

88. For the Chinese Passengers Act, 1855 and other emigration-related local ordinances up to 1876, see *HKGG* 1875, pp. 399–401.

89. 'Harbour Master's Report for 1870', *HKGG* 1871, pp. 97–110, p. 98. This was suggested by the Emigration Board to Frederick Rogers at the Colonial Office, 29 July 1869: CO 129/140, because there had been too many cases of abuse.

90. Rutherford Alcock (1809–97) became Consul at Fuzhou, 1844 and Shanghai in 1846. After serving as Britain's first Consul-General in Japan 1858–65, he became Minister-Plenipotentiary at Peking, 1865–71. See Alexander Michie, *The Englishman in China*, 2 volumes (Edinburgh: Blackwood, 1900).

91. MacDonnell to Alcock, 3 August 1869, enclosed in MacDonnell to Granville, 4 August 1869, #767: CO 129/139.

92. 'Report accompanying the Blue Book', *Blue Book* 1852, pp. 136–7.

93. MacDonnell to Alcock, 3 August 1869, enclosed in MacDonnell to Granville, 4 August 1869. #767: CO 129/139.

94. Irick, *Coolie Trade*, pp. 257–63; for Ruilin's attitude, see Campbell, *Coolie Emigration*, pp. 148–9.

95. *Report of the Commission sent by China to Ascertain the Conditions of Chinese Coolies in Cuba* (Taipei: 1970; 1st published Shanghai: Imperial Maritimes Customs Press, 1876) gives the most heart-rending accounts of the hardship suffered there. See also Campbell, *Coolie Emigration*, p. 135.

96. This is the main thesis of Robert Irick's book.

97. Norton-Kyshe, *Laws and Courts*, Vol. II, pp. 186–7, 210.

98. John Jackson Smale, a well-known reporter in Chancery, arrived in Hong Kong as Attorney General in 1861 and became Chief Justice in 1866. He retired in 1881. His career as Chief Justice was colourful, and his opposition to both the emigration business and slavery, which he equated, provides insight to the nature of Hong Kong society and the struggle between Chinese customary law and cultural attitudes and English law. See Norton-Kyshe, *Laws and Courts*.

99. Norton-Kyshe, *Laws and Courts*, Vol. II, p. 186.

100. *DP*, 9 September 1871.

101. *DP*, 13 May 1871; for an account of the mutiny on the *Dolores Uqarte*, see extract from the *Globe*, 30 December 1870, enclosed in Granville to Sir C. Murray, 17 January 1871, in 'Correspondence respecting Emigration of Chinese Coolies from Macao' 1871, [C.–403] *BPP* IV, pp. 256–7.

102. *DP*, 20 May 1871; *ZW*, 27 May 1871.

103. *ZW*, 27 May 1871.

104. *XH*, 9 June 1874.

105. *DP*, 7 October 1871.

106. 'A Correct Statement of the Wicked Practice of Decoying and Kidnapping, Respectfully laid before His Excellency' enclosed in Kennedy to Kimberley, 7 June 1872, in 'Papers relative to the Measures taken to Prevent the Fitting out of Ships at Hong Kong for the Macao Coolie Trade' [C.–829] presented July 1873, *BPP*, Vol. IV, pp. 309–62 (hereafter Papers on Macao Coolie Trade, July 1873), pp. 313–16.

107. Campbell, *Coolie Emigration*, p. 157; Norton-Kyshe, *Laws and Courts*, Vol. II, p. 207.

108. *DP*, 15 May 1873. In his '*Dai shang Guangzhou taishou Feng Zili douzhuan*', Wang Tao also mentioned that the Tung Wah Directors had employed detectives to investigate kidnapping with a special subscription before they asked the Governor to pay for it. Unfortunately he did not say when the practice started.

109. *DP*, 22, 24 May 1873.

110. *DP*, 15 May 1873.

111. *DP*, 12 July 1873.

112. Campbell, *Coolie Emigration*, p. 152; 'Police Reports' for 1868, 1870, 1873, and 1877, *HKGG* 1869, pp. 209–12; *HKGG* 1871, pp. 281–87; *HKGG* 1874, pp. 84–90; *HKGG* 1878, pp. 125–30; and 'Harbour Master's Report for 1888', p. 636; all emphasize the difficulty of detecting kidnapping cases which were often falsely reported and difficult to prove. It was strongly felt that Chinese officials should fight their own crimes.

113. See Tung Wah to Lockhart, 4 October 1899 in Tung Wah *'Xinbu'* I, p. 81, in which it informed him that 200 workers recruited for Manila were supposedly kidnapped, and offered to send them home. The information had come from the China Association in San Francisco and from gentlemen of the Siyi counties.

114. Cases of kidnapping decreased because of cessation of contract emigration from Macao in late 1874, see 'Police Report for 1874', *HKGG* 1875, pp. 45–50, p. 46; Hennessy's Reply to Chinese Deputation, *HKGG* 1880, pp. 185–92, p. 190; for the Protector of Chinese, see Eunice Thio, 'The Singapore Chinese Protectorate: Events and Conditions Leading to its Establishment, 1823–1877', *Journal of the South Seas Society* XVI (1970), pp. 40–80, and R. N. Jackson, *Pickering: Protector of Chinese* (Kuala Lumper: 1965).

115. See Guangxing tang (廣行堂) of Dongguan city, 26 March 1884 to Po Leung Kuk and Tung Wah (Po Leung Kuk *'Xinbu'* I) informing it that a woman would come to Hong Kong for a girl saved by the Po Leung Kuk and their reply that the girl had been sent home, instructing the Guangxing tang to ensure that her husband would provide for her; Guangxing tang to Po Leung Kuk and Tung Wah, 7 April 1884 (Po Leung Kuk *'Xinbu'* I) asking it to find a supposedly kidnapped girl; Guangzhao gongsuo, Cholon, to Tung Wah, 11 April 1887 (Po Leung Kuk *'Xinbu'* I) thanking it for work with kidnapped girls; —— to Tung Wah, (April–May?) 1884 (Po Leung Kuk *'Xinbu'* I); the writer had been sold as a 'pig' but had escaped, and was writing to ask the Tung Wah to find him a job, and to plead with the Registrar General; Chenjia Gongsuo (陳家公所) of San Francisco, to the Tung Wah, 18 December 1887 (Po Leung Kuk *'Xinbu'* III) on women kidnapped from Hong Kong to San Francisco and asking the Tung Wah to make sure that kidnappers got their due; Yu Hu youshizi (寓滬憂時子) to Tung Wah, 12 August 1888 (Po Leung Kuk *'Xinbu'* IV) reporting a man dealing with the human trade and hoping that it would detain girls on a ship to Singapore travelling through Hong Kong who might have been kidnapped; Zhang Zhendong to Tung Wah, 17 September, 1889 (Po Leung Kuk *'Xinbu'* VI) informing it that since it had found his maid, who had been decoyed to Hong Kong, it could try to marry her off to a suitable man; Xiqiao Chongzheng shantang (西樵崇正善堂), 13 March 1890 (Po Leung Kuk, *'Jichou nian gebu laiwangxin di bu* (2)' (己丑年各埠來往信底簿) ('Copies of letters to and from abroad for 1889–1890') (hereafter *'Xinbu'* VIII) requesting help for people believed to be kidnapped for Borneo; Zheng Jizhong (鄭繼宗), General in Command of the Marine Forces, to the Tung Wah, 31 May 1890 (Po Leung Kuk, *'Gengyin nian gebu laiwangxin bu'* (庚寅年各埠來往信簿) ('Copies of letters to and from abroad for 1890') (hereafter *'Xinbu'* IX) informing it of a woman decoyed to Hong Kong and detained next to the Man Mo Temple, and asking it to take her husband there to find her and let the yamen runners coming from China take her back; Haifeng Bao'anju (海豐保安局) to the Tung Wah, 10 June 1890 (Po Leung Kuk *'Xinbu'* VIII) informing it of a child suspected to have been kidnapped from Hong Kong and requesting information; Po Leung Kuk to Zhang Peilin (張沛霖) of Annam, 9 August 1890, for Tung Wah (Po Leung Kuk *'Xinbu'* IX) on the sale of girls from

Annam; Provincial Commander-in-Chief Feng to Tung Wah and Po Leung Kuk, 3 June 1891 (Po Leung Kuk '*Xinbu*' X) reporting on a Chinese officer implicated in robbery and kidnapping; Qiongtai Hui'ai yiyuan (瓊台惠愛醫院) to Tung Wah, 6 October 1891 (Po Leung Kuk '*Xinbu*' X) asking it to send up two women guilty of kidnapping; Danshui Bao'an gongju (淡水保安公局) to Tung Wah, 25 October 1891 (Po Leung Kuk '*Xinbu*' X) asking it to investigate an alleged case of decoying; Shanghai Guangzhao gongsuo to Tung Wah, 31 October, 1891 (Po Leung Kuk '*Xinbu*' X) asking it to find and repatriate a woman and her son decoyed from Shanghai, sought by grandmother; a lawyer in Singapore to Tung Wah, 7 October 1895 (Po Leung Kuk, '*Yiwei nian gebu laixin bu*' (乙未年各埠來信簿) ('Letters from abroad, 1895–96') (hereafter '*Xinbu*' XVI) asking it to help release a girl detained by the Protector of Chinese in Singapore; Qingyuan Lianhe gongju (清遠聯合公局) to Tung Wah and Po Leung Kuk, 25 February, 1896 (Po Leung Kuk, '*Bingshen nian jie gebu laixin bu*' (丙申年接各埠來信簿) ('Letters from abroad, 1896') (hereafter '*Xinbu*' XVIII) informing them of women kidnapped to Annam but not being helped by the Guangzhao gongsuo there; Guangzhao gongsuo (廣肇公所) of Cholon to Tung Wah, 2 April 1896 (Po Leung Kuk '*Xinbu*' XVIII) asking them to arrest kidnappers who would be travelling through Hong Kong and to send them on to Qingyuan; Simiao zengyiju (四廟贈醫局) of Canton to Po Leung Kuk and Tung Wah, 11 October 1899 (Po Leung Kuk, '*Jihai nian jie gebu xinbu*' (己亥年接各埠信簿) ('Incoming letters from abroad, 1899') (hereafter '*Xinbu*' XXII) asking them to locate a kidnapped friend; Guangzhou huiguan (廣州會館), 6 July 1899 (Po Leung Kuk '*Xinbu*' XXII) on kidnapped persons; Tung Wah to Guangji Hospital, 15 November 1899 (Tung Wah '*Xinbu*' I, p. 98) on two kidnapped men to be fetched; Tung Wah to Lockhart, 4 October 1899 (see Note 142); Tung Wah to Guangren shantang (廣仁善堂), 26 March 1900 (Tung Wah '*Xinbu*' I, p. 139) on returning kidnapped destitutes; Sheng Mou Hao (生茂號) to Tung Wah, 31 January 1901 (Tung Wah '*Xinbu*' I, p. 285) asking it to investigate the family for which a boy kidnapped to Hong Kong from Canton had worked because his testimony was suspect; also Tung Wah to Sheng Mou Hao, 4 February 1901 (Tung Wah '*Xinbu*' I, p. 286) on the same subject; Hall of Sustaining Love to Tung Wah and Po Leung Kuk, 5 September 1888 (Po Leung Kuk '*Xinbu*' IV), asking them to help a father find a boy lost in Canton; Guangxing tang to Tung Wah, 17 October 1890 (Po Leung Kuk '*Xinbu*' IX) on a stray boy to be collected by the uncle. See also Chapter 3, Note 125.

116. Governor's speech on his visit to the Tung Wah Hospital, 8 February 1878, *HKGG* 1878, pp. 47–9, p. 48; for correspondence regarding emigration to Hawaii, see *HKGG* 1880, pp. 958–60.

117. 'Harbour Master's Report for 1881', *HKGG* 1882, pp. 387–409, p. 389; *DP*, 27 September and 14 December 1880.

118. *DP*, 22 and 23 October 1875.

119. *CM*, 5 November 1875; see letter from the Consul of the Netherlands at Hong Kong to Kennedy, 20 August 1875 on his intention to recruit labour from Hong Kong for Acheen for the government there, *HKGG* 1875, pp. 501–2; a similar case occurred in 1889 when mutiny broke out when emigrants discovered that they were going to Deli instead of Singapore, 'Harbour Master's Report for 1889', p. 492.

120. *CM*, 8 November 1875.

121. *CM*, 8 November 1875.

122. *DP*, 23 October 1875.

123. Lucie Cheng Hirata, 'Free, Indentured, Enslaved: Chinese Prostitutes in Nineteenth-Century America', *Signs* 5:1 (Autumn 1979), pp. 3–29, 12.

124. 'Memorandum on Subject of slavery in Hong Kong on the State of the

Law as Applicable to such Slavery' by J. J. Francis, and Further Report by E. J. Eitel, sub-enclosed in 'Correspondence respecting the Alleged Existence of Chinese Slavery in Hong Kong' [C.–3185] LIX, March 1882, *BPP* XXVI, pp. 213–21 (hereafter Correspondence: Chinese Slavery, March 1882).

125. 'Report of the Commissions appointed by His Excellency John Pope Hennessy to inquire into the Working of the Contagious Diseases Ordinance, 1867' [C.–118] XLIX in *BPP* XXV, 508–70, p. 562.

126. Hirata, 'Chinese Prostitutes', pp. 26–7 analyses the complex reasons behind the attempt by Chinese merchants to curb emigration of Chinese prostitutes, offering explanations in the conflicts between the tongs and the allied forces of the Chinese consulate and Six Companies and to minimize the target of anti-Chinese antagonism. But it is also possible that respectable Chinese were genuinely ashamed of the degradation of Chinese women abroad; see Chinese Consolidated Benevolent Association of Victoria, B. C. to Tung Wah, 8 September 1887 (Po Leung Kuk '*Xinbu*' III). The Association was founded in 1884. See Edgor Wickberg (ed.), *From China to Canada: A History of the Chinese Communities in Canada* (Toronto: Minister of Supply and Services, 1982), pp. 24–26, 37–40.

127. Kennedy to Kimberley, 7 June 1872, #24: CO 129/158.

128. 'Harbour Master's Report 1874', *HKGG*, pp. 120–39, p. 122.

129. Harbour Master's Report 1874, p. 123.

130. For the Act of U. S. Congress Supplementary to Acts in relation to Immigration, 1875, See *HKGG* 1875, pp. 306–7.

131. C. C. Smith to D. H. Bailey, 12 August 1875, enclosed in Bailey to Cadwalader, 38 August 1875, #307: United States National Archives, Despatches from U. S. Consuls in Hong Kong 1844–1906 (M 108); 'Harbour Master's Report 1875', *HKGG* 1876, pp. 124–40, p. 126 also expresses the opinion that female emigration should not be prohibited.

132. Bailey to Cadwalader, 28 August 1875, #307.

133. *DP*, 10 August 1875; *CM*, 11 August 1875. Letter from Leong On and the 'Enquiry Committee' to Bailey, dated [?] August 1875, enclosed Bailey to Cadwalader, 28 August 1875, #307.

134. Rules of the Procedure, see Bailey to Cadwalader, 28 August 1875 #307, and Appendix V.

135. *CM*, 3 December 1875.

136. Chinese Consolidated Benevolent Association, Victoria, B. C. to Tung Wah, 9 September 1887.

137. *DP*, 20 October 1873; Zhang Yinhuan, *Riji, juan* 5:7b, 5:20.

138. '*Yangcheng Ping'antang ge shanshi changjuan Shanghai laiwang huochuan yuzhi taipingguan xiaoyin*' (羊城平安堂各善士倡捐上海來往火船預置太平棺小引) ('A note on the proposal by benevolent persons at Canton to raise funds for coffins to be placed on ships going to Shanghai'), 1877. This is accompanied by a cumulative list of accounts in the Tung Wah's *Zhengxinlu* each year after 1877.

139. Zhang Zhidong (張之洞) (1837–1909) was one of the most important officials of the late Qing period. In 1884 he became Governor-General of Guangdong and Guangxi, taking a very strong stand against the French during Sino-French hostilities 1884–86. He was also famous as a modernizer, and advocate of sending students abroad. See Li Guoqi (李國祁), *Zhang Zhidong de waijiao zhengze* (張之洞的外交政策) (*Zhang Zhidong's Foreign Policy*) (Taipei: 1970); William Ayers, *Chang Chih-tung and Education Reform in China* (Cambridge, Mass.: Harvard University Press, 1971); Daniel H. Bays, *China Enters the 20th Century: Chang Chih-tung and the Issues of a New Age, 1895–1909* (Ann Arbor, Michigan: University of Michigan Press, 1978).

140. See Taiping guan accounts in *Zhengxinlu* 1885.
141. Chinese Consolidated Benevolent Association, Victoria, B. C. to Tung Wah, 9 September 1887.
142. The Great Northern Telegraph Co. opened a branch in Hong Kong in 1869 after completing the cable from Shanghai to Hong Kong. The Shanghai-Amoy line opened for traffic in 1870. It was linked to Singapore via Saigon in 1871, to Manila in 1880, and to Canton in 1882. See Wright, *Impressions*, p. 134.
143. Wright, *Impressions*, p. 134.
144. For the development of English-language newspapers in Hong Kong and the China Coast, see Frank H. H. King and Prescott Clarke, *A Research Guide to China-Coast Newspapers 1822–1911* (Cambridge, Mass.: Harvard University Press, 1965).
145. *DP*, 30 May, 5th June 1873; 6 April, 2 May, 25 May 1876; 20 February 1880; 6 March 1882; *XH*, 6 March 1882; 18, 22 January 1886; *Zhengxinlu* 1877, 55b; *Zhengxinlu* 1885, Part 4:27b; Zhengxinlu 1886, Part 4:30a. Telegram from 'Chinese Guild or Club' and from the Chinese Consul-General in San Francisco, to the Tung Wah Hospital, 21 February 1886, enclosed in Seymour to Porter, 3 March 1886: #97. United States National Archives, Despatches from U. S. Consuls in Canton, 1790–1906 (M 101). In fact the matter was complicated by the Exclusion Act which banned Chinese labourers but allowed non-labourers and others who had a special claim for entering the United States, for example, those who had been there before 1882 and their relatives. The result was much impersonating, leading to abuse, corruption, and suffering.
146. The Six Companies (*liu gongxi*) (六公司) were the six most powerful *huiguan* in San Francisco. See Gunther Barth, *Bitter Strength: A History of the Chinese in the United States, 1850–1870* (Cambridge, Mass.: Harvard University Press, 1965), Chapter IV, 'Chinese California'; S. Y. Wu, *One Hundred Years of Chinese in the United States and Canada* (美國華僑百年紀實) (bilingual) (Hong Kong: 1954), pp. 14–16.
147. U. S. Senate, *Chinese Exclusion* (Washington, D. C.: Government Printing Office, 1902); Chang Tsun-wu (張存武), *Zhong Mei Gongyue fengchao* (中美工約風潮) (*The Chinese Boycott of American Goods, Exclusion Against 1905–1906*) (Taipei: 1982). Chapter One gives the background to the Movement. Aying, *Fan Mei Huagong jinyue wenxue ji (Literature on the Movement against the United States' Exclusion Act)* (Peking: 1960); *Zhengxinlu* 1885, Part 4:27b; *Zhengxinlu* 1887, Part 4:30b.
148. Zhang Yinhuan, *Riji, juan* 4:99, 6:67, 8:55; Liu Fuqian (劉福謙), Chinese Consul at Lima to Tung Wah, 21 October 1889 (Po Leung Kuk '*Xinbu*' VI) asking it to prevent Chinese from proceeding to Peru.
149. Clarence E. Glick, *Sojourners and Settlers: Chinese Migrants in Hawaii* (Honolulu: University of Hawaii Press, 1980), p. 12.
150. *DP*, 21 October 1875.
151. *DP*, 14 December 1880.
152. *DP*, 14 December 1880.
153. Liu Kunyi, '*Fu Li Zhongtang*' (覆李中堂) ('Reply to Li Hongzhang'), 16 June 1879 in *LYJ*, Vol. V, p. 2459.
154. Liu Kunyi, '*Fu Li Zhongtang*'.
155. Liu Kunyi, (劉坤一) (1830–1902) made a name by fighting the Taipings. He served in many provincial governorships before becoming Governor-General of Guangdong and Guangxi from 1875–79. See Hummel, *Eminent Chinese*, Vol. I, p. 523.
156. Liu Kunyi, '*Fu Chen Liqiu*' (覆陳荔秋) ('Reply to Chen Lanbin'), 18 October 1881, *LYJ*, Vol. V, p. 2521. Hawaii introduced the passport system to restrict the number of arrivals from China; see *Zhengxinlu* 1885, Part 4:27b, for

evidence of Tung Wah warning people not to proceed to Hawaii; Steven B. Zuckermann, 'Pake in Paradise, A Synthetic Study of Chinese Immigration to Hawaii', *Bulletin of the Institute of Ethnology, Academia Sinica* 45 (Spring 1978) pp. 39–80.

157. Hance to Tenterdon, 5 November 1878 enclosed in F.O. to C.O., 30 December 1878: CO 129/183.

158. See 'Statement of Hennessy', *HKGG* 1881, pp. 421 and 426. Also see *DP*, 28 February 1877, Chinese Deputation to Kennedy. Chan was also interpreter of the Commission to investigate the work of the Contagious Diseases Ordinance, and was appreciated as 'an interpreter of the highest value' and for his 'intimate and thorough knowledge of his countrymen and of their modes of thought and feelings', without which the Commission would not have reached them. (*BPP* XXV, p. 523). See Chapter 3, Note 30.

159. '*Zhu Riben Li shi laidian*' (駐日本黎使來電) ('Telegram from Minister in Japan, Li Shuchang'), 11 May 1882 (*LQJ*, Vol. VI, p. 1:6b); 'Fu Li shi' (覆黎使) ('Reply to Minister Li'), 13 May 1882 (*LQJ*, Vol. VI, 1:7a); Registrar General to acting Colonial Secretary, 17 June 1882, enclosed in Marsh to Kimberley, 20 June 1882, confidential: CO 129/201.

160. James Russell (1843–93) started as a cadet and became a Police Magistrate in 1870, acting Registrar General in 1874, and Registrar General, 1881. He became acting Chief Justice in 1884 and Chief Justice in 1888. See H. J. Lethbridge, *Hong Kong: Stability and Change* (Hong Kong: Oxford University Press, 1978), p. 47, n. 16.

161. Registrar General to acting Colonial Secretary, 17 June 1882.

162. Char Tin-yuke, *The Sandalwood Mountains* (Honolulu: University Press of Hawaii, 1975), p. 320, n. 43. Chun Fong was appointed commercial agent and not Consul in 1879 because China had no treaty relation with Hawaii.

163. MacDonnell to Granville, 13 May 1869, #701: CO 129/137. The problem of establishing a Chinese Consul in Hong Kong is treated in my paper 'A Chinese Consul for Hong Kong: China-Hong Kong relations in the Late Qing Period', presented at the International Conference on the History of the Ming–Ch'ing Periods, 12–15 December 1985, University of Hong Kong, to be published by the University.

164. Zhang Yinhuan (1837–1900) became Minister to the United States in 1885, and to Britain, France, Germany, and Russia in 1897. His diary *Sanzhou riji*, written during his ministership, is one of the most valuable sources of information on the history of Overseas Chinese and Chinese emigration as well as Chinese diplomacy. See Hummel, *Eminent Chinese*, Vol. I, pp. 60–4.

165. Memorial of Chinese Merchants Praying to be allowed to form an Association for suppressing Kidnapping and Traffic in Human Beings, 9 November 1878 in 'Correspondence: Chinese Slavery, March, 1882', pp. 190–2. For a history of the Po Leung Kuk, see Po Leung Kuk, Board of Directors 1977–1978, *Centenary History of the Po Leung Kuk, Hong Kong 1878–1978* (香港保良局百年史略) (bilingual) (Hong Kong: The Board, 1978); for an analytical account, see J. H. Lethbridge, 'The Evolution of a Chinese Voluntary Association: the Po Leung Kuk', *Journal of Oriental Studies* 10 (1972), pp. 33–50, reprinted in his *Stability and Change*, pp. 71–103.

166. Po Leung Kuk, '*Yishibu*' (議事簿) ('Minutes of meetings' from 1880–1885) reveals much about the Po Leung Kuk's operations and planning at the early stage, especially the intimate involvement of the Tung Wah Hospital. The meetings related to the founding of the Kuk are recorded in *XH*, 14, 16 and 20 August 1880.

167. Memorial of Chinese Merchants, 9 November 1878.

168. J. J. Francis, 'Memorandum on the subject of Slavery'. See also Smale's

exposition on the sale of human beings in Chief Justice to acting Colonial Secretary, 26 August 1880 and 24 November 1880, enclosed in Hennessy to Kimberley, 28 July 1881, enclosed in 'Correspondence: Chinese Slavery, March 1882', pp. 258–60, 261–4.

169. Merchant's Petition and Statement, 25 October 1879 enclosed in Hennessy to Kimberley, 23 January 1880 in 'Correspondence: Chinese Slavery, March 1882', pp. 208–213, p. 212.

170. 'Correspondence: Chinese Slavery, March 1882', pp. 208–213.

171. 'Correspondence: Chinese Slavery, March 1882', p. 209.

172. Report by the acting Police Magistrate and acting Police Superintendent of Police, 28 June 1880, enclosed in Hennessy to Kimberley, 3 September 1880 in 'Correspondence: Chinese Slavery, March 1882', pp. 84–5.

173. Some cases are enclosed in 'Correspondence: Chinese Slavery, March 1882', pp. 170–90, 198–9, 200–8.

174. Merchants' Petition and Statement, 25 October 1879.

175. Chief Justice to acting Colonial Secretary, sub-enclosed in 'Correspondence: Chinese Slavery, March 1882', pp. 251–2.

176. Notes of Suggested Amendment [to the proposed rules of the Society] by the Attorney General, Edward O'Malley, enclosed in Hennessy to Kimberley, 31 August 1881, in 'Correspondence: Chinese Slavery, March 1882', pp. 282–3.

177. Kimberley to Hennessy, 3 November 1881 in 'Correspondence: Chinese Slavery, March 1882', p. 284. Minutes of a meeting held at the Magistracy, 28 November 1878 in 'Correspondence: Chinese Slavery, March 1882', pp. 195–6.

178. Hennessy to Hicks-Beach, 23 January 1880, #8: CO 129/187; for his belief in the freedom of women, see his reply to Chinese Deputation, HKGG 1880, pp. 185–92, p. 190.

179. For the muitsai question, see Lethbridge, Stability and Change, pp. 93–6; Fan xubi hui (反蓄婢會) (Anti-Muitsai Society), Xianggang xubi wenti (香港蓄婢問題) (The Problem of muitsai) (Hong Kong: The Society, 1923); Great Britian Colonial Office, Hong Kong: Papers relative to the Muitsai Question (London: H.M.S.O., 1929); Hugh Lyttleton Hastelwood, Child Slavery in Hong Kong and the Muitsai System (London: Sheldon Press, 1930); British Commission on Muitsai in Hong Kong and Malaya, Muitsai in Hong Kong and Malaya, [London, 1936], I, pp. 73–300; Hong Kong, Muitsai Committee, Muitsai in Hong Kong: Report of the Committee... (London: H.M.S.O., 1936). Norman Miners, Hong Kong Under Imperial Rule, 1912–1945 (Hong Kong: Oxford University Press, 1987), especially Chapters 8 and 9; Carl Smith, 'The Chinese Church, Labour and Elites and the Mui Tsai Question in the 1920s', JHKBRAS 21 (1981), pp. 91–113.

180. 'Civil Establishment', Blue Book 1872, pp. 64, 66, 76.

181. 'Civil Establishment', Blue Book 1876, pp. 67, 88, 90, 109.

182. Hennessy to Hicks-Beach, 2 August 1878, confidential: CO 129/181.

183. C. C. Smith to Hennessy, enclosed in Hennessy to Hicks-Beach, 24 September 1878, #89: CO 129/182; see also the minute on it.

184. 'Minute by the acting Colonial Secretary on the Secretary of State's Despatch no. 105 of 29th May, 1882, dated 19th July, 1882,' enclosed in Marsh to Kimberley, 20 July 1882, #136: CO 129/202.

185. 'Minute by the acting Colonial Secretary'.

186. Hennessy to Kimberley, 7 March 1882, #56: CO 129/198; Hennessy to Hicks-Beach, 16 November 1878, #116: CO 129/182.

187. Hennessy to Hicks-Beach, 16 November 1878, #116.

188. Minute on Hennessy to Hicks-Beach, 2 August 1878, confidential: CO 129/181.

189. Minute on Hennessy to Hicks-Beach, 16 November 1878, #116: CO 129/182.
190. Minute on Hennessy to Hicks-Beach, 16 November 1878, #116. John Bramston was Attorney General at Hong Kong, 1873–76 and became Under-Secretary of State for the Colonies in 1876. See Norton-Kyshe, *Laws and Courts*, Vol. II, p. 229n; Brian L. Blakeley, *The Colonial Office 1886–1892* (Durham, N. C.: Duke University Press, 1972), p. 80.
191. Minute on Hennessy to Hicks-Beach, 16 November 1878, #116: CO 129/182.
192. *DP*, 12 July 1873.
193. Irish Distress Fund Committee and Subscription Lists, enclosed in Hennessy to Kimberley, 9 July 1880, #98: CO 129/189. The European contribution was $12,000 while the Chinese contribution was $118,000.
194. *CM*, 29 September 1881.
195. *DP*, February 1882.
196. Marsh to Kimberley, 14 April 1882, #21: CO 129/199. This subject will be discussed more fully in Chapter 5.
197. *DP*, 28 February 1882.
198. Wang Tao, '*Chuangjian Donghua Yiyuan xu*'.

Notes to Chapter 5

1. *DP*, 19 May 1873.
2. *DP*, 2 June, 20 October 1873.
3. *CM*, 29 September 1881.
4. *DP*, 5 June 1873
5. *DP*, 21 May, 1 July, 25 July, 1873; 25 July 1875; *CM*, 13 November 1875 and May 1879.
6. *DP*, 23 May, 9 September 1871.
7. *CM*, 13 November 1875.
8. *CM*, 8 November 1875.
9. *CM*, 13 November 1875.
10. *ZW*, 14 October 1871.
11. *ZW*, 13 April 1874.
12. *CM*, 15 November 1875
13. *CM*, 16 November 1875, reports on notices in Chinese newspapers.
14. *CM*, 15 November 1875.
15. *CM*, 15 November 1875.
16. Marsh to Kimberley, 14 April 1882, #21: CO 129/199.
17. Wei will be discussed below; Woo Sing Lim (吳醒廉), *Prominent Chinese in Hong Kong* (香港華人名人史略) (bilingual) (Hong Kong: 1937), p. 4; see also Arnold Wright (ed.), *Twentieth Century Impressions of Hong Kong, Shanghai and Other Treaty Ports* (London: Lloyd's Greater Britain Publishing, 1908), p. 109.
18. Marsh to Kimberley, 14 April 1882, #21: CO 129/199: See petition from 'the Chinese Mercantile Community of Hong Kong', presented to Hennessy on 19 February 1880, *HKGG* 1880, pp. 185–92.
19. Marsh to Kimberley, 14 April 1882, #21: CO 129/199.
20. William Marsh (1827–1906) served in Mauritius 1848–79 and became Auditor General in 1876; Colonial Secretary and Attorney General of Hong Kong 1879–87. Administered the government of Hong Kong 1882–83, September to October 1883, and 1885-87. He retired in 1887 and was knighted. See G. B.

Endacott, *Government and People in Hong Kong* (Hong Kong: Hong Kong University Press, 1964), p. 97, n. 2.

21. Marsh to Kimberley, 14 April 1882, #21.

22. Osbert Chadwick was the son of Edwin Chadwick, whose Report on sanitation had persuaded the British government to introduce the first Public Health Act in 1848. Osbert was sent out to Hong Kong in 1881 to investigate the sanitary conditions, and his *Report on the Sanitary Condition of Hong Kong: with Appendices and Plans* (London: H.M.S.O., 1882) is one of the most important sources of information on the colony's housing and social conditions.

23. Marsh to Kimberly, 14 April 1882, #21: CO 129/199.

24. One of the best indicators of this is the number of letters addressed jointly to the Tung Wah and Po Leung Kuk in the latter's archives. Some were addressed to the Tung Wah, but forwarded to the Po Leung Kuk.

25. Minute on Hicks-Beach to Hennessy, 20 February 1879, confidential: CO 129/183.

26. *DP*, 12 July 1873.

27. *HKGG* 1876, p. 30.

28. Hance to Foreign Office, 5 November 1878, #37, enclosed in F.O. to C.O., 30 December 1878: CO 129/183.

29. Hicks-Beach to Hennessy, 20 February 1879, confidential: CO 129/183.

30. Marsh to Kimberley, 20 June 1882, confidential: CO 129/201.

31. Eitel's Report on Paupers, enclosed in Hennessy to Kimberley, 26 May 1881, #73: CO 129/193.

32. Hennessy to Kimberley, 9 April 1881, telegram: CO 129/192.

33. Minute on Hennessy to Kimberley, 9 April 1881, telegram.

34. Kimberley to Marsh, 29 May 1882, #105: CO 129/198.

35. Hennessy to Kimberley, 7 March 1882, #56: CO 129/198.

36. Kimberley to Marsh, 29 May 1882, #105: CO129/198. He crossed out this phrase in the draft.

37. Marsh to Kimberley, 20 June 1882, confidential: CO 129/201.

38. Registrar General's Report, 5 June 1882, enclosed in Marsh to Kimberley, 20 June 1882, confidential.

39. Registrar General's Report, 7 June 1882, enclosed in Marsh to Kimberley, 20 June 1882, confidential.

40. Attorney General's minute on Registrar General's report, 5 June 1882.

41. Marsh to Kimberley, 20 June 1882, confidential: CO 129/201.

42. Marsh to Kimberley, 20 June 1882, confidential.

43. Kimberley to Marsh, 29 May 1882, #105: CO 129/198; Kimberley to Marsh, 4 September 1882, confidential: CO 129/201.

44. Marsh to Kimberley, 14 August 1882, #161: CO 129/202.

45. Registrar General to acting Colonial Secretary, 2 August 1882, enclosed in Marsh to Kimberley, 14 August 1882, #161.

46. Registrar General to acting Colonial Secretary, 2 August 1882.

47. Acting Colonial Secretary to Chairman of the Tung Wah Hospital Committee, enclosed in Marsh to Kimberley, 14 August 1882, #161.

48. Marsh to Kimberley, 20 July 1882, #136: CO 129/202.

49. Minute by the acting Colonial Secretary on Secretary of State's Despatch #105 on 29 May 1882, dated 19 July 1882, enclosed in Marsh to Kimberley, 20 July 1882, #136.

50. Fung Ming-shan (Feng Mingshan) (馮明珊) was compradore of A. H. Hogg & Co., and later Chartered Mercantile Bank. He was educated at St Paul's College. A member of the Tung Wah's Founding Committee, Director in 1872, and Chairman of 1879, he was the chief promoter of the Po Leung Kuk.

51. Marsh to Kimberley, 20 July 1882, #136: CO 129/202.

52. Minute by the acting Colonial Secretary, enclosed in Marsh to Kimberley, 20 July 1882, #136.

53. Marsh to Kimberley, 17 August 1882, #166: CO 129/202.

54. Marsh to Kimberley, 28 August 1882, #174: CO 129/202.

55. Minute on Marsh to Kimberley, 28 August 1882, #174.

56. Marsh to Bowen, enclosed in Bowen to Derby, 9 April 1883, #17: CO 129/208.

57. Minute on Bowen to Derby, 11 April 1883, telegram: CO 129/208.

58. Derby to Bowen, 30 April 1883, #75: CO 129/208.

59. Registrar General's memorandum enclosed in Bowen to Derby, 18 April 1884, #126: CO 129/215.

60. Bowen to Derby, 18 July 1884, #263: CO 129/217.

61. Lin Youlan, *'Jindai Zhongwen baoye xianqu — Huang Sheng'* (現代中文報業先驅—黃勝) ('Huang Sheng, pioneer in modern Chinese journalism'), *Baoxue* 4:3 (December 1969), pp. 108-11; Smith, 'The Emergence of a Chinese Élite', in his *Chinese Christians: Élite, Middlemen and the Church in Hong Kong* (Hong Kong: Oxford University Press, 1985), pp. 122-3, 134-5.

62. Bowen to Derby, 28 December 1883, #355: CO 129/213.

63. *HKGG* 1878, p. 599.

64. Bowen to Derby, 3 December 1883, #324: CO 129/213.

65. Bowen to Derby, 3 December 1883, #324. There were 20 English, one American, six Germans and other Continental Europeans, two Chinese, three Jews, and two Parsees and Armenians.

66. For naturalizations, see lists in *HKGG* for respective years.

67. Marsh to Derby, 22 January 1883, #13: CO 129/207.

68. Bramston's minute on Bowen to Derby, 4 April 1883, #4: CO 129/208.

69. Derby to Bowen, 9 March 1883, #57: CO 129/207.

70. The Contagious Diseases Ordinance was introduced in 1867 to protect British troops; see 'Report of the Commission...to enquire into the working of the Contagious Diseases Ordinance', *BPP* XXV.

71. Registrar General to acting Colonial Secretary, 19 September 1882, enclosed in Marsh to Kimberley, 27 September 1882, #209: CO 129/202.

72. Marsh to Derby, 21 September 1883, #240: CO 129/211.

73. Bowen to Derby, 25 August 1884, #298: CO 129/217.

74. For the 1884 strike-riot, see Fang Hanqi (方漢奇) *'Yiba basi nian Xianggang renmin de fan di douzheng'* (一八八四年香港人民的反帝鬥爭) ('The anti-imperialist struggle of the Hong Kong people in 1884'), *Jindaishi ziliao* 近代史資料 (*Sources on Modern China*) 57:6 (December 1957), pp. 20-30; Li Mingren (李明仁), *'Yiba basi nian Xianggang bagong yundong'* (一八八四年香港罷工運動) ('The strike in Hong Kong, 1884'), *Lishi yanjiu* (歷史研究) (*Historical Studies*) 1958:3 (March 1958), pp. 89-90; Lewis M. Chere, 'The Hong Kong Riots of October, 1884: Evidence for Chinese Nationalism', *JHKBRAS* 20 (1980), pp. 54-65; Elizabeth Sinn, 'The Strike and Riot of 1884 — A Hong Kong Perspective', *JHKBRAS* 22 (1982), pp. 65-98; Ts'ai Jung-fang, 'The 1884 Hong Kong Insurrection: Anti-Imperialist Popular Protest during the Sino-French War', *Bulletin of Concerned Asian Scholars* 16:1 (January-March 1984), pp. 2-14.

75. A translated version of the proclamation is enclosed in Marsh to Derby, 25 September 1884 #336: CO 129/217; another is in *DP*, October 1884. The original is in Hu Quanzhao (胡傳釗), *Tunmo liufen* (盾墨留芬) (*Notes on the [Sino-French] War*), 2 volumes, 8 *juan* (Taipei: 1973, photographic reprint; original preface dated 1898), *juan* 2:28b-29b.

76. *DP*, 19 September 1884.

77. *CM*, 2 October 1884.

78. Sinn, 'The Strike and Riot of 1884', pp. 77-80.

79. Minute by Robert Herbert on *Standard* to C.O., 16 October 1884: CO 129/218.

80. Marsh to Derby, 25 September 1884, #336: CO 129/217.

81. *DP*, 4 October 1884.

82. Marsh to Derby, 6 October 1884, #340: CO 129/217.

83. *CM*, 29 September 1 and 2 October 1884; *DP*, 9 October 1884.

84. *CM*, 5 October 1884.

85. Marsh to Derby, 6 October 1884, #340: CO 129/217.

86. Minute by the acting Colonial Secretary of a conference held with certain members of the native community regarding the strike and riot, enclosed in Marsh to Derby, 6 October 1884, #340.

87. Marsh to Derby, 6 October 1884, #340.

88. Memorandum by the Colonial Secretary, 5 December 1884, enclosed in Bowen to Derby 5 December 1884, #399: CO 129/218.

89. T. Jackson's speech at Legislative Council, 9 October 1884, reported in *DP*, 10 October 1884.

90. Zhang Zhidong, 'Zhi Zongshu' (致總署) ('To the Tsungli Yamen'), 9 October 1884, telegram in *ZQJ juan* 73:7a–7b.

91. Sir Thomas Jackson, Bt., was appointed chief manager of the Hong Kong & Shanghai Banking Corporation in 1876, retired in 1902, and served on the London Committee of the Bank until his death in 1915. Knighted in 1899, he became a baronet in 1902. He was appointed to the Legislative Council in 1884 and resigned 1887. See Endacott, *Government and People*, p. 101, n. 1. See also Frank H. H. King, *The Hong Kong Bank in Late Imperial China 1864–1902* (Cambridge: Cambridge University Press, 1987).

92. T. Jackson's speech at the Legislative Council, 9 October 1884.

93. T. Jackson's speech at the Legislative Council, 9 October 1884.

94. P. Ryrie's speech at the Legislative Council, 9 October 1884, reported in *DP*, 10 October 1884.

95. Zhang Zhidong, '*Huichou baohu qiaoshang shiyi zhe*' (會籌保護僑商事宜摺) ('Joint memorial for the protection of Chinese traders overseas'), 30 March 1886, in *ZQJ, juan* 15: 7b–14a.

96. Hu, *Tunmo liufen*, (Notes on the [Sino-French] war), *juan* 2: 16b.

97. See Chapter 3, Note 36.

98. Marsh to Parkes, 4 October 1884, enclosed in F.O. to C.O., 2 February 1885: CO 129/224; *DP*, 4 October 1884.

99. Zhang Zhidong, 'Zhi Zongshu' (致總署) ('To Tsungli Yamen'), 9 October 1884, *ZQJ* pp. 7a–7b. The term '*shi ke ji zhi*' (適可即止) is more commonly expressed as '*shi ke er zhi*' (適可而止).

100. Zhang Zhidong, 'Zhi Zongshu', 9 October 1884.

101. *CM*, 14 October 1884.

102. Marsh to O'Conor, 20 January 1886, #13/G enclosed in Marsh to Stanley, 25 January 1886, confidential: CO 129/225.

103. *Weixin ribao* (維新日報), 31 December 1885; the clipping is enclosed in Marsh to O'Conor, 20 January 1886, FO 228/842; and a translated version is in CO 129/225.

104. Zhang Zhidong, 'Huichou baohu qiaoshang shiyi zhe'; Michael Godley, *The Mandarin-Capitalists from Nanyang: Overseas Chinese Enterprise in the Modernization of China 1893–1911* (Cambridge, Mass.: Harvard University Press, 1981), p. 72.

105. The Chinese telegram from the 'Chinese Guild or Club' and from the Chinese Consul-General in San Francisco to the Tung Wah Hospital Committee, 21 February 1886, enclosed in Seymour to Porter, 3 March 1886, #97, United

States, National Archives, Despatches from U. S. Consuls in Canton 1790–1906 (M101).

106. Seymour to Porter, 3 March 1886, #97.

107. Zhang Zhidong, '*Lichen Huaqiao bi hai Yuesheng banli qingxing bing chicui cheng ban zhe*' (瀝陳華僑被害粵省辦理情形並勒催懲辦摺) ('Memorial reporting on the victimization of Overseas Chinese and Canton conditions, and urging immediate action'), 19 May 1886, *ZQJ, juan* 16: 18a–25a.

108. Lin Xiaosheng (林孝勝), '*Qingchao zhu Xing lingshi yu Haixia zhimindi zhengfu de juifen (1877–1894)*' (清朝駐星領事與海峽殖民地政府的糾紛) ('The controversy between the Chinese Consul at Singapore and the Straits Settlements Government') in Ke Mulin (柯木林) and others, *Xingjiapo Huazu shi lunji* (星加坡華族史論集) (*Collection of Essays on the History of the Chinese People in Singapore*) (Singapore: 1972), pp. 13–47.

109. Hicks-Beach to Hennessy, 20 February 1879, confidential: CO 129/183.

110. Kimberley to Marsh, 4 September 1882, confidential: CO 129/201.

111. Report by the acting Registrar General enclosed in Marsh to Stanley, 25th January, 1886, confidential: CO 129/225, *XH*, 6 June, 1, 2, 4, 6, 7, 12, 13, July 1885.

112. Zhang Yinhuan, *Riji, juan* 4:33a.

113. Zhang Zhidong, undated letter to Jiang daren (蔣大人) in *Zhang Wenxiang shuhan mobao* (張文襄書翰墨寶) (*Calligraphy of Zhang Zhidong*) (Shanghai: 1924), pp. 1–6.

114. Report by the acting Registrar General enclosed in Marsh to O'Conor, 20 January 1886.

115. 'Petition from Kwan Hoi-chun', Chairman of the Tung Wah Hospital, enclosed in Marsh to Granville, 24 March 1886, #91: CO 129/225.

116. This idea is suggested by Michael Godley and though there is no evidence, it is highly plausible. See his *The Mandarin-Capitalists from Nanyang*, p. 72.

117. 'Petition from Mr Kwan Hoi-chun'.

118. Report by the acting Registrar General enclosed in Marsh to O'Conor, 20 January 1886; Provincial Treasurer's original dispatch, dated 8 December is in FO 228/842. See Appendix VI.

119. Marsh to O'Conor, 20 January 1886, enclosed in Marsh to Stanley, 25 January 1886, confidential: CO 129/225.

120. Report by the acting Registrar General, enclosed in Marsh to Stanley, 25 January 1886; *XH*, 2 January 1886.

121. Report by the acting Registrar General.

122. Report by the acting Registrar General. Ho Amei's note to Kwan informing him of the arrival of the tablet is enclosed in Marsh to O'Conor, 20 January 1886: FO 228/842. The dispatch accompanying the tablet scroll was addressed to the Tung Wah Hospital Committee but was apparently sent in care of Ho. This is also enclosed in Marsh to O'Conor, 20 January 1886.

123. Report by the acting Registrar General, sub-enclosed in Marsh to Stanley, 25 January 1886, confidential: CO 129/225.

124. Report by the acting Registrar General.

125. Marsh to O'Conor, 20 March 1886, #47/G, enclosed in Marsh to Granville, 24 March 1886, #91: CO 129/225.

126. Report by the Registrar General, sub-enclosed in Marsh to Stanley, 25 January 1886, confidential: CO 129/225.

127. Ho Amei's article in *Huazi ribao*, sub-enclosed in Marsh to O'Conor, 20 January 1886: FO 228/842.

128. Ho Amei's article in *Huazi ribao*.

129. This is the '*shen wei pu you*' plaque; see Chapter 4.

130. Marsh to O'Conor, 20 January 1886, #13/G, enclosed in Marsh to Stanley, 25 January 1886, confidential: CO 129/225; the original documents are enclosed in Marsh to O'Conor, 20 January 1886: FO 228/842.
131. Minute on Marsh to Stanley, 25 January 1886, confidential: CO 129/225.
132. Minute on Marsh to Granville, 24 March 1886, #91: CO 129/225.
133. 'Petition from Mr Kwan Hoi-chun'.
134. The *shan hou ju* (善後局) (Board of Reorganization) was a committee established after rebellions, warfare, or physical calamities to pacify or to restore order. It comprised of the Governor-General, the Governor, Treasurer, the Judicial Commission, the Salt Controller, and Grain Intendant.
135. 'Petition from Mr Kwan Hoi-chun'.
136. 'Petition from Mr Kwan Hoi-chun.
137. Marsh to O'Conor, 20 March 1886, #47/G enclosed in Marsh to Granville, 24 March 1886, #91: CO 129/225.
138. Board of Reorganization to the Tung Wah Directors, 5 February 1886, authenticated copy enclosed in Marsh to O'Conor, 20 March 1886, #47/G: FO 228/842. See Appendix VII.
139. Board of Reorganization to the Tung Wah Directors, 5 February 1886.
140. Marsh to Granville, 24 March 1886, #91: CO 129/225.
141. Marsh to Granville, 24 March 1886.
142. Zhang Yinhuan, *Riji, juan* 4:33a.
143. Zhang Yinhuan, *Riji, juan* 4:33a.
144. O'Conor to Ministers of the Tsungli Yamen, 5 April 1886, enclosed in F.O. to C.O., 3 June 1886: CO 129/230.
145. Minute on Marsh to Granville, 1 May 1886, #138: CO 129/226.
146. Marsh to Stanley, 25 January 1886, confidential: CO 129/225.
147. F.O. to C.O., 26 April 1886: CO 129/230; F.O. to O'Conor, 8 November 1886, #294: FO 228/822.
148. Tsungli Yamen to O'Conor, 8 April 1886, enclosed in O'Conor to Marsh, 8 April 1886, enclosed in Marsh to Granville, 1 May 1886, #138: CO 129/226.
149. Marsh to Granville, 1 May 1886, #138.
150. Minute on Marsh to Granville, 1 May 1886, #138.
151. F.O. to C.O., 26 October 1886: CO 129/230.
152. Preface to *Zhengxinlu* 1886.
153. Zhang Zhidong, *'Qing cuishe Xianggang lingshi zhe'* (請催設香港領事摺) ('Memorial urging the establishment of a Consul at Hong Kong') of 20 March 1886, in *ZQJ, juan* 15:14a–15b. Compare *'Yuedong Zhang Zhidong zouqing cuishe Xianggang lingshi yi qi annei yuwai zhe* (粵東張之洞奏請催設香港領事以期安內馭外摺) ('Zhang Zhidong's memorial urging the establishment of a Consul at Hong Kong in order to bring internal and external order'), submitted to the Tsungli Yamen on 26 April 1886, in *Qingji waijiao shiliao* (清季外交史料) (*Historical Materials Relating to Late Qing Diplomacy), 164 juan* (Peking: 1935), *juan* 69: 9b–12a.
154. Ho Kai's 'Memorandum on the Hong Kong Chinese Chamber of Commerce', 30 May 1888, enclosed in Stewart to Knutsford, 11 December 1888, #360: CO 129/239.
155. Stewart to Knutsford, 11 December 1888, #360.
156. Ho Kai's 'Memorandum on the Hong Kong Chinese Chamber of Commerce'.
157. Ho Kai's 'Memorandum on the Hong Kong Chinese Chamber of Commerce'.
158. Ho Kai's 'Memorandum on the Hong Kong Chinese Chamber of Commerce'.

159. Rule no. 4, in Rules and Regulations, sub-enclosed in Stewart to Knutsford, 11 December 1888, #360.

160. Lockhart to Stewart, 5 June 1888, enclosed in Stewart to Knutsford, 11 December 1888, #360.

161. Lockhart to Stewart, 5 June 1888.

162. Stewart to Knutsford, 11 December 1888, #360: CO 129/239.

163. See Sinn, 'A Chinese Consul for Hong Kong: China–Hong Kong Relations in the Late Qing Period'.

164. Bowen to Derby, 28 December 1883, #355: CO 129/213.

165. Dr Ho Kai's Protest against the Public Health Bill, submitted to the government by the Sanitary Board, and the Board's Rejoinder thereto, *HKSP* 30/1887, pp. 403–12.

166. Dr Ho kai's Protest. Ho wrote in English, but his friend Hu Liyuan (see Note 177) translated many of his works into Chinese to give them wider circulation. Several of the most important of Ho's reformist writings are translated and compiled into *Xinzheng zhenchuan* (新政眞詮) (*The True Meaning of the New Politics*) in *Hu Yinan xiansheng quanji* (胡翼南先生全集) (*The Collected Works of Hu Liyuan*) 60 *juan* (Hong Kong: 1920). One of Ho's first works is a review of Zeng Jize's 'China: the Sleep and the Awakening', which first appeared in the *China Mail* in 1887 and is appended in Chiu Ling Yeong, 'Sir Kai Ho Kai', pp. 314–38. To Ho, the real weakness of China lay in her loose morality and evil habits, both social and political, but his concepts of reform were inspired by Britain.

167. Bowen to Derby, 22 January 1883, #13; CO 129/207.

168. 'Registrar General's Report, 1891', p. 365.

169. 'Registrar General's Report, 1892', pp. 442–3.

170. Ho Fuk (He Fu) was the brother of Ho Tung (see Chapter 7). He was educated at the Central School in Hong Kong and worked as interpreter for the government before succeeding Ho Tung as compradore of Jardine's in 1900.

171. Thomas Henderson Whitehead of Chartered Bank of India, Australia, and China, was unofficial Legislative Councillor, 1890–1902.

172. See Hong Kong, *Report of the Po Leung Kuk*.

173. Hong Kong, *Report of the Po Leung Kuk*, pp. V–X.

174. Ng Lun Ngai-ha, *Interactions of East and West: Development of Public Education in Early Hong Kong* (Hong Kong: Chinese University Press, 1984), pp. 165–6; See also her 'The Role of Hong Kong Educated Chinese in the Shaping of Modern China', *MAS* 17 (1983), pp. 137–63. For the Central School/Queen's College, see Gwenneth Stokes, *Queen's College* (Hong Kong: Queen's College, 1987, 1st published 1962) and Yan Woon Yin, 'Hong Kong and the Modernization of China (1862–1911). The Contributions of Central School Graduates' (B.A thesis, University of Hong Kong, 1980).

175. For Wang Tao, see his 'Xianggang luelun' (香港略論) ('Brief discussion on Hong Kong'), *Taoyuan wenlu waibian*, pp. 177–81; for Guo Songdao, see *Riji*, III, pp. 108–9; for Kang Youwei, see Kang Tongbi (康同璧) (ed.), *Nanhai Kang xiansheng zibian nianpu* (南海康先生自編年譜) (*Chronological Autobiography of Kang Youwei*) (Peking: 1958), p. 5a; for Sun Yat-sen, see Ng Lun Ngai-ha, 'The Hong Kong Origins of Dr Sun Yat-sen's Address to Li Hung-chang', *JHKBRAS* 21 (1981), pp. 168–78.

176. (See Note 166). Satisfaction with the British political system and the opportunities offered by Hong Kong's are manifest throughout Ho Kai and Hu Liyuan's writings, and particularly in '*Xinzheng lunyi*' (新政論議) ('Discourse on new politics') (1895) and '*Kang shuo shu hou*' (康說書後) ('Review of Kang

Youwei's speech'), (*Hu Yinan xiansheng quanji, juan* 4-6, 13-14; see especially *juan* 13:16a-19a).

177. Hu Liyuan (胡禮垣) (1847-1916) was a student of the Central School and later taught Chinese there. After working at the *Xunhuan ribao* as translator, he entered business, but retained academic interests, translating many of Ho Kai's works into English. See Ts'ai, 'Comprador Ideologists'.

178. This theme is developed throughout Joseph Levenson, *Liang Ch'i-ch'ao and the Mind of Modern China* (Berkeley, Los Angeles: University of California Press, 1970; first published 1953)

179. Wang Xingrui (王興瑞), 'Qingchao Furen Wenshe yu geming yundong de guanxi' (清朝輔仁文社與革命運動的關係) ('The Furen literary society and the revolutionary movement in the Qing period'), *Shixue zaji* (史學雜誌) (*Historical Journal*), (*Chungking*) 1:1 (December 1945); *The Chinese Republic — the Secret History of the Chinese Revolution* (Hong Kong: South China Morning Post, 1924) by Tse Tsan Tai, one of its founders, gives some interesting insights into the thinking of the members; for Tse, see Chapter 6.

180. See reports of the Registrar General after 1891, in both the *HKGG* and *HKSP*. In 1892, for instance, there were 37 petitions related to the disappearance of wives, 13 to the disappearance of children and young girls, 33 to domestic disputes, and 15 to business disputes. (*HKGG* 1893, p. 465.)

181. H. J. Lethbridge, 'Sir James Haldane Stewart Lockhart' in his *Hong Kong Stability and Change, A Collection of Essays* (Hong Kong: Oxford University Press, 1978), pp. 133-4.

182. Ch'ü T'ung-tsu, *Local Government in China under the Ch'ing* (Cambridge, Mass.: Harvard University Press, 1962).

Notes to Chapter 6

1. Robinson to Ripon, 17 May 1894, #115: CO 129/263; a report by Dr Alex Rennie of Canton on the epidemic is given in *Hong Kong Telegraph* (hereafter *HKT*), 10 May 1894. For the Plague in Hong Kong, see *Blue Books 1894-1904, Regarding the Bubonic Plague in Hong Kong*, collection bound together for the Government Secretariat's Library; 'Colonial Surgeon's Report, 1894', *HKSP* 1895, pp. 473-520; Wilfred William Pearce, *Plague in Hong Kong* (Hong Kong: Government Printers, 1905); Charles J. H. Halcombe, *The Mystic Flowery Land* (London: 1896), Chapter XXVIII, 'The Great Plague of Hong Kong'; James Dalziel, *Chronicles of a Crown Colony* (Hong Kong: South China Morning Post, 1907), pp. 1-15, 'The Case of John Dyer: Hero,' is a touching fictional account of the plague; E. G. Pryor, 'The Great Plague of Hong Kong', *JHKBRAS* 15 (1975), pp. 61-70; William McNeil, *Plagues and Peoples* (Oxford: Blackwell Press, 1976).

2. James A. Lowson, 'The Epidemic of Bubonic Plague in Hong Kong, 1894' (hereafter Lowson's Plague Report, 1894) enclosed in *HKSP* 16, 1895, pp. 178-236, p. 179.

3. Lowson's Plague Report, 1894, p. 178.

4. 'Report of the Colonial Surgeon on his Inspection of the Town of Victoria and on the Pig Licensing System, Hong Kong, April, 1874, in 'Correspondence relating to the Working of the Contagious Diseases Ordinance of the Colony of Hong Kong' [C. -3093] LXV, 1881, *BPP* XXV, pp. 573-639, pp. 621-624; G. B. Endacott, *A History of Hong Kong* (Hong Kong: Oxford University Press, 1983), pp. 183-5.

5. The Chadwick Report, see Chapter 5, Note 22.

6. James William Norton-Kyshe, *The History of the Laws and Courts of Hong Kong* (Hong Kong, Vetch & Lee, 1971), Vol. I, pp. 408–10.

7. Dr Ho Kai's Protest against the Public Health Bill,' *HKSP* 30, 1887, pp. 403–12.

8. Endacott, *History*, pp. 200–1.

9. *HKT*, 10 May 1894.

10. Lau Wai Chuen (劉渭川) was a Director of the Tung Wah Hospital in 1884, Chairman of the Po Leung Kuk in 1887, and appointed to the District Watch Committee in 1892. He was compradore of the Hong Kong and Shanghai Bank from 1892, but had his own. Australia and California trade. He went bankrupt in 1907.

11. *HKT*, 10 May 1894.

12. James Alfred Lowson, M.B.C.M., a graduate of the University of Edinburgh, arrived in 1889 to become the Assistant Surgeon in the government.

13. Lowson's Report, 16 May 1894, enclosed in Robinson to Ripon, 17 May 1894, #115: CO 129/263.

14. Lowson's Report, 16 May 1894.

15. Ayres and Lowson to Lockhart, Secretary of the Sanitary Board, enclosed in Lowson's Report, 16 May 1894.

16. *HKT*, 10 May 1894.

17. Lowson's Report, 16 May 1894.

18. J. J. Francis was admitted as an attorney in the Hong Kong court in 1869, after being articled to Mr William Gaskell. In 1886 he was appointed Q.C. for Hong Kong and was elected to the Sanitary Board in 1888, when elections were first held. See Norton-Kyshe, *Laws and Courts*, Vol. II; G. B. Endacott, *Government and People in Hong Kong* (Hong Kong: Hong Kong University Press), pp. 152–3. For Francis, see Walter Greenwood, 'John Joseph Francis, Citizen of Hong Kong. A Biographical Note', *JHKBRAS* 26 (1986), pp. 17–45.

19. Lowson's Report, 16 May 1894.

20. C. Fraser Brockington, *A Short History of Public Health* (London: J. & A. Churchill Ltd, 1966), p. 38.

21. *CM*, 11 May 1894.

22. *HKT*, 12 May 1894.

23. *CM*, 13 June 1894.

24. Lowson's Plague Report, 1894, p. 203.

25. *HKT*, 12 May 1894.

26. Report on interview with Lowson, *HKT*, 22 May 1894.

27. Letter of 'Heathen Chinese' in *HKT*, 12 May 1894.

28. *HKT*, 12 May 1894.

29. *DP*, 21 May 1894.

30. *DP*, 15 May 1894.

31. Letter of 'Heathen Chinese', *HKT*, 23 May 1894.

32. Interview with Lowson, *HKT*, 22 May 1894.

33. Robinson to Ripon, 23 May 1894, #122: CO 129/263; Consul Brenan to O'Conor, 11 June 1894, enclosed in O'Conor to Kimberley, 22 June 1894, in FO 17/1227: China Riots, confidential 40, section 1 (hereafter 'China Riots'), p. 2.

34. Lowson's Evidence, *TWR*, pp. 38–48, p. 42.

35. *CM*, 14 May 1894.

36. Jean Cantlie Stewart, *The Quality of Mercy: The Lives of Sir James and Lady Cantlie* (London: George Allen & Unwin, 1983), p. 67.

37. *HKT*, 18 May 1894.

38. *DP*, 21 May 1894.

39. Jeanne L. Brand, *Doctors and the State: The British Medical Profession*

and Government Action in Public Health, 1870–1912 (Baltimore: Johns Hopkins Press, 1965), p. 7.

40. Letter from 'A Chinaman' to *DP*, 13 June 1894; Robinson to Ripon, 20 June 1894, #21, *HKSP* 1894, pp. 283–292, p. 284.

41. Compare India, 1897, when plague broke out in Poona. The Plague Committee President, on whose instructions and authority the sanitary operations were carried out, was murdered. See R. C. Majumdar and others, *British Paramountcy and Indian Renaissance* (Bombay: 1963–65), pp. 591–2. I am grateful to Mrs Coonoor Kripalani-Thadani for this information. *HKT*, 28 June 1894, compares the situation to Glasgow where owners of houses declared uninhabitable had a chance to challenge orders to close them whereas in Hong Kong there was no recourse.

42. *DP*, 19 May 1894.

43. Francis Henry May (1860–1922), cadet officer in Hong Kong in 1881 and Colonial Secretary 1902–10; he was Governor of Fiji and High Commissioner of Western Pacific 1910, and Governor of Hong Kong 1912–19. See Endacott, *Government and People*, p. 137.

44. *Hong Kong Weekly Press* (hereafter *HKWP*), 24 May 1894, p. 403, enclosed in Robinson to Ripon, 23 May 1894, #122: CO 129/263.

45. *HKWP*, 24 May 1894, p. 403.

46. *HKWP*, 24 May 1894, p. 403.

47. *DP*, 22 May 1894.

48. K. C. Wong and Wu Lien-teh, *History of Chinese Medicine* (Tientsin: The Tientsin Press, 1932), p. 357.

49. *DP*, 22 May 1894.

50. William Robinson (1836–1912) joined the Colonial Office as a clerk in 1854. In 1874 he became Lieutenant-Governor of the Bahamas and Governor in 1875; he was Governor of the Windward Islands from 1880, of Trinidad from 1885, and of Hong Kong 1891–98. See Endacott, *Government and People*, p. 109, n. 21.

51. *HKWP*, 24 May 1894, pp. 404–5.

52. *HKWP*, 24 May 1894, p. 404.

53. *HKWP*, 24 May 1894, p. 404.

54. Robinson to Ripon, 20 June 1894, #21, *HKSP* 1894, p. 284.

55. Robinson to Ripon, 20 June 1894, #21, p. 284.

56. Robinson to Ripon, 20 June 1894, #21, p. 284.

57. Robinson to Ripon, 20 June 1894, #21, p. 284.

58. Tse Tsan Tai (Xie Zuantai) (謝纘泰) (1872–1938) began his career as a government clerk and later became a compradore, first of the Boyd Kaye & Co., exports and imports merchants, then of the Shewan Tomes & Co., and, in 1902, the South China Morning Post. His other activities were far more interesting. A social reformer and revolutionary, he was also the inventor of what he claimed to be the first airship, an art appreciator, and artist. He wrote prolifically on many subjects. See his *The Chinese Republic — the Secret History of the Chinese Revolution* (Hong Kong: South China Morning Post, 1924); W. Feldwick, *Present Day Impressions of the Far East* (London: 1917), pp. 583–5; Huang Jiaren (黃嘉仁), '*Cai Xianggang gao geming de Xie Zuantai*' (在香港搞革命的謝纘泰), ('Revolutionary in Hong Kong, Tse Tsai Tai'), *Da Hua* 1:3 (1970), pp. 13–15; Vincent H. G. Jarrett, 'Old Hong Kong', Vol. I, p. 23; *SCMP*, 5, 6 April 1938.

59. In 1890 he advocated the abolition of the evil practice of *fengshui* in the Chinese Empire in order to prepare the way for building railways and mines. He opposed opium smoking (see his letter to *DP*, 18 May 1894, signed 'A Chinaman'). In 1898 he took a leading part in the formation of the Anti-Opium Society of South China; he also advocated forming a society for the suppression

of footbinding in China. (See chronology presumably compiled by himelf, located among the Lockhart Papers at University of Edinburgh.) He had compiled various such autobiographical works and was obviously a self-advertizer.

60. Tse's letter to *DP*, 30 May 1894. He was reprimanded by the Colonial Secretary for 'dabbling in politics' for this. See Tse, *The Chinese Republic*, p. 8.

61. Tse's letter to *DP*, 30 May 1894.

62. 'A Chinaman's' letter to *HKT*, 23 May 1894; see also letter from 'Heathen Chinese', *HKT*, 23 May 1894.

63. 'A Chinaman's' letter, *HKT*, 23 May 1894; compare Chinese defence of the Hospital Committee in Chapter 5.

64. *CM*, 23 May 1894.

65. *HKT*, 23 May 1894.

66. *HKT*, 23 May 1894.

67. Robinson to Ripon, 20 June 1894, #21, *HKSP* 1894, p. 285.

68. Robinson to Ripon, 20 June 1894, #21; Brenan to O'Conor, 11 June 1894: 'China Riots', p. 2; *DP*, 25 May 1894.

69. See Note 33.

70. *HKT*, 24 May 1894.

71. Robinson to Ripon, 20 June 1894, #21, p. 284.

72. Robinson to Brenan, 24 May 1894, telegram, and Robinson to Brenan, 24 May 1894, #95, enclosed in Robinson to Ripon, 29 May 1894, #128: CO 129/263.

73. Li Hanzhang (李瀚章), brother of Li Hongzhang. Before becoming Governor-General of Guangdong and Guangxi (1889–95) he had served as Governor of Jiangsu, Zhejiang, and Sichuan. See Cai Guanlo (ed.), *Qindai qibai mingren zhuan (Biographies of 700 Prominent Qing Personalities* (Hong Kong: 1963), Vol. I, pp. 402–5.

74. Brenan to O'Conor, 11 June 1894: 'China Riots', p. 2.

75. Brenan to O'Conor, 11 June 1894.

76. Brenan to O'Conor, 11 June 1894, confidential: 'China Riots', p. 7.

77. Li Hanzhang to Tsungli Yamen, 18 June 1894, enclosed in O'Conor to Kimberley, 22 June 1894: 'China Riots', pp. 1–2. In the letter, the Tung Wah Directors were referred to as 'Directors of the Benevolent Society at Hong Kong'.

78. Proclamation by Nanhai and Panyu magistrates, dated [?] May 1894, enclosed in O'Conor to Kimberley, 22 June 1894: 'China Riots', p. 3.

79. Brenan to O'Conor, 11 June 1894, confidential: 'China Riots', p. 7.

80. Brenan to O'Conor, 11 June 1894, confidential.

81. Lockhart to Brenan, 4 June 1894, enclosed in O'Conor to Kimberley, 22 June 1894: 'China Riots' pp. 4–5.

82. O'Conor to Kimberley, 22 June 1894.

83. O'Conor to Kimberley, 22 June 1894, p. 5.

84. Lowson's Plague Report, 1894, p. 204.

85. *CM*, 28 May 1894.

86. Ho Amei to Sanitary Board, 2 June 1894, enclosed in his letter to *HKT*, 7 June 1894.

87. Ho's letter to Sanitary Board, 2 June 1894.

88. Ho's letter to Sanitary Board, 2 June 1894.

89. Robinson to Ripon, 20 June 1894, #21, *HKSP* 1894, p. 286.

90. Robinson to Ripon, 20 June 1894, #21, p. 288.

91. G. R. Sayer, *Hong Kong 1862–1919* (Hong Kong: Hong Kong University Press, 1975), p. 73. The population in 1894 was 240,000. Robinson reported that 80,000 had left while Sayer claimed that there might have been as many as 100,000. See Robinson to Ripon, 20 June 1894, p. 288.

92. *DP*, 2 July 1894.

93. *CM*, 9 June 1894.

94. *CM*, 11 June 1894.
95. *HKT*, 13 June 1894.
96. *DP*, 13 June 1894; *CM*, 13 June 1894.
97. *HKT*, 13 June 1894.
98. Robinson to Ripon, 20 June 1894, #21, p. 286.
99. Government notification #208, 1894, enclosed in 'Correspondence relative to the Outbreak of Bubonic Plague at Hong Kong' [C.–7461] *BPP* XXVI, pp. 383–405, pp. 404–5.
100. Robinson to Ripon, 20 June 1894, #21, p. 288.
101. Report on riot in Honam, *CM*, 12 June 1894; *DP*, 14 June 1894.
102. *DP*, 14 June 1894.
103. Li Hanzhang to Tsungli Yamen, 18 June 1894: 'China Riots', pp. 1–2.
104. Tsungli Yamen to O'Conor, 19 June 1894, enclosed in O'Conor to Robinson, no date, enclosed in O'Conor to Kimberley, 11 July 1894, #182, enclosed in F.O. to C.O., 11 September 1894: CO 129/265.
105. O'Conor to Robinson, 20 June 1894, telegram, enclosed in Robinson to Ripon, 21 June 1894, #152: CO 129/263.
106. Robinson to Ripon, 21 June 1894, #152.
107. Robinson to Ripon, 21 June 1894, #152.
108. Proclamation enclosed in Robinson to Ripon, 21 June 1894, #152.
109. Lowson's Plague Report, 1894, pp. 203–6.
110. *HKT*, 26 June 1894; *DP*, 27 June 1894.
111. Robinson to Ripon, 11 July 1894, #168: CO 129/263.
112. Minute by G. W. Johnson on F.O. to C.O., 20 September 1894: CO 129/265.
113. *HKT*, 30 June 1894.
114. *DP*, 2 July 1894.
115. *DP*, 2 July 1894.
116. *DP*, 2 July 1894.
117. *DP*, 2 July 1894.
118. *CM*, 2 July 1894.
119. *DP*, 3 July 1894.
120. *CM*, 3 July 1894; the 'Battle' was reported in *CM*, 5 July 1894; the English papers took sides: *DP*, 7 July 1894; *CM*, 7 July 1894; and *HKT*, 7 July 1894.
121. *DP*, July 1894.
122. *DP*, 5 July 1894.
123. *HKT*, 10 July 1894.
124. *HKT*, 12 July 1894.
125. *CM*, 17 July 1894.
126. *HKT*, 12 July 1894.
127. Robinson to Ripon, 4 September 1894, #203: CO 129/264; *DP*, 4 September 1894.
128. Robinson to Ripon, telegram, received 29 August 1894 in 'Further Correspondence relative to the Bubonic Plague at Hong Kong', [C.–7545] 1894, *BPP* XXVI, pp. 407–426, p. 407. For an analysis of the death statistics in relation to race and age, see G. H. Choa, *The Life and Times of Sir Kai Ho Kai* (Hong Kong: Chinese University Press, 1981), pp. 201–2.
129. Sayer, *Hong Kong*, p. 75.
130. *HKT*, 22 May 1894.
131. Robinson's speech at the Legislative Council, 11 June 1894, in *Hong Kong Hansard*, 1893–94, p. 47.
132. Quoted by Brenan in Brenan to O'Conor, 28 June 1894, enclosed in O'Conor to Kimberley, 11 July 1894, enclosed in F.O. to C.O., 11 September 1894: CO 129/265.

133. Choa, *Sir Kai Ho Kai*, p. 201.
134. *DP*, 25 May 1894.
135. *HKT*, 11 June, 1894.
136. *HKT*, 24 May 1894.
137. *DP*, 18 June 1894.
138. *HKT*, 21 June 1894.
139. Robinson to Ripon, 4 September 1894, #203: CO 129/264. Ironically, Francis refused to accept his reward — an inkstand — considering it too slight. See Greenwood, 'J. J. Francis', pp. 38–42.

Notes to Chapter 7

1. Jeanne L. Brand, *Doctors and the State: The British Medical Profession and Government Action in Public Health, 1870–1912* (Baltimore: Johns Hopkins Press, 1965), p. 15.
2. Brand, *Doctors and the State*, p. 2.
3. *DP*, 11 May 1894; Lowson's Report, 16 May 1894.
4. U I-kai (Hu Erjie) (胡爾楷) (1865–1898) was for many years senior native apothecary at the Government Civil Hospital. While doing his work there he attended lectures at the Hong Kong College of Medicine, and passed in 1893 as a native doctor. He was the father of Drs Arthur and Kitty Woo, two prominent Hong Kong residents. (*TWR*, p. 55; 'Colonial Surgeon's Report for 1894', *HKSP* 1895, pp. 473–530, p. 477; Timothy David Woo, *To Spread the Glory* (Honolulu: Transcultural Press of the East and West, 1977), p. 16.)
5. The evidence of Lo Chi-t'in (盧芝田), *TWR*, pp. 48–9, p. 48. In 1893 the Colonial Surgeon had proposed a scheme to secure more reliable returns of the 'real causes' of death — in other words, to use Western pathological standards, but it appears not to have been carried out. For the problem of death registration, see 'Registrar General's Report, 1891', *HKGG* 1892, p. 362. See 'Report on the subject of securing more reliable returns of the real causes of death and furnishing medical aid to the poorer classes of the colony', 'Registrar General's Report, 1892', *HKGG* 1893, Table IX.
6. Lowson's Report on the Plague, 17 May 1894, reproduced in *TWR*, pp. 40–3, p. 40. Lowson included this report in his 1895 Report on Bubonic Plague, but this and other sections on the Tung Wah Hospital were omitted before the report was published and forwarded to London. This section was reproduced for the Tung Wah Commission.
7. Lowson's Plague Report, 1894, p. 204.
8. Li Hanzhang to Tsungli Yamen, 18 June, 1894, enclosed in O'Conor to Kimberley, 22 June 1894: 'China Riots', pp. 1–2.
9. Lowson's Plague Report, 1894, p. 204; *DP*, 15 June 1894.
10. Lowson's Plague Report, 1894, p. 204.
11. Lowson's Plague Report, 1894, p. 204, p. 212.
12. Lowson's Report on the Pague, *TWR*, p. 41.
13. Lowson's Report on the Plague, *TWR*, p. 41.
14. *HKT*, 7 June 1894.
15. Lowson to Ayres, 1 May 1895, covering letter to his Plague Report, 1894, *HKSP*, p. 177.
16. Lowson to Ayres, 1 May 1895.
17. Lowson's Report on the Plague, *TWR*, p. 42.
18. Lowson to Ayres, 1 May 1895.
19. Lowson's evidence, *TWR*, p. 48.
20. Ripon to Robinson, 31 May 1895: CO 129/267.

21. Hugh McCallum's evidence, *TWR*, p. 22.
22. Report of the Secretary of the Sanitary Board, 8 April 1895, Appendix VI, *TWR*, pp. LIX–LX.
23. Report of the Secretary of the Sanitary Board, 8 April 1895.
24. Lowson to Lockhart, 8 August 1895, *TWR*, p. LIII; Atkinson's evidence, *TWR*, pp. 8–18, p. 14.
25. John Mitford Atkinson (1856–1917) became Superintendent of the Government Civil Hospital, Hong Kong in 1887 and acting Colonial Surgeon in 1895. In 1897 he became Colonial Surgeon and President of the Sanitary Board. See Arnold Wright (ed.), *Twentieth Century Impressions of Hong Kong, Shanghai and Other Treaty Ports* (London: Lloyd's Greater Britain Publishing Co., 1908), p. 107; *Hong Kong Hansard*, 1917B, p. 45.
26. *TWR*, p. 17.
27. *TWR*, p. 17.
28. *TWR*, p. 15.
29. *TWR*, p. 13.
30. *TWR*, p. 13.
31. *TWR*, p. 14.
32. *TWR*, p. 9.
33. *TWR*, p. 9.
34. *TWR*, p. 9.
35. Ku Fai-shan's evidence, *TWR*, pp. 25–30, p. 30.
36. Deacon to Colonial Surgeon, 6 November 1895, *TWR*, p. LII.
37. Wei Yuk's evidence, *TWR*, pp. 32–5, p. 35; Dr Thomson's evidence, *TWR*, pp. 55–9, p. 56.
38. *TWR*, p. 11.
39. *TWR*, p. 10.
40. *TWR*, p. 12.
41. *TWR*, p. 12.
42. *TWR*, p. 33.
43. *TWR*, p. 33.
44. *TWR*, p. 29.
45. *TWR*, p. 65.
46. *TWR*, p. 49.
47. *Huazi ribao*, 17, 18 January 1896; *DP*, 20, 28, 29 January 1896. A brief history of the Chinese Chamber of Commerce is given in Lu Yan (魯言) 'Xianggang Huaren shetuan de fazhan shi — san yi qi ming de Xianggang Zhonghua zong shang hui' (香港華人社團發展史 — 三易其名的香港中華總商會) ('The history of the development of Chinese social organization in Hong Kong — the Hong Kong Chamber of Commerce which changed its name three times'), *Xianggang Zhanggu*, Vol. V (September 1982), pp. 35–58; Elizabeth Sinn, 'A Preliminary History of Regional Associations in Pre-War Hong Kong', conference paper presented at the Centre of Asian Studies, December, 1986, to be published by the Centre.
48. *DP*, 24 December 1895.
49. *DP*, 24 December 1895; *Huazi ribao*, 24, 25 December 1895.
50. *Huazi ribao*, 24, 25 December 1895.
51. *Huazi ribao*, 24 December 1895.
52. *Huazi ribao*, 24 December 1895.
53. *Huazi ribao*, 25 December 1895; *DP*, 24 December 1895.
54. James William Norton-Kyshe, *The History of the Laws and Courts of Hong Kong* (Hong Kong: Vetch & Lee, 1971), Vol. II, pp. 456–7; *Huazi ribao*, 2, 7, 9, 16 December 1895.
55. Ho Amei's speech, *DP* 23 December 1895.
56. For Ho Tung (He Dong) (何東), see Woo Sing Lim, *Prominent Chinese in*

Hong Kong (Hong Kong: 1937), pp. 1-3; and his daughter, Irene Cheng's *Clara Ho Tung: A Hong Kong Lady, Her Family and Her Times* (Hong Kong: Chinese University Press, 1976).

57. Record of the meeting is in *DP*, 23 December 1895 and *Huazi ribao*, 24 December 1895.

58. *DP*, 23 December 1895.

59. *DP*, 23 December 1895.

60. *DP*, 24 December 1895.

61. Ho Tung's Letter to the *Daily Press*, 28 December 1895.

62. *Huazi ribao*, 24 December 1895.

63. *Huazi ribao*, 4 January 1896.

64. *Huazi ribao*, 4 January 1896.

65. *Huazi ribao*, 7 January 1896; *DP*, 7 January 1896.

66. Robinson to Chamberlain, 24 January 1896, confidential: CO 129/271.

67. The Commission, *TWR*, Appendix I, p. III. The Commission was dated 5 February, but Robinson had already mentioned appointing one in his letter to Chamberlain, 24 January 1896, confidential: CO 129/271.

68. Paul Chater (1846-1926) was of Armenian extraction from Calcutta. He came to Hong Kong in 1864 as assistant in the Bank of Hindustan, China, and Japan. He resigned in 1866 to become an exchange and bullion broker; was unanimously elected to the Legislative Council 1887, and again in 1893 and 1899, retiring at the end of the third term in 1906. He was a member of the Executive Council 1896-1926, and was one of Hong Kong's most successful business men. See G. B. Endacott, *Government and People in Hong Kong* (Hong Kong: Hong Kong University Press, 1964), p. 103, n. 1; see also Wright, *Impressions*, pp. 107-8.

69. *TWR*, pp. 17, 43.

70. *TWR*, p. 45.

71. *TWR*, p. 42.

72. *TWR*, p. 36.

73. *TWR*, pp. 36-7.

74. Ku Fai-shan (Gu Huishan) (古輝山) was a California Trade merchant; Chairman of the Tung Wah 1895; Director of the Po Leung Kuk in 1894 and 1905, and its Chairman in 1901.

75. *TWR*, p. 28.

76. *TWR*, p. 28.

77. *TWR*, p. 64.

78. *TWR*, p. 48.

79. Report by J. H. Stewart Lockhart, A. M. Thomson, and Ho Kai, *TWR*, pp. *v–xiii*.

80. *TWR*, pp. *ix–xiii*.

81. Report by C. P. Chater, *TWR*, p. *xv*.

82. Report by T. H. Whitehead, *TWR*, pp. *xvii–xxxii*, pp. *xxviii–xxix*.

83. *TWR*, p. *xxx*.

84. *TWR*, p. *xxviii*.

85. H. J. Lethbridge, 'The Evolution of a Chinese Voluntary Association: The Po Leung Kuk' in *Hong Kong: Stability and Change, A Collection of Essays* (Hong Kong: Oxford University Press, 1978), pp. 71-103, p. 86.

86. *TWR*, pp. *xxx–xxxii*.

87. Robinson to Chamberlain, 6 May 1896, 117: CO 129/272.

88. Robinson to Chamberlain, 16 August 1895, confidential: CO 129/268; G. B. Endacott, *A History of Hong Kong* (Hong Kong: Oxford University Press, 1983), p. 225.

89. See Chapter 5, Note 17.

90. *CM*, 2 December 1896.

91. *CM*, 2 December 1896.

92. Robinson to Chamberlain, 29 December 1896, #294: CO 129/273; for Dr John C. Thomson, see K. C. Wong and Wu Lien-teh, *History of Chinese Medicine* (Tientsin: The Tientsin Press, 1932), Book II, pp. 320–2.

93. *CM*, 14 December 1896.

94. For the post-war development and decline of kaifongs, see Lau Siu-kai, *Society and Politics in Hong Kong* (Hong Kong: Chinese University Press, 1982), pp. 131–5.

95. Fung Wa Chuen (Feng Huachuan) (馮華川) was compradore of China National Bank, and later of the Shewan Tomes & Co. See Smith, *Chinese Christians: Élites, Middlemen and the Church in Hong Kong* (Hong Kong: Oxford University Press, 1985), p. 166. Also see William Meigh Goodman, 'Reminiscences of a Colonial Judge' (printed for private circulation by the Kingsgate Press, no date; preface dated 1907), p. 260.

96. *CM*, 14 December 1896.

97. Robinson to Chamberlain, 29 December 1896, #294: CO 129/273.

98. *CM*, 21 December 1896.

99. *CM*, 21 December 1896.

100. Dr Chung Boon-chor (Zhong Penchu) (鍾本初) was appointed Resident Surgeon at the Tung Wah at $150 a month without private practice. See Robinson to Chamberlain, 29 December 1896, #294: CO 129/273.

101. 'Report by Dr Thomson on the Tung Wa Hospital', 8 April 1897, enclosed in Robinson to Chamberlain, 21 April 1897, #83: CO 129/275.

102. 'Report by Dr Thomson on the Tung Wa Hospital', 8 April 1897.

103. Thomson, 'Quarterly report of the Tung Wa Hospital', 1 October to 31 December 1897, enclosed in Black to Chamberlain, 18 February 1898, #47: CO 129/281.

104. Thomson, 'Quarterly report of the Tung Wa Hospital', 1 October to 31 December 1897.

105. 'Report by Dr Thomson on the Tung Wa Hospital', 8 April 1897.

106. Dr Chung performed an amputation on a thigh in 1899, the first major operation performed in the Tung Wah Hospital. See minutes for 28 March 1899, 'Hong Kong Medical Society Minutes, 1886–1891' (photographic copy of manuscript, at the University of Hong Kong Library). Dr Chung also attended other meetings at the Society and showed cases of interest from the Tung Wah Hospital.

107. Dr Thomson to Dr Atkinson, 13 July 1898, enclosed in Robinson to Chamberlain, 21 July 1898, #201: CO 129/284.

108. 'Report by acting Registrar General, A. W. Brewin', enclosed in Black to Chamberlain, 20 May 1898, #147: CO 129/283. He reported very active canvassing against Fung who represented the 'progressive party', and the conservatives managed to prevent his appointment as one of the three Principal Directors because in 1896 he had recommended engaging a Chinese trained in Western medicine for the Hospital.

109. H. J. Lethbridge, 'The District Watch Committee', in his *Hong Kong: Stability and Change*, pp. 104–29, p. 113.

110. 'Report by acting Registrar General A. W. Brewin' in Black to Chamberlain, 20 May 1898, #147: CO 129/283.

Notes to Epilogue

1. C. A. Middleton Smith, *The British in China and the Far Eastern Trade* (London: 1926) quoted by H. J. Lethbridge, 'The Tung Wah', in *Hong Kong: Stability and Change, A Collection of Essays* (Hong Kong: Oxford University Press, 1978), p. 63. For its fund-raising work, see Tung Wah Board of Directors, 1960–1961, *Development of the Tung Wah Hospitals (1870–1960)*, Part 3, pp. 1–32.

2. Alistair MacMillan, *Seaports of the Far East* (London: 1923), p. 218.

3. Lo Man Kam's speech recorded in Vincent H. G. Jarrett, 'Old Hong Kong', Vol, II, 534.

4. 'Registrar General's Report, 1903', *HKSP* 1904, pp. 355–82.

5. Tung Wah, *'Dongshiju huiyi lu'*, 1904, meetings on 7 July and 14 August; 'Registrar-General's Report for 1906', *HKSP* 1907, pp. 331–64, p. 337.

6. 'Registrar General's Report for 1906', p. 337; membership of the Advisory Board can be seen in the Civil List of subsequent years.

7. For Chinese nationalism as a form of anti-imperialism, see Li Enhan (李恩涵), 'Zhongguo jindai zhi shou hui tielu liquan yundong' (中國近代之收回鐵路利權運動) ('The movement of retrieving railway rights in modern China'), *Zhongguo jindaishi zhuanti yanjiu baogao* (中國近代史專題研究報告) (*Report at Seminar on Modern Chinese history*) (Taipei: August, 1972), pp. 1–33; his *'Lun Qingji Zhongguo de minzu chuyi'* (論清季中國的民族芻義) ('Chinese nationalism in late Qing') in his *Jindai Zhongguo shishi yanjiu lunji* (近代中國史事研究論集) (*Essays on Modern Chinese History*) (Taipei: 1982), pp. 45–67; Liao Kuang-sheng, *Antiforeignism and Modernization in China 1860–1980* (Hong Kong: Chinese University Press, 1984); Mary Backus Rankin, *Early Chinese Revolutionaries: Radical Intellectuals in Shanghai and Chekiang 1902–1911* (Cambridge, Mass.: Harvard University Press, 1971); Chow Tse-tsung, *The May Fourth Movement* (Stanford: Stanford University Press, 1967; 1st published 1960); Ernest P. Young, 'Nationalism, Reform and Republican Revolution: China in the Early Twentieth Century' in James B. Crowley (ed.), *Modern East Asia: Essays in Interpretation* (New York: 1970) pp. 151–179. For the development of the Chinese labour movement, see Nym Wales (pseudonum), *The Chinese Labour Movement* (New York: The John Day Co., 1945); S. K. Sheldon Tso, *The Labour Movement in China* (Shanghai: 1928); Deng Zhongxia (鄧中夏), *Zhonguo zhigong yundong jianshi* (中國職工運動簡史) (*A Brief History of the Chinese Labour Movement*) (Tientsin: 1949).

8. Lugard to Harcourt, 23 November 1911, #397: CO 129/381; A. E. Wood, *Report on the Chinese Guilds of Hong Kong Compiled from Materials Collected by the Registrar General* (Hong Kong: Noronha, 1912); for a historical account, see Ming K. Chan, 'Perspectives on the Chinese Labour Movement: the Hong Kong Connection', paper presented at the 'Hong Kong and China: Influence and Interaction' Seminar, 26–28th February 1981, Centre of Asian Studies, University of Hong Kong; Ming K. Chan and others, *Zhongguo yu Xianggang gongyun congheng* (中國與香港工運縱橫) (*Dimensions of the Chinese and Hong Kong Labour Movement*) (Hong Kong: Christian Industrial Committee, 1986).

9. For the Seamen's Strike, see Zhang Hong (章洪), *Xianggang haiyuan da bagong* (香港海員大罷工) (*The Seamen's Strike of Hong Kong*) (Canton: 1979); Yi Bin (宜彬), *Xianggang haiyuan da bagong* (香港海員大罷工) (*The Seamen's Strike of Hong Kong*) (Shanghai: 1955); Gary Wallace Glick, 'The Chinese Seamen's Union and the Hong Kong Seamen's Strike of 1922' (Ph.D. thesis, Columbia University, 1969).

10. *Huazi ribao*, 25 February 1922.

11. Deng, *Zhongguo zhigong yundong jianshi*, p. 42; see pp. 42-5 for the strike negotiations.

12. Great Britain: Colonial Office, Confidential Prints Eastern, Series 882, #144, 'Hong Kong. Correspondence (1925-1926) relating to the Strike and Boycott'; Cai Luo (蔡洛) and Lu Quan (盧權), *Sheng Gang da bagong* (省港大罷工) *(The Great Strike of Hong Kong and Canton)* (Canton: 1980); Earl John Motz, 'Great Britain, Hong Kong and Canton: the Canton-Hong Kong Strike and Boycott of 1925-1926' (Ph.D. thesis, Michigan State University, 1972); Rosemary Chung Lu-cee, 'A Study of the 1925-26 Canton-Hong Kong Strike-Boycott' (M. A. thesis, University of Hong Kong, 1969).

13. Letter from 'A Patriot', Hong Kong, 22 June 1925, in Tung Wah, '*Gechu xinbu*' (各處信簿) ('Incoming letters') 1925; also telegram dated 28 August 1925 from Makassar, '*Gechu xinbu*'. This album contains many other letters relating to the strike-boycott; the correspondence of 1925-26 is bound in several albums bearing various titles.

14. Clementi to Amery, 24 September 1926, confidential: CO 129/498.

15. See Chapter 4. The Tung Wah's passive role can be seen in Mai Meisheng (麥梅生), *Fandui xubi shilue* (反對蓄婢史略) (*A History of the Anti-Muitsai Movement*) (Hong Kong: 1933), pp. 152-61.

16. T. C. Cheng, 'Chinese Unofficial Members of the Legislative and Executive Councils in Hong Kong up to 1941', *JHKBRAS* 9 (1969), pp. 7-30.

17. Hong Kong, *The City District Office Scheme: Report by the Secretary for Chinese Affairs* (Hong Kong: [1969]), p. 12.

18. G. H. Choa, 'Chinese Traditional Medicine and Contemporary Hong Kong', *Symposium Paper*, October 1966 (Hong Kong: Hong Kong Branch of the Royal Asiatic Society, 1967), pp. 31-5; Rance P. L. Lee, *Problems of Integrating Chinese and Western Health Services in Hong Kong: Topia and Utopia* (Hong Kong: Social Research Centre, Chinese University, 1974); his 'Towards a Convergence of Modern Western and Traditional Chinese Medical Services in Hong Kong' in S. R. Ingram and A. E. Thomas (eds.), *Topias and Utopias in Health* (The Hague: Mouton, 1975), pp. 393-412; his 'Interaction between Chinese and Western Medicine in Hong Kong: Modernization and Professional Inequality' in A. Kleinman and others, *Medicine in Chinese Cultures: Comparative Studies of Health Care in Chinese and other Societies* (U. S. Department of Health, Education, Welfare, 1975), pp. 219-40; his *Perceptions and Uses of Chinese and Western Medical Care in Hong Kong* (Hong Kong: Social Research Centre, Chinese University, 1977).

Appendix I

The Chinese Hospital Ordinance No. 3 of 1870

SIR RICHARD GRAVES MACDONNELL,
Knight, C.B.,
Governor and Commander-in-Chief.

No. 3 OF 1870.

An Ordinance enacted by the Governor of Hongkong, with the Advice of the Legislative Council thereof, for establishing a Chinese Hospital to be supported by Voluntary Contributions, and for erecting the same into an Eleemosynary Corporation. Title.

[30th March, 1870.]

WHEREAS it has been proposed by the said Governor His Excellency SIR RICHARD GRAVES MACDONNELL to found a Chinese Hospital for the Care and Treatment of the indigent Sick to be supported by Voluntary Contributions; And Whereas Her Majesty Queen VICTORIA has been graciously pleased by Way of Endowment of the said Hospital to grant a Piece of Crown Land as a Site for the Erection thereof and also to authorize the Payment out of the Public Funds of the Colony of a Donation of Fifteen thousand Dollars towards the Cost and Expenses of erecting and maintaining the same; And Whereas the several Persons whose Names are set out and contained in the Schedule to this Ordinance are Donors to the Funds of the said intended Hospital, and have formed themselves into a Committee for the Purpose of carrying out the Objects aforesaid; And Whereas for the better Accomplishment thereof they have applied to His Excellency the Governor to grant to them an Ordinance of Incorporation which His said Excellency has consented to do under and subject to the Conditions and Provisions hereinafter contained; Be it therefore enacted by the Governor of Hongkong, with the Advice of the Legislative Council thereof, as follows:— Preamble.

Short Title.

I. This Ordinance may be cited for all Purposes as "The Chinese Hospital Incorporation Ordinance, 1870."

Grant of Incorporation.

II. The said several Persons whose Names are set out and contained in the Schedule to this Ordinance together with such and so many other Persons being of Chinese Origin as shall from Time to Time become Donors of any Sum not under Ten Dollars to the Funds of the said Hospital and whose Names shall be entered upon the Register of Members hereinafter provided, shall be One Body Politic and Corporate, in Name and in Deed by the Name of "The Tung Wa Hospital," with Perpetual Succession and a Common Seal, and with Power to purchase, hold, take,

Power to hold Lands and sue and be sued in Corporate Name.

and enjoy to themselves and their Successors all Houses, Buildings, Lands and Hereditaments which they may require for the Purposes of the said Hospital; and shall and may sue and be sued in their Corporate Name in all Courts whether of Law or of Equity.

Object and Purpose of Incorporation

III. The Corporation is erected for the Purpose of establishing and maintaining a Public Free Hospital for the Treatment of the Indigent Sick among the Chinese Population to be supported by Voluntary Contributions, and governed by a Board of Direction; Provided nevertheless that it shall be lawful for the Board of Direction to admit any Chinese Patients into the said Hospital upon Payment of such Charges and upon such Conditions as may be specified in and by any Regulations to be hereafter made in that Behalf under Section X.

Preliminary Board of Direction. Its Constitution and Duration.

IV. For the First Two Years after the Passing of this Ordinance, the Board of Direction shall consist of the several Persons, whose Names are set out and contained in the Schedule thereto; and in Case any such Person shall die or desire to be relieved of his Duties, or shall cease to reside within the Colony before the Expiration of the said Term, it shall be lawful for the Governor in Council to appoint in his Stead some other fit Person to be a Member of the said Board, during the Residue of the said Term.

Its Powers.

V. All the Provisions of this Ordinance relating to the permanent Board of Direction to be hereafter elected by the Members of the Corporation and all the Powers and Authorities thereby vested in such Board, shall so far as the Case permits be deemed to apply to and shall be vested in the Preliminary Board of Direction appointed under this Ordinance.

Permanent Board of Direction. Its Constitution and Term of Office of Members.

VI. At the Expiration of the said Term of Two Years, a permanent Board of Direction shall be formed consisting of not less than Six, and not more than Twelve Members of the Corporation, to be elected as hereinafter mentioned, who shall from Time to Time appoint One of their Body to be President; and every Member of the said Board shall hold Office for the Term of One Year only, but shall be re-eligible at the Expiration thereof.

VII. The Members of the said Board shall be elected from Time to Time as Occasion shall require by a Majority of Votes of Members of the Corporation, who shall be within the Colony at the Time of such Election, and every such Member of the Corporation shall, until otherwise provided by any Regulation to be hereafter made under Section X, be entitled to One Vote only. *Its Election.*

VIII. The Board of Direction shall, subject to the Provisions of this Ordinance, have full Power and Authority generally to govern, direct and decide all Matters whatsoever connected with the Administration of the Affairs of the Corporation and the Accomplishment of the Object and Purposes thereof and may appoint a Board of Management consisting of so many Members of the Corporation as they shall think fit, who shall, under such Regulations as may from Time to Time be made by the Board of Direction in that Behalf, undertake and exercise the immediate Supervision and Management of the Hospital. *Its general Powers.* *Board of Management.*

IX. The Board of Direction shall have Power, with the Consent of the Governor in Council, to change or vary the Corporate Name and the Common Seal of the Corporation, and the Amount of the Donation to the Funds of the Hospital hereinbefore prescribed as a Qualification for becoming a Member thereof, and the Term of Office of Members of the Board of Direction, and also may, for reasonable Cause and with such Consent as aforesaid, refuse to admit any Person as a Member of the Corporation or may expel any existing Member, and cause his Name to be erased from the Register. *Special Powers to be exercised with Consent of Governor in Council.*

X. The Board of Direction shall have Power to frame Regulations for their Procedure in the Transaction of Business and the Maintenance of Good Order at their Meetings, the Mode of Voting for the Election of Members of the Board of Direction and the Appointment of the President thereof, and for the Guidance of the Board of Management and generally for all Matters relating to the Administration and Discipline of the Hospital: Provided always that a Copy of such Regulations shall, from Time to Time, be furnished to the Colonial Secretary and every such Regulation shall be subject to Disallowance at any Time by the Governor in Council. *Power to frame Regulations subject to Disallowance by Governor in Council.*

XI. All Questions which may arise at any Meeting of the Board of Direction shall be decided by a Majority of Votes, and in Case of an Equality of Votes, the President in Addition to his original Vote shall have a Casting Vote. *Questions to be decided by Majority.*

XII. In Case any Doubt or Ambiguity shall arise and any Controversy shall take place among the Members of *Questions of Doubt or Ambiguity.*

the Board of Direction as to the Interpretation of this Ordinance the same shall be referred to the Governor in Council whose Decision thereon shall be final.

Preliminary Board of Direction to erect Hospital on the Site granted by Her Majesty. Provisional Extension of Office.

XIII. The Preliminary Board of Direction appointed under this Ordinance shall, with all convenient Despatch after the Passing thereof, proceed to elect a President, and shall cause all Buildings and Works required for the Purposes of the said Hospital to be erected and executed out of the Funds of the Corporation upon the Site granted by Her said Majesty as aforesaid, and the Members of the said Board shall continue to hold Office provisionally after the Expiration of the said Term of Two Years, until the Permanent Board of Direction shall have been elected under the Provisions hereinbefore contained.

Inspection by Public Officers.

XIV. The Hospital and all Buildings and Premises of the Corporation shall be open at all reasonable Times to the Inspection of the Register General, the Colonial Surgeon and of any other Person whom the Governor may appoint in that Behalf.

Register of Members, and Books of Account to be kept. Annual Statement to be furnished.

XV. The Board of Direction shall cause a Register to be kept in which every Person desiring to become a Member of the Corporation and being duly qualified shall, subject to the Provisions of Section IX, be entitled to have his Name inscribed, and also shall cause proper Books of Account to be kept which shall be open at all reasonable Times to the Inspection of Members of the Corporation and of any Person whom the Governor in Council may appoint in that Behalf, and also shall within One Month after the Expiration of every Year of the Chinese Calendar transmit to the Colonial Secretary a true Statement of the Assets and Liabilities of the Corporation and an Account of their Receipts and Disbursements during the previous Year and such Statement shall if required be verified on Oath or by Declaration before a Justice of the Peace by Two Members of the Board.

Provision for Repeal of Ordinance in certain Cases.

XVI. In Case it shall at any Time be shown to the Satisfaction of the Governor in Council that the Corporation have ceased or neglected or failed to carry out in a proper Manner the Object and Purposes of this Ordinance or to fulfil the Conditions thereof, or that sufficient Funds cannot be obtained by Voluntary Contributions to defray the necessary Expenses of Maintaining the said Hospital, or that the Corporation is unable for any Reason to pay its Debts, it shall be lawful for the Governor, with the Advice of the Legislative Council of the Colony by an Ordinance to be passed for that Purpose, to repeal this Ordinance and to declare that the Incorporation hereby granted shall cease and determine and become absolutely void; Provided always that Six Months' Notice of the Governor's Intention to pass such as Ordinance shall be previously given to the Corporation.

XVII. In case the Incorporation hereby granted shall cease under the Provisions of the last preceding Section, all the Property and Assets of the Corporation shall become vested in the Crown subject to the rateable Payment thereout of the just Debts and Liabilities of the Corporation, to the Extent of such Property and Assets and in such Manner as shall be provided by the Repealing Ordinance or by any Order to be made in that Behalf by the Governor in Council.

In Case of Repeal of Ordinance, Property of Corporation to vest in Crown. Proviso for Payment of Debts.

SCHEDULE.

梁鶴巢	Leung Hok Chau,[1]	買辦
何斐然	Ho Fí In,[2]	建南
李玉衡	Lí Yuk Hang,[3]	和興
吳振揚	'Ng Chan Yeung,	福隆
羅堯基	Lo Iu Kí,	買辦
蔡龍之	Ts'oi Lung Chí,	買辦
陳瑞南	Ch'an Sui Nám,	買辦
陳定之	Ch'an Ting Chí,	買辦
黃勝	Wong Shing,	英華書院
楊瓊石	Yeung K'ing Shek,	美隆
高滿和	Ko Mún Wo,	元發行
鄧鑑之	Tang Kam Chí,	廣利源行

Key: 1. Leung On.
2. Ho Asik.
3. Li Sing.

Note: Subsequently a thirteenth director was added.

Source: *Hong Kong Government Gazette* 1870.

Appendix II

Tung Wah Hospital Ground Plan, 1870

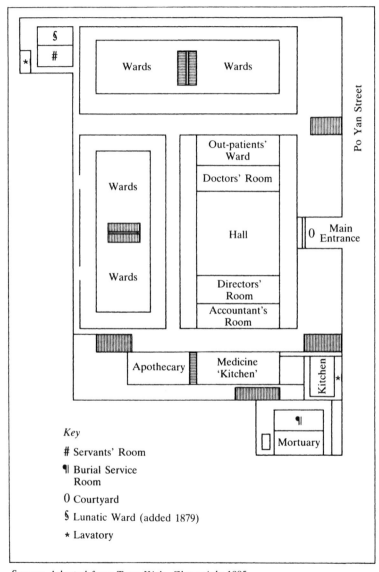

Key

\# Servants' Room

¶ Burial Service Room

0 Courtyard

§ Lunatic Ward (added 1879)

* Lavatory

Source: Adapted from Tung Wah, *Zhengxinlu* 1885.

The Pattern of Guild Representation on the Tung Wah Hospital Board 1869–1896

Years	Compradore	California Traders	Piecegoods	Nam Pak Hong	Rice	Opium	Yarn Dealers	Pawn Brokers	Insurance	Unspecified	Yinhu	Others	Total
1869–71	xxxxx	x	x	xx	x	x				x		x	13
1872	xxx	x	x	xxx	x	xx				x			12
1873	xxx	x	x	xx	x	x	x	x		x			12
1874	xxx	x	x	xx	x	x	x			xx			12
1875	xxx	x	x	xx	x	x	x	x			x		12
1876	xxx	x	x	xx	x	x	x	x			x		12
1877	xxx	x	x	xx	x	x	x	x			x		12
1878	xxx	x	x	xx	x	x	x	x		x			12
1879	xxx	x	x	xx	x	x	x	x		x			12
1880	xx	x	x	xx	x	x	x	x		xx			12
1881	xxx	x	x	xx	x	x	x	x		x			12
1882	xxx	x	x	xx	x	x	x	x	x				12
1883	xx	x	x	xx	x	x	x	x	x	x			12
1884	xxx	x	x	xx	x	x	x	x		x			12
1885	xxx	x	x	xx	x	x	x	x		x			12
1886	xxx	x	x	xx	x	x	x	x		x			12
1887	xxx	x	x	xx	x	x	x	x			x		12
1888	xxx	x	x	xx	x	x	x	x			x		12
1889	xxx	x	x	xx	x	x	x	x			x		12
1890	xxx	x	x	xx	x	x	x	x			x		12
1891	xxx	x	x	xx	·x	x	x	x			x		12
1892	xxx	x	x	xx	x	x	x	x			x		12
1893	xxx	x	x	xx	x	x	x	x			x		12
1894	xxx	x	x	xx	x	x	x	x				x	12
1895	xxx	x	x	xx	x	x	x	x		x			12
1896	xxx	x	x	xx	x	x	x	x				x	12

Source: Based on material from Tung Wah, *Zhengxinlu* 1933.

Appendix IV

Subscribing Guilds, 1873

Guilds	Amount ($)	Remarks
Nam Pak Hong	1,500	#
Compradores	1,000	#
Piecegoods	700	#
Ji Zheng Gongsi¶	600	* 1874
Rice dealers	500	#
Opium dealers	500	#
California traders	500	#
Yarn dealers	400	§
Medicine dealers	400	#
Matting dealers	250	#
Metal goods dealers	200	#
Pawn brokers	200	#
Foreign goods importers/exporters	200	#
Pig dealers	200	* 1895
Salt fish dealers	200	#
Goldsmiths	200	#
Dry food dealers	200	#
Wood dealers	200	* 1874
Silversmiths	200	§
Wood dealers (Masters)	150	* 1895
Provisioners	200	#
Tailors (Masters)	100	§ * 1877
Haberdashers	40	#
Pork dealers	200	§ * 1895

* Discontinued in the year given.
# Continued until 1896, paying same amounts.
§ Amounts varying from year to year.
¶ Nature of guild unknown.

Source: Based on material from Tung Wah, Zhengxiulu, various dates.

Appendix V

Application Form for Women Emigrants to the United States

Enclosure No. 9.

DECLARATION OF CHINESE FEMALES

who intend to go to California, or any other place in the United States of America.

Surname, name, ...

Residence in HongKong, and story of house, ...

Names of the people in the same house,......................

When and from what place I came to HongKong,...............

Person or Persons with whom I came,........................

Name, country and occupation of my father,.................

Name, country and occupation of my husband,................

Names, and addresses of the Sureties. ....

Relatives or Friends from whom enquiries may be made,.......

Person or Persons with whom I am going,....................

Object of my going, ...

Place to which I am going, ...

To whom I am going, Street and No: of house,...............

I do hereby declare that the above statements are true, and that I am not kidnapped decoyed or forced to emigrate to the United States; that I have not entered into a contract or agreement for a term of service within the United States for lewd and immoral purposes; nor am I going for the purpose of prostitution, and I do herewith submit my photographs as required by the United States Consul.

Signature of Surety.   *Signature.*

華人婦女往舊金山及美國屬地註冊式

選例將實赴舊婦人　門　氏現年　歲住港

就寓　頂樓　中樓　樓下全居男人

門牌第

於　年　月　日由

父名　係　省　府　縣　郡人現在　做　事業

夫名　係　省　府　縣　郡人現在　做　事業

男人

觀勵戚友作證詢查間　與我全去往

婦人

並非爲娼及被人誘拐或勢迫等弊　祖保人保　准因　行店　事

所報確係實情道無詐僞如有則歸任從送　官究辦

凡良家婦女係自港或由外埠到港赴港內無觀勵可保者有行店人等熟識可爲可問

花牌氏水身影像紙呈粘處

年　月　日婦人　代領人　的華　摸模

及蓮担保落船或官醫驗冊內以便各紳董易於稽查

一影和三個註册册預早七日交送英國領事署隨錄此紙給金山之日即交囘此相

一個與原人收一個存於金山關口一個留任香港領事署爲據

各紳董精于無疑或必須覓見指報册婦女之前方蓮巷間明白該婦女報册時須註明

允否見面查問字樣如欲紳董見面則明載册底倘若囘註明在何處見面如不欲紳董見面亦書明册內不允字樣以便預蓮認法查檢

Note: It is indicated in the Chinese section that these forms would be examined by Tung Wah Directors.

Source: Enclosure #9 in Bailey to Cadwalader, 28 August 1875, #307, Despatches from U.S. Consuls in Hong Kong, 1844–1906, United States, National Archives.

Appendix VI

Letter from the Guangdong Provincial Treasurer to the Directors of the Tung Wah Hospital, dated 8 December 1885, enclosing memorial to the throne

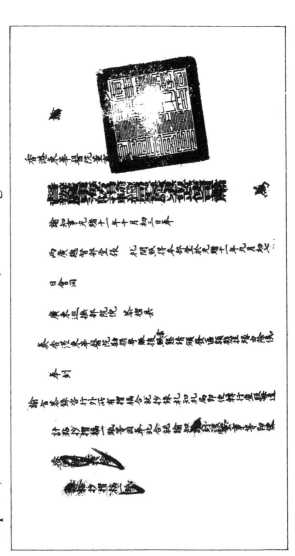

Appendix VI (continued)

奏為商民游歷身販遷奏懇請

須簽遊歷護照恭憑仰祈

聖鑒事竊商民本年五月間據天台沿海沿途然放武遷奉奉等小順商
流離為販自販牽子奏懇建接身愿奏本舉股兵事呵販遷牽勒尚遷商
民情販助販查毛照上途懇想全舉舉奉商修廣助為奉洗舉四兵舉兵子
除元申最冠冰司事直及放水免所奉亮廉經宜職之像洋身家民不氽
故民所經病雖量廣埃埃總批埃病条捐照以全舉稜垂皇不孩氽
路有隱泰祀

神為本聲進堂稀堂捐韻嗣道詳讀具
奉旨

慶都奉本通用承情前泉旦手亦查泰四兵間廣東春志會中申春申埔
事君陟遵速通牽手為廣民身捐批號緊一為申百春元絶絶洪春號氽速
明奉子牽奉會情條泰祀

聞奉奏敬
須給通清奉
會懇泰本泰今奉遷史本最臨奉最助聯事同一低你遙稀尚通最隱泰祀

神奉灸奉典懿
人最情准准

須簽通類一方申且奉臨絡洧稀奉春茂設遷隨遷讀承
神麻所激勉谷今詞明其陳狀亡

皇太后
皇上聖奉理

奏

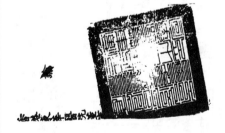

Source: Enclosed in Marsh to O'Conor, 20 January 1886: FO 228/842.

Appendix VII

Authenticated copy of the letter from the Board of Reorganization of Guangdong Province to the Directors of the Tung Wah Hospital, dated 5 February 1886

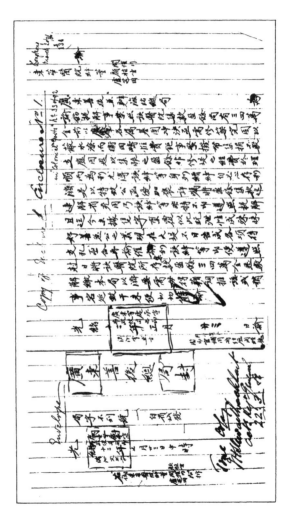

Source: Enclosed in Marsh to O'Conor, 20 March 1886, #47/G: FO 228/842.

Glossary

Aiyutang 愛育堂
baojia 保甲
baozhang 保長
bashi 罷市
Beihai 北海
Chan Ayin (Chen Axian) 陳阿賢
Ch'an Sui-nam (Chen Ruinan) 陳瑞南
Chaozhou 潮州
Chen Aiting 陳靄亭
Chen Lanbin 陳蘭彬
Chung Boon-chor (Zhong Penchu) 鍾本初
Chuang jian zongli 創建總理
dibao 地保
Ding Richang 丁日昌
Dong Bao *ijia* 東保一家
Donghua Yiyuan [of San Francisco] 東華醫院
Dongguan 東莞
Fan A-wye (Fan Awei) 范阿為
Fan Mo (fenmo) [Street] 墳墓
Fushan 福善
Fung Ming Shan (Feng Mingshan) 馮明珊
Fung Wa Chuen (Feng Huachuan) 馮華川
Furen Wenshe 輔仁文社
Gao Tingjie 高廷楷
Guan di 關帝
Guangji yiyuan 廣濟醫院
Guangxu yubi zhi bao 光緒御筆之寶
Guangzhao 廣肇
Guangzhou [prefecture] 廣州
Guo Songdao 郭嵩燾
Haikou 海口
he Gang hangshang 閩港行商
he Gang jiefang tongren 閩港街坊同人
he Gang Wenwu Miao 閩港文武廟
He Xianchi 何獻墀
Ho Amei (He Amei) 何阿美
Ho Asik (He Axi) 何阿錫
Ho Fuk (He Fu) 何福
Ho Fuk Tong (He Futang) 何福堂

Ho Kai (He Qi) 何啓
Ho Tung (He Dong) 何東
Hu Liyuan 胡禮垣
Huazi ribao 華字日報
huiguan 會館
Huizhou 惠州
huizhou haiwai 惠周海外
I-ts'z (*yici*) 義祠
Jinghu yiyuan 鏡湖醫院
jinshen 縉紳
jushen 局紳
kaifong (*jiefang*) 街坊
Kang Youwei 康有爲
Kao Manhua (Gao Manhua) 高滿華
Kinan (Jiannan) 建南
Ku Fai-shan (Gu Huishan) 古輝山
kung-so (*gongsuo*) 公所
kungsuh (*gongsuo*) 公所
Kwan Hoi-chun (Guan Kaichuan) 關愷川
Kwok Asing (Guo Yasheng) 郭亞勝
Kwong Fook (Guangfu) 廣福
Lai-chi-kok (Lizhijiao) 荔枝角
Lau Wai Chuen (Liu Weichuan) 劉渭川
Leung On (Liang An) 梁安
Li Hanzhang 李瀚章
Li Hongzhang 李鴻章
Li Shuchang 黎庶昌
Li Sing (Li Sheng) 李昇
Liu Kunyi 劉坤一
Lo Ch'i-t'in (Lu Zhitian) 盧芝田
Lo Man Kam (Lo Wenjian) 羅文錦
Loo Aqui (Lu Agui) 盧阿貴
mahjong (*majiang*) 麻將
Man Mo [Temple] (Wenwu miao) 文武廟
Nam Pak Hong (Nan bei hang) 南北行
Ng Choy (Wu Cai) 伍才
O Chun-chit (Ke Chenjie) 柯振捷
On Tai (Antai) 安泰
Paouchong (*baozhang*) 保長
Paoukea (*baojia*) 保甲
Po Leung Hui (Bao liang hui) 保良會
Po Leung Kuk (Bao liang ju) 保良局
Po Yan (puren) [Street] 普仁
qiao'an 僑安

Qiying 耆英
Sanon ooi kuan (Xin'an huiguan) 新安會館
Sanwan *zhong puhu zhumin* 三環眾舖戶居民
shen 紳
'*Shen shi du shi lun*' 審時度勢論
shen wei pu you 神威普佑
shendong 紳董
Shennong 神農
shenshang 紳商
Sheung-wan (Shanghuan) 上環
shi ke ji zhi 適可即止
shou zongli 首總理
Sin Tak Fan (Xian Defan) 冼德芬
Taiping 太平
taiping guan 太平棺
Tai-ping-shan (Taipingshan) 太平山
Tam Achoy (Tan Acai) 譚阿才
Tamsui (Danshui) 淡水
tang 堂
tanyuan 探員
Tepo (*dibao*) 地保
Tiandi hui 天地會
Tianhua 天華
Tongji 同濟
Tse Tsan Tai (Xie Zuantai) 謝纘泰
Tso Ping-lun (Zuo Binglong) 左秉隆
Ts'o U-t'ing (Cao Yuting) 曹雨亭
U I-kai (Hu Erjie) 胡爾楷
Wa T'o (Huatuo) 華陀
Wah Hop (Huahe) 華合
wan wu xian li 萬物咸利
Wang Tao 王韜
Wei Yuk (Wei Yu) 韋玉
Weixin ribao 維新日報
Wong Kwan Tong (Huang Juntang) 黃筠堂
Wong Shing (Huang Sheng) 黃勝
Wu Tingfang 伍廷芳
Xiangshan 香山
xieli 協理
Xunhuan ribao 循環日報
yang 陽
yangdou 洋痘
yangnu 洋奴
Yantai 煙台

yi yi Xi fa wei zhi 一依西法爲之
yin 陰
yinhu 殷戶
yinshang 殷商
yiyuan 醫院
yuanbu 緣部
yulan 盂蘭
yongyue tongxin 踴躍同心
Zeng Guoquan 曾國荃
Zhang Shusheng 張樹聲
Zhang Yinhuan 張蔭桓
Zhang Zhidong 張之洞
Zhengxinlu 徵信錄
zhili 值理
Zhongwai xinwen qiri bao 中外新聞七日報
zongli 總理

Bibliography

Materials in Private Archives

The Tung Wah Group of Hospitals' Archives

Research on the Tung Wah Hospital would have been impossible without these archieves. For the pre-1896 period, materials consist primarily of the *Zhengxinlu* (徵信錄) (Annual Reports), photographs, plaques, and other inscriptions. The *Zhengxinlu* are extant from 1873 but the series is incomplete. Correspondence is extant from 1899, and is bound in volumes variously named. For this study, the most valuable is the one marked '*Fachu xinbu* (發出信簿) (Outward Letters) 1900–1907' which actually contains copies of letters from 1899 to 1904, and from 1906 to 1907, numbering almost 1,000. Another useful source is the '*Dongshiju huiyi lu*' (董事局會議錄) ('Minutes of board meetings') even though the series begins only in 1904. A particularly important document in these archives is the '*Wenwu Miao zhengxinlu*' (文武廟徵信錄) ('Annual Report of the Man Mo Temple') 1911, which contains essays on its history and a simplified cumulative account of expenditures and incomes from 1873.

For a more detailed description of the Tung Wah and Po Leung Kuk Archives, see my paper 'Materials for Historical Research: Source Materials on the Tung Wah Hospital 1869–1941 — the Case of a Historical Institution' in Alan Birch, Y. C. Jao, and Elizabeth Sinn (eds.), *Research Materials for Hong Kong Studies* (Hong Kong: Centre of Asian Studies, University of Hong Kong, 1984), pp. 195–223.

The Po Leung Kuk Archives

For the nineteenth century, materials here are more complete than the Tung Wah Archives and are equally valuable. I have relied on the '*Yishibu*' (議事簿), a one-volume collection of minutes from 1880 to 1885. The volumes of correspondence, extant from 1884, are given various titles, but are basically classified into incoming and outgoing letters for each year.

Materials in Public Archives

Great Britain, Colonial Office, Original Correspondence: Hong Kong, 1841–1951, Series 129 (CO 129).

Great Britain, Foreign Office, General Correspondence: China 1815–1905, Series 17 (FO 17).

284 BIBLIOGRAPHY

Great Britain, Foreign Office, Embassy and Consular Correspondence, 1834–1930, Series 228 (FO 228).
Great Britain, Foreign Office, Miscellanea, 1759–1935, Series 233 (FO 233).
United States, National Archives, Despatches from U.S. Consuls in Hong Kong, 1844–1906 (M108).
United States, National Archives, Despatches from U.S. Consuls in Hong Kong, 1844–1906 (M108).

Official Publications

British Commission on Muitsai in Hong Kong and Malaya, *Muitsai in Hong Kong and Malaya* ([London: 1936]).
Great Britain, Parliament, *Parliamentary Papers: China* (Shannon: Irish University Press, 1971–) (*BPP*).
Hong Kong Blue Book
Hong Kong Government Gazette (*HKGG*)
Hong Kong Hansard
Hong Kong Sessional Papers (*HKSP*)
Hong Kong, Muitsai Committee, *Muitsai in Hong Kong: Report of the Committee...* (London: H.M.S.O., 1936).
Hong Kong, *Report of the Commission appointed by H. E. Sir William Robinson, K.C.M.G. . . . .to enquire into the Working and Organization of the Tung Wa [sic] Hospital together with the Evidence taken before the Commission and other Appendices, 1896* (*TWR*).
Hong Kong, *The City District Office Scheme, Report by the Secretary for Chinese Affairs* (1969).

Newspapers

English-language newspapers

China Mail (*CM*), 1845 onwards
Hong Kong Daily Press, (*DP*), 1870 onwards
Hong Kong Telegraph (*HKT*), 1881 onwards

Chinese-language newspapers*

Huazi ribao (華字日報) (*Chinese Mail*), 1895 onwards
Xunhuan ribao (循環日報) (*Universal Circulating Herald*) (*XH*), 1874 onwards

---

* Chinese newspapers provide a very different perspective on the development of the Chinese community; unfortunately, for the nineteenth century they are fragmentary.

Zhongwai xinwen qiri bao (中外新聞七日報) (*China and World News Weekly*) (*ZW*), March 1871–March 1872.

Selected Books, Papers, and Articles

Alice Ho Mui Ling Nethersole Hospital 1887–1967 (Hong Kong: the Hospital, 1967).

Aying (阿英) (pseudonym), *Fan Mei Huagong jinyue wenxue ji* (反美華工禁約文學集) (*Literature on the Movement against the United States' Exclusion Act*) (Peking: 1960).

Balme, Harold, *China and Modern Medicine, A Study in Medical Mission Development* (London: United Council for Missionary Education, 1921).

Barth, Gunther, *Bitter Strength: A History of the Chinese in the United States, 1850–1870* (Cambridge, Mass.: Harvard University Press, 1965).

Bastid, Marianne, 'The Social Context of Reform', in Paul A. Cohen and John E. Schrecker (eds.), *Reform in Nineteenth-Century China* (Cambridge, Mass.: Harvard University Press, 1976), pp. 117–27.

Bird, Isabella, *The Golden Chersonese* (Kuala Lumpur: Oxford University Press, 1967; first published 1883).

Blakeley, Brian L., *The Colonial Office 1868–1892* (Durham, N.C.: Duke University Press, 1972).

Brand, Jeanne L., *Doctors and the State: The British Medical Profession and Government Action in Public Health, 1870–1912* (Baltimore: Johns Hopkins Press, 1965).

Brockington, C. Fraser, *A Short History of Public Health* (London: J. & A. Churchill, 1966).

Cai Guanlo (蔡冠洛) (ed.), *Qingdai qibai mingren zhuan* (清代七百名人傳) (*Biographies of 700 Prominent Qing Personalities*), 3 volumes (Hong Kong: 1963; preface dated 1936).

Campbell, Persia Crawford, *Chinese Coolie Emigration to Countries within the British Empire* (New York: Negro University Press, 1969; first published 1923).

Cantlie Stewart, Jean, *The Quality of Mercy: The Lives of Sir James and Lady Cantlie* (London: George Allen & Unwin, 1983).

Cell, John W., *British Colonial Administration in the Mid-nineteenth Century: the Policy Making Process* (New Haven and London: Yale University Press, 1970).

Chan, Ming K., 'Perspectives on the Chinese Labour Movement: the Hong Kong Connection', paper presented at the 'Hong Kong and China: Influence and Interaction' Seminar, 26–28 February 1981, Centre of Asian Studies, University of Hong Kong.

Chan, Ming K. (陳明銶) and others, *Zhongguo yu Xianggang gongyun congheng* (中國與香港工運縱橫) (*Dimensions of the Chinese and Hong Kong Labour Movement*) (Hong Kong: Christian Industrial Committee, 1986).

Chan, Wellingt on K. K., *Merchants, Mandarins and Modern Enterprise in Late Ch'ing China* (Cambridge, Mass.: East Asian Research Centre, Harvard University Press, 1977).

Chang Chung-li, *The Chinese Gentry: Studies in Their Role in Nineteenth-century Chinese Society* (Seattle and London: University of Washington Press, 1955).

Chang Hao (張灝) and others, *Wan Qing sixiang* (晚清思想) (*Thought in the Late Qing Period*) (Taipei: 1971).

Chen Bangxian (陳邦賢), *Zhongguo yixue shi* (中國醫學史) (*History of Medicine in China*) (Shanghai: 1955; first published 1937).

Chen Hansheng (陳翰笙) (ed.), *Huagong chuguo shiliao huibian* (華工出國史料彙編) (*A Compilation of Historical Materials on the Emigration of Chinese Labourers*), Vol. 1– (Peking: 1980–).

Chen Yongliang (陳永亮), *Zhongguo yixueshi gangyao* (中國醫藥史綱要) (*An Outline History of Medicine in China*) (Canton: 1947).

Cheng, Irene, *Clara Ho Tung: A Hong Kong Lady, Her Family and Her Times* (Hong Kong: Chinese University Press, 1976).

Cheng T. C., 'Chinese Unofficial Members of the Legislative and Executive Councils in Hong Kong up to 1941', *Journal of the Hong Kong Branch of the Royal Asiatic Society*, 9 (1969), pp. 7–30.

Chesneaux, J. (ed.), *Popular Movements and Secret Societies in China, 1840–1950* (Stanford: Stanford University Press, 1972).

Choa, G. H., 'Chinese Traditional Medicine and Contemporary Hong Kong', *Symposium Paper*, October 1966 (Hong Kong: Hong Kong Branch of the Royal Asiatic Society 9 (1969), pp. 7–30.

——'A History of Medicine of Hong Kong' in *Medical Directory of Hong Kong* (Hong Kong: 1970), pp. 12–26.

——*The Life and Times of Sir Kai Ho Kai* (Hong Kong: Chinese University Press, 1981).

Chouban yiwu shimo (籌辦夷務始末) (*The Complete Account of the Management of Barbarian Affairs*), *juan* 260 (photographic reprint) (Peking: 1930).

Chow Tse-tsung, *The May Fourth Movement* (Stanford: Stanford University Press, 1967; first published 1967).

Chuan, S. H. 'Chinese Patients and their Prejudices', *China Medical Journal*, Vol. XXXI: 5 (October 1917), pp. 504–10.

Ch'ü T'ung-tsu, 'Chinese Class Structure and its Ideology' in John K. Fairbank, *Chinese Thought and Institution* (Chicago: University of Chicago, 1957), pp. 235–50.

——*Local Government in China under the Ch'ing* (Cambridge, Mass.: Harvard University Press, 1962).

——*Law and Society in Traditional China* (Paris: Mouton, 1965).

Cohen, Paul A., 'Wang T'ao and Incipient Chinese Nationalism', *Journal of Asian Studies* XXVI:4 (August 1967), pp. 559–74.

——*Between Tradition and Modernity: Wang T'ao and Reform in Late Ch'ing China* (Cambridge, Mass.: Harvard University Press, 1974).

Crissman, Lawrence W., 'The Segmentary Structure of Urban Overseas Chinese Communities', *Man* 2:2 (June 1967), pp. 185–204.

de Glopper, Donald Robert, 'Temple, Faction and Loan Club: Voluntary Associations in a Taiwanese Town', paper prepared for the 23rd Annual Meeting, Association for Asian Studies, Washington, D.C., March 1971.

Deng Zhongxia (鄧中夏), *Zhongguo zhigong yundong jianshi* (中國職工運動簡史) (*A Brief History of the Chinese Labour Movement*) (Tientsin: 1949).

des Voeux, G. William, *My Colonial Service*, 2 volumes (London: 1903).

Ding You (丁又), *Xianggang chuqi shihua (1841–1907)* (香港初期史話) (*Early History of Hong Kong 1841–1907*) (Peking: 1983; first published 1958).

'The Districts of Hong Kong and the Name Kwan Tai Lo', *China Review* 1 (1872–73), pp. 333–4.

Dou Jiliang (竇季良), *Tongxiang zushi zhi yanjiu* (同鄉組織之研究) (*The Study of Regional Organizations*) (Chungking: 1943).

Eitel, E. J., *Europe in China* (Hong Kong: Oxford University Press, 1983; first published 1895), with an introduction by H. J. Lethbridge.

Elvin, Mark, and Skinner, G. W. (eds.), *The Chinese City Between Two Worlds* (Stanford: Stanford University Press, 1974).

Endacott, G. B., *A Biographical Sketchbook of Early Hong Kong* (Hong Kong: Eastern Universities Press, 1962).

——*Government and People in Hong Kong* (Hong Kong: Hong Kong University Press, 1964).

——*A History of Hong Kong* (Hong Kong: Oxford University Press, 1983; first published 1958).

England, Joe, and Rear, John, *Chinese Labour under British Rule* (Hong Kong: Oxford University Press, 1975).

Evans, Dafydd M. Emrys, 'Chinatown in Hong Kong: The Beginnings of Taipingshan', *Journal of the Hong Kong Branch of the Royal Asiatic Society* 10 (1970), pp. 69–78.

——*Constancy of Purpose* (Hong Kong: Hong Kong University Press, 1987).

Fairbank, John King, *Trade and Diplomacy on the China Coast* (Stanford: Stanford University Press, 1968; first published 1953).

Fei Xiaotong (費孝通), *Xiangtu Zhongguo* (鄉土中國) (*Rural China*) (Shanghai: 1947).

Fei Xiaotong and others (eds.), *Huangquan yu shenquan* (皇權與紳權)

(*Imperial Power and Gentry Power*) (Hong Kong: 1981; first published 1948).

Feldwick, W., *Present Day Impressions of the Far East and Prominent and Progressive Chinese at Home and Abroad: The History, People, Commerce, Industries and Resources of China, Hong Kong and Indo-China, Malaya and Netherlands Indies* (London: 1917).

Fieldhouse, D. K., *The Colonial Empires, A Comparative Study from the Eighteenth Century* (London: Weidenfeld & Nicolson, 1966; first published 1965).

Freedman, Maurice, 'Immigrants and Associations: Chinese in 19th Century Singapore', *Comparative Studies in Social History* 3 (1961), pp. 25–48.

Furnivall, J. S., *Colonial Policy and Practice: A Comparative Study of Burma and Netherlands India* (New York: New York University Press, 1956; first published 1948).

Gao Zhenbai (高貞白), 'Xianggang Donghua yiyuan yu Gao Manhe [*sic*] (香港東華醫院與高滿和) ('The Tung Wah Hospital of Hong Kong and Gao Manhe'), *Da Hua* (大華) 1:4 (October 1970), pp. 2–6.

——'Cong Xianggang de Yuan Fa Hang tan qi' (從香港的元發行說起) ('On Yuan Fa Hang of Hong Kong'), *Da cheng* (大成) 117 (August 1983), pp. 47–52; 118 (September 1983), pp. 45–51; 119 (October 1983), pp. 34–9; 120 (November 1983), pp. 46–54.

Ge Gongzhen (戈公振), *Zhongguo baoye shi* (中國報業史) (*The History of Chinese Journalism*) (Hong Kong: 1964).

Godley, Michael, 'The Late Ch'ing's Courtship of the Chinese in Southeast Asia', *Journal of Asian Studies* 34:2 (February 1975), pp. 361–85.

——*The Mandarin-Capitalists from Nanyang: Overseas Chinese Enterprise in the Modernization of China 1893–1911* (Cambridge, Mass.: Harvard University Press, 1981).

Glick, Clarence E., *Sojourners and Settlers: Chinese Migrants in Hawaii* (Honolulu: University Press of Hawaii, 1980).

Graham, Gerald, *The China Station, War and Diplomacy, 1830–1860* (Oxford: Oxford University Press, 1978).

Gray, John Henry, *China, A History of the Law, Manners and Customs of the People*, 2 volumes (London: Macmillan, 1878).

Guo Songdao (郭嵩燾), *Yangzhi shuwu yiji* (養知書室遺集) (*Works from the Yangzhi Studio*) 28 *juan* (photographic reprint) (Taipei: 1964).

——*Guo Songdao riji* (郭嵩燾日記) (*The Diary of Guo Songdao*), 4 volumes (Zhangsha: 1981–).

Gutzlaff, Charles, 'On the Secret Triad Society of China, Chiefly from Papers Belonging to the Society found at Hong Kong', *Journal of the Royal Asiatic Society* 8 (1846), pp. 361–7.

Halcombe, Charles J. H., *The Mystic Flowery Land* (London: 1896).

Hao Yen-p'ing, *The Comprador in Nineteenth-Century China — Bridge between East and West* (Cambridge, Mass.: Harvard University Press, 1970).

Hayes, James, *The Hong Kong Region 1850–1911: Institutions and Leadership in Town and Countryside* (Hamden, Connecticut: Archon Books, Dawson, 1977).

Hirata, Lucie Cheng, 'Free, Indentured, Enslaved: Chinese Prostitutes in Nineteenth-century America', *Signs* 5:1 (Autumn 1979), pp. 3–29.

Hiroaki, Kani (可兒明弘), *Kindai Chūgoku no kuri to choka* (近代中國の苦力と「豬花」) (*The Coolies and 'Slave Girls' of Modern China*) (Tokyo: 1979).

A History of the Sam Yup Benevolent Association in the United States 1850–1974 (旅美三邑總會館簡史) (bilingual) (San Francisco: Sam Yup Benevolent Association, 1975).

Ho Ping-ti, *The Ladder of Success in Imperial China: Aspects of Social Mobility, 1368–1911* (New York: Columbia University Press, 1962).

Ho Ping-ti (何炳棣), *Zhongguo huiguan shilun* (中國會館史論) (*A Historical Survey of Landsmannschaften in China*) (Taipei: 1966).

Hobson, Benjamin, 'Reports', *China Repository* XIII (1844), pp. 377–82.

Hsiao Kung-chuan, *Rural China: Imperial Control in the Nineteenth Century* (Seattle: University of Washington Press, 1960).

Hsu, Immanual, *China's Entry into the Family of Nations* (Cambridge, Mass.: Harvard University Press, 1960).

Hu Liyuan (胡禮垣), *Hu Yinan xiansheng quanji* (胡翼南先生全集) (*Collected Works of Hu Liyuan*) 60 *juan* (Hong Kong: 1920).

Hu Quanzhao (胡傳釗), *Tunmo liufen* (盾墨留芬) (*Notes on the* [Sino-French] *War*), 2 volumes, 8 *juan* (Taipei: 1973, photographic reprint; original preface dated 1898).

Huaqiao zhi zongzuan weiyuan hui (華僑誌總纂委員會) (ed.), *Huaqiao zhi zongzhi* (華僑誌總誌) (*Records of Overseas Chinese, A Summary*) (Taipei: 1964; first published 1956).

Huazi ribao qishiyi zhounian jinian kan (華字日報七十一周年紀念刊) (*Publication to Commemorate the 71st Anniversary of the 'Huazi ribao'*) (Hong Kong: 1934).

Huessler, Robert, *Yesterday's Rulers: The Making of the British Colonial Service* (New York: Syracuse University Press, 1963).

Hummel, Arthur W. (ed.), *Eminent Chinese of the Ch'ing Period (1644–1912)*, 2 volumes (Washington: Government Printing Office, 1943–4).

Irick, Robert Lee, *Ch'ing Policy towards the Coolie Trade, 1847–1878* (Taipei: Chinese Materials Centre, 1980).

Jarrett, Vincent H. G., 'Old Hong Kong', a series of articles on the history of Hong Kong taken from the *South China Morning Post* from 17 June 1933 to 13 April 1935, re-organized alphabetically by subject. Photographic copy of a typed copy is deposited at the University of Hong Kong Library, in four volumes.

Jaschok, Maria H., *Concubines and Bondservants* (London: Zed Books, 1988).

Jia Dedao (賈得道), *Zhongguo yixue shilue* (中國醫學史略) (*Brief History of Medicine in China*) (Taiyuan: 1979).

Jin Rihong (金日紅), '*Liji Yixuetang shimo ji jiaoxue gaikuang*' (利濟醫學堂始末及教學概況) ('A brief account of the Liji medical school'), *Zhonghua yishi zazhi* (中華醫史雜誌) (*Chinese Journal of Medical History*) 12:2 (February 1982), pp. 90–2.

Jinghu Yiyuan jiushi zhouji jinian tekan (鏡湖醫院九十周季紀念特刊) (*Special 90th Anniversary Memorial Magazine of the Jinghu Hospital*) (Macao: [1961]).

Kerr, John, 'The Native Benevolent Institutions of Canton', part 1: *China Review* 2 (1873), pp. 88–95; part 2: 3 (1874–5), pp. 108–14.

King, Frank H. H., and Prescott Clarke, *A Research Guide to China-coast Newspapers 1822–1911* (Cambridge, Mass.: Harvard University Press, 1965).

Knaplund, Paul, *James Stephen and the British Colonial System 1813–1847* (Madison: University of Wisconsin Press, 1933).

Kubicek, Robert V., *The Administration of Imperialism: Joseph Chamberlain at the Colonial Office* (Durham, N.C.: Duke University Press, 1969).

Lai Guanglin (賴光臨), 'Wang Tao yu *Xunhuan ribao*' (王韜與循環日報) ('Wang Tao and *Xunhuan ribao*'), *Baoxue* (報學) (*Journalism*) 3:9 (Taipei: December 1967) pp. 52–64.

Lane-Poole, Stanley, *Thirty Years of Colonial Government: Selections from the Despatches and Letters of the Right Honourable Sir George Ferguson Bowen, G.C.M.G.*, 2 volumes, (London: Longmans, Green, 1887).

Lau Siu-kai, *Society and Politics in Hong Kong* (Hong Kong: Chinese University Press, 1982).

Lee, Rance P. L., *Problems of Integrating Chinese and Western Health Services in Hong Kong: Topia and Utopia* (Hong Kong: Social Research Centre, Chinese University, 1974).

Legge, James, 'Lecture on Reminiscences of a Long Residence in the East', *China Review* 1 (1872), pp. 163–76.

Lethbridge, H. J., *Hong Kong: Stability and Change; A Collection of Essays* (Hong Kong: Oxford University Press, 1978).

Li Wenzhong Gong quanji (李文忠公全集) (*Complete Works of Li Hongzhang*), 7 volumes (Hong Kong: 1967) (*LQJ*).

Lin Qianliang (林乾艮), 'Wo guo jindai caoji de Zhongyi xuexiao' (我國近代早期的中醫學校) ('Early Chinese medical schools in modern times'), Zhonghua yishi zashi 10:2 (February 1980), pp. 90–91.

Lin Youlan (林友蘭), 'Xianggang baoye fazhan shilue' (香港報業發展史略) ('A brief history of the development of journalism in Hong Kong'), Baoxue 2:10 (August 1962), pp. 100–15.

—— 'Jindai Zhongwen baoye xianqu — Huang Sheng' (近代中文報業先驅 — 黃勝) ('Huang Sheng, pioneer in modern Chinese journalism'), Baoxue 4:3 (December 1969), pp. 108–11.

Liu Kunyi yiji (劉坤一遺集) (Works of Liu Kunyi), 6 volumes (Shanghai: 1959) (LYJ).

Liu Pei-ch'i (劉伯驥), Meiguo Huaqiao shi (美國華僑史) (A History of the Chinese in the United States of America) (Taipei: 1976).

Liu, William, 'The Legal Person of the Hong Kong Chinese in British Law', Asian Profile 4:3 (June 1976), pp. 195–203.

Liu Xiaobin (劉小斌), 'Guangdong jindai de Zhongyi jiaoyu — tiyao' (廣東近代的中醫教育－提要) ('Chinese medical education in modern Guangdong — abstract'), Zhonghua yishi zazhi 12:3 (March 1982), pp. 133–137.

Lo Hsiang-lin (羅香林), Xianggang yu Zhong Xi wenhua zhi jiaoliu (香港與中西文化之交流) (Hong Kong and East-West Cultural Exchange) (Hong Kong: 1961).

Lockhart, William, The Medical Missionary in China, A Narrative of Twenty Years' Experience (London: Hurst & Blackett, 1861).

Lu Yan (魯言) and others, Xianggang zhanggu (香港掌故) (Hong Kong Tales), 10 volumes (Hong Kong: 1977–).

Mai Meisheng (麥梅生), Fandui xubi shiliao (反對蓄婢史料) (A History of the Anti-Muitsai Movement) (Hong Kong: 1933).

MacMillan, Alistair, Seaports of the Far East (London: 1923).

Manning, Helen Taft, 'Who Ran the Empire — 1830–1850?', Journal of British Studies 5 (1965), pp. 88–121.

Manson-Bahr, Philip A., and A. Alcock, The Life and Work of Sir Patrick Manson (London: Cassell, 1927).

Martin, Robert Montgomery, 'Report on the Island of Hong Kong' in his Reports, Minutes and Despatches on the British Position and Prosperity in China (London: [1846]).

McNeil, William, Plagues and Peoples (Oxford: Blackwell Press, 1976).

Miners, Norman, Hong Kong Under Imperial Rule, 1912–1941 (Hong Kong: Oxford University Press, 1988).

Morgan, W. P., Triad Societies in Hong Kong (Hong Kong: Government Printer, 1982; first published 1960).

Morrell, W. P. British Colonial Policy in the Age of Peel and Russell (Oxford: Clarendon Press, 1930).

Morse, Hosea Ballou, *The Gilds of China with an Account of the Gild Merchant or Co-hong of Canton* (New York: Russell & Russell, 1967; first published 1932).

Nanbei hang gongsuo (南北行公所), *Xinsha luocheng ji chengli bashiliu nian jinian tekan* (新廈落成暨成立八十六年紀念特刊) (*Special Publication Commemorating the 86th Anniversary and the Completion of the New Building*) (Hong Kong: 1954).

——*Chengli yibai zhounian jinian tekan* (成立一百周年紀念特刊) (*Centenary Publication*) (Hong Kong: 1968).

New Cambridge Modern History, Vol. X, The Zenith of European Power 1830–70 (Cambridge: Cambridge University Press, 1967; first published 1960); Vol. XI, *Material Progress and World Wide Problems 1870–98* (Cambridge: Cambridge University Press 1967; first published 1962).

Nanhai xianzhi (南海縣志) (*Nanhai Gazetteer*) (1910).

Nishisato Yoshiyuki (西里喜行), '*Ō Tō to Junken nippo ni tsuide*' (王韜と循環日報について) ('Wang Tao and the *Xunhuan ribao*'), *Tōyōshi kenkiū* (東洋史研究) (*Chinese Historical Studies*) 43:3 December 1985), pp. 508–547.

Ng Lun Ngai-ha, *Interactions of East and West: Development of Public Education in Early Hong Kong* (Hong Kong: Chinese University Press, 1984).

Norton-Kyshe, James William, *The History of the Laws and Courts of Hong Kong*, 2 volumes (Hong Kong: Vetch & Lee, 1971; first published 1898).

Paterson, E. H., *A Hospital for Hong Kong 1887–1987* (Hong Kong: the Nethersole Hospital, 1987)

Pearce, Wilfred William, *Plague in Hong Kong* (Hong Kong: Government Printers, 1905).

Po Leung Kuk, Committee for 1966/67, 1967/68, and 1968/69, *History of the Po Leung Kuk Hong Kong 1878–1968* (香港保良局史料) (bilingual) (Hong Kong: [1968]).

——Board of Directors, 1977–78, *Centenary History of the Po Leung Kuk Hong Kong 1878–1978* (香港保良局百年史略) (bilingual) (Hong Kong: [1978]).

Pope-Hennessy, James, *Verandah: Some Episodes in the Crown Colonies, 1867–1889* (London: George Allen & Unwin, 1964).

——*Half-Crown Colony: A Hong Kong Note Book* (London: Jonathan Cape, 1969).

Pryor, E. G., 'The Great Plague of Hong Kong', *Journal of the Hong Kong Branch of the Royal Asiatic Society* 15 (1975), pp. 61–70.

Purcell, Victor, *The Chinese in Malaya* (Kuala Lumpur, Hong Kong, and London: Oxford University Press, 1967; first published 1948).

Quan Hansheng (全漢昇), *Zhongguo hanghui zhidu shi* (中國行會制度史)

(*The Guild System of China*) (Taipei: 1978; first published 1935).

Qingji waijiao shiliao (清季外交史料) (*Historical Materials Relating to Late Qing Diplomacy*) 164 juan (Peking: 1935).

Ren Yingqiu (任應秋), '*Yiyuan de jianli — bingfang*' (醫院的建立 — 病坊) ('The establishment of hospitals') reprinted in *Ming bao yuekan* (明報月刊) (*Ming Pao Monthly*) 57 (September 1970), p. 19.

Report of the Commission sent by China to Ascertain the Conditions of Chinese Coolies in Cuba (Taipei: 1970: first published, Shanghai: Imperial Maritime Customs Press, 1876).

Sangren, P. Steven, 'Traditional Chinese Corporations: Beyond Kinship', *Journal of Asian Studies* XLIII:3 (May 1984), pp. 391–415.

Sayer, G. R., *Hong Kong 1862–1919* (Hong Kong: Hong Kong University Press, 1975).

Sinn, Elizabeth, 'The Strike and Riot of 1884 — A Hong Kong Perspective', *Journal of the Hong Kong Branch of the Royal Asiatic Society* 22 (1982), pp. 65–98.

——'Materials for Historical Research: Source Materials on the Tung Wah Hospital 1869–1941 — the Case of a Historical Institution' in Alan Birch, Y. C. Jao, and Elizabeth Sinn (eds.), *Research Materials for Hong Kong Studies* (Hong Kong: Centre of Asian Studies, University of Hong Kong, 1984), pp. 195–223.

——'A Chinese Consul for Hong Kong: China-Hong Kong Relations in the Late Qing Period', paper presented at the 'International Conference on the History of the Ming-Ch'ing Periods', 12–15 December 1985, University of Hong Kong.

Skinner, G. W., *Chinese Society in Thailand, An Analytical History* (Ithaca, New York: Cornell University Press, 1957).

——*Leadership and Power in the Chinese Community of Thailand* (Ithaca, New York: Cornell University Press, 1958).

——'Overseas Chinese Leadership: Paradigm for a Paradox' in Gehan Wijeyewardene, *Leadership and Authority: A Symposium* (Singapore: University of Malaya Press, 1968), pp. 191–207.

——*The City in Late Imperial China* (Stanford; Stanford University Press, 1977).

Smith, Carl T., 'The Chinese Settlement of British Hong Kong', *Chung Chi Bulletin* 48 (May, 1970) pp. 26–32.

——'Notes on Chinese Temples in Hong Kong', *Journal of the Hong Kong Branch of the Royal Asiatic Society* 13 (1973), pp. 133–9.

——'Visit to Tung Wah Group of Hospitals Museum, 2nd October, 1976' (Notes and Queries), *JHKBRAS* 16 (1976).

——'Sun Yat-sen's School Days in Hong Kong: The Establishment of the Alice Memorial Hospital', *Ching Feng*, XXI:2 (1978), pp. 78–94.

——*Chinese Christians: Élites, Middlemen and the Church in Hong Kong* (Hong Kong: Oxford University Press, 1985).

Stewart, Watt, *Chinese Bondage in Peru: A History of the Chinese Coolie in Peru 1849–1874* (Westport, Connecticut: Greenwood Press, 1951).

Thong Chai Medical Institution Opening Ceremony Souvenir Magazine (同濟醫院大廈落成紀念特刊) (bilingual) (Singapore: [1979]).

Ticozzi, Sergei, *Xianggang Tianzhujiao zhanggu* (香港天主教掌故) (*Stories of the Catholic Church in Hong Kong*) translated by You Liqing (游麗清) (Hong Kong: 1983).

Tongji Yiyuan yibai zhounian jinian tekan (同濟醫院壹佰周年紀念特刊) (Centenary publication of the Thong Chai Medical Institution) (Singapore: [1968]).

Topley, Marjorie, 'Chinese Traditional Etiology and Methods of Cure in Hong Kong', in Charles Leslie (ed.), *Asian Medical Systems* (Berkeley: University of California Press, 1976), pp. 243–65.

Tse Tsan Tai, *The Chinese Republic — the Secret History of the Chinese Revolution* (Hong Kong: South China Morning Post, 1924).

Tung Wah Board of Directors, 1960–1961, *Development of the Tung Wah Hospital (1870–1960)* (東華三院發展史略) (bilingual) (Hong Kong: [1961]).

Tung Wah Board of Directors, 1870–1970, *One Hundred Years of the Tung Wah Hospital 1870–1970* (香港東華三院百年史略), 2 volumes (bilingual) (Hong Kong: [1970]).

Turnbull, C. M., *A History of Singapore* (Kuala Lumpur: Oxford University Press, 1977).

Wang Ermin (王爾敏), *Wan Qing zhengzhi sixiang shilun* (晚清政治思想史論) (*Political Thought in the Late Qing Period*) (Taipei: 1969).

Wang Gungwu, *A Short History of the Chinese in Nanyang* (Singapore: Eastern Universities Press, 1959).

Wang Tao (王韜), *Taoyuan wenlu waibian* (弢園文錄外編) (*Additional essays of Wang Tao*), 12 juan (Peking: 1959; first published Hong Kong, 1883).

——*Manyu suilu* (漫遊隨錄) (*A Record of Travels*) (Zhangsha: 1982; first published 1887).

——*Taoyuan zhidu* (弢園尺牘) (*Letters of Wang Tao*), 12 juan (Shanghai: no. date; first published 1893).

Wang Xiji (王錫祺), *Xiao fanghu cai yudi zong cao* (小方壺齋輿地叢鈔) (*Collected Texts on Geography from the Xiao fanghu cai Study*) (Shanghai: preface 1877; second supplement 1897).

Waung, W. S. K., *The Controversy: Opium and Sino-British Relations 1858–1887* (Hong Kong: Lungmen Press, [1977]).

Wei Qingyuan (韋慶遠) and others, *Qingdai nubi zhidu* (清代奴婢制度) (*The Slavery System in Qing*) (Peking: 1984; first published 1982).

Wickberg, Edgar (ed.), *From China to Canada: A History of the Chinese*

Communities in Canada (Toronto: Ministry of Supply and Services, 1982).

Willmott, W. E., *The Political Structure of the Chinese Community in Cambodia* (London: London School of Economics, Monographs on Social Anthropology, no. 42, 1970).

Wong, J. Y., 'The Cession of Hong Kong: a Chapter of Imperial History', *Journal of Oriental Society of Australia* 2 (1976), pp. 49–61.

——*Anglo-Chinese Relations 1839–1860* (London: The British Academy, 1983).

Wong, K. C., *The Lancet and the Cross* (Shanghai: Council of Christian Medical Work, 1950).

Wong, K. C., and Wu Lien-teh, *History of Chinese Medicine* (Tientsin: The Tientsin Press, 1932).

Wong Sing-wu, *The Organization of Chinese Emigration, 1848–1888, with Special Reference to Chinese Emigration to Australia* (San Francisco: Chinese Materials Centre, 1978).

Woo Sing Lim (吳醒廉), *Prominent Chinese in Hong Kong* (香港華人名人史略) (bilingual) (Hong Kong: 1937).

Wood, A. E., *Report on the Chinese Guilds of Hong Kong compiled from Materials Collected by the Registrar General* (Hong Kong: Noronha, 1912).

Wright, Arnold (ed.), *Twentieth Century Impressions of Hong Kong, Shanghai and Other Treaty Ports* (London: Lloyd's Greater Britain Publishing, 1908).

Xunhuan ribao liushi zhounian jinian tekan (循環日報六十周年紀念特刊) (*Special Publication to Commemorate the 60th Anniversary of the 'Xunhuan ribao'*) (Hong Kong: 1932).

Yen Ching-Hwang, 'Ch'ing's Sale of Honours and the Chinese Leadership in Singapore and Malaya, 1877–1912', *Journal of Southeast Asian Studies* 1:2 (September 1970), pp. 20–32.

——'Changing Images of the Overseas Chinese (1644–1912)', *Modern Asian Studies* 15:2 (1981), pp. 261–85.

——*Coolies and Mandarins* (Singapore: Singapore University Press, 1985).

Yu Ch'i-hsing (余啓興), '*Wu Tingfang yu Xianggang zhi guanxi*' (伍廷芳與香港之關係) ('Wu Tingfang and Hong Kong') in *Shou Luo Xianglin jiaoshou lunwen ji* (壽羅香林教授論文集) (*Essays in Chinese Studies presented to Professor Lo Hsiang-lin*) (Hong Kong: 1970), pp. 255–78.

Yu Shenchu (俞慎初), *Zhongguo yixue jianshi* (中國醫學簡史) (*Brief History of Medicine in China*) (Fuzhou: 1983).

Zhang Yinhuan (張蔭桓), *Sanzhou riji* (三洲日記) (*Diary of Three Continents*) 8 *juan* (no publisher, no date).

Zhang Wenxiang Gong quanji (張文襄公全集) (*Complete Works of Zhang*

Zhidong), 228 *juan*, 6 volumes, photographic reprint (Taipei: 1963) (*ZQJ*).

Zhang Wenxiang Gong shuhan mobao (張文襄公書翰墨寶) (*Calligraphy of Zhang Zhidong*) (Shanghai: 1924).

Zhongguo shixue hui (中國史學會) (Chinese History Society) (ed.), *Yapian zhanzheng* (鴉片戰爭) (*The Opium War*), 6 volumes (Shanghai: 1954).

Zhu Shijia (朱士嘉), *Meiguo pohai Huagong shiliao* (美國迫害華工史料) (*Materials on American Persecution of Chinese Labour*) (Shanghai: 1958).

Zuckermann, Steven B., 'Pake in Paradise, A Synthetic Study of Chinese Immigration to Hawaii', *Bulletin of the Institute of Ethnology, Academia Sinica*, 45 (Spring 1978), pp. 39–80.

Unpublished Theses

Arensmeyer, Elliott C., 'British Merchant Enterprise and the Chinese Coolie Labour Trade, 1850–1874' (Ph.D. thesis, University of Hawaii, 1979).

Chang Yun-chao, 'Wu T'ing-fang's Contribution Towards Political Reform in Late Ch'ing Period' (Ph.D. thesis, University of Hong Kong, 1982).

Chiu Ling-yeong, 'The Life and Thought of Sir Kai Ho Kai' (Ph.D. thesis, University of Sydney, 1968).

Chung, Rosemary Lu-cee, 'A Study of the 1925–26 Canton–Hong Kong Strike–Boycott' (M.A. thesis, University of Hong Kong, 1969).

de Glopper, Donald Robert, 'City on the Sands: Social Structure in a Nineteenth-century Chinese City' (Ph.D. thesis, Cornell University, 1973).

Shin, Linda Pomerantz, 'China in Transition: The Role of Wu Ting-fang (1842–1922)' (Ph.D. thesis, University of California, Los Angeles, 1970).

Ts'ai Jung-fang, 'Comprador Ideologists in Modern China: Ho Kai (Ho Ch'i) (1859–1914) and Hu Li-yuan (1847–1916)' (Ph.D. thesis, University of California, 1975).

Index